D1565905

# ADVANCES IN HUMAN GENETICS

**1**

# CONTRIBUTORS TO THIS VOLUME:

**J. H. Edwards**
*Department of Human Genetics*
*University of Birmingham*
*Birmingham, England*

**Jean Frézal**
*Unité de Recherches de Génétique Malade*
*Hôpital des Enfants Malades*
*Paris, France*

**H. Hugh Fudenberg**
*Department of Medicine*
*University of California, San Francisco*
*Department of Bacteriology and Immunology*
*University of California, Berkeley*

**Peter Hechtman**
*The deBelle Laboratory for Biochemical Genetics*
*McGill University — Montreal Children's Hospital Research Institute*
*Montreal, Canada*

**Orlando J. Miller**
*Department of Obstetrics and Gynecology*
*College of Physicians and Surgeons, Columbia University*
*New York City*

**Jean Rey**
*Unité de Recherches de Génétique Malade*
*Hôpital des Enfants Malades*
*Paris, France*

**Charles R. Scriver**
*The deBelle Laboratory for Biochemical Genetics*
*McGill University — Montreal Children's Hospital Research Institute*
*Montreal, Canada*

**Noel L. Warner**
*The Walter and Eliza Hall Institute of Medical Research*
*Royal Melbourne Hospital*
*Victoria, Australia*

# ADVANCES IN HUMAN GENETICS

# 1

**Edited by**

# Harry Harris

Galton Professor of Human Genetics
University College London
London, England

**and**

# Kurt Hirschhorn

Arthur J. and Nellie Z. Cohen Professor of Genetics and Pediatrics
Mount Sinai School of Medicine of The City University of New York

ℚ PLENUM PRESS·NEW YORK-LONDON·1970

First Printing - February 1970
Second Printing - October 1974

Library of Congress Catalog Card Number 77-84583

SBN 306-39601-7

© 1970 Plenum Press, New York
A Division of Plenum Publishing Corporation
227 West 17th Street, New York, N.Y. 10011

United Kingdom edition published by Plenum Press, London
A Division of Plenum Publishing Company, Ltd.
Donington House, 30 Norfolk Street, London W.C.2, England

Printed in the United States of America

## ARTICLES PLANNED FOR FUTURE VOLUMES:

04967

# Preface

During the last few years the science of human genetics has been expanding almost explosively. Original papers dealing with different aspects of the subject are appearing at an increasingly rapid rate in a very wide range of journals, and it becomes more and more difficult for the geneticist and virtually impossible for the nongeneticist to keep track of the developments. Furthermore, new observations and discoveries relevant to an overall understanding of the subject result from investigations using very diverse techniques and methodologies and originating in a variety of different disciplines. Thus, investigations in such various fields as enzymology, immunology, protein chemistry, cytology, pediatrics, neurology, internal medicine, anthropology, and mathematical and statistical genetics, to name but a few, have each contributed results and ideas of general significance to the study of human genetics. Not surprisingly it is often difficult for workers in one branch of the subject to assess and assimilate findings made in another. This can be a serious limiting factor on the rate of progress.

Thus, there appears to be a real need for critical review articles which summarize the positions reached in different areas, and it is hoped that "Advances in Human Genetics" will help to meet this requirement.

Each of the contributors has been asked to write an account of the position that has been reached in the investigations of a specific topic in one of the branches of human genetics. The reviews are intended to be critical and to deal with the topic in depth from the writer's own point of view. It is hoped that the articles will provide workers in other branches of the subject, and in related disciplines, with a detailed account of the results so far obtained in the particular area, and help them to assess the relevance of these discoveries to aspects of their own work, as well as to the science as a whole. The reviews are also intended to give the reader some idea of the nature of the technical and methodological problems involved, and to indicate new directions stemming from recent advances.

The contributors have not been restricted in the arrangement or organization of their material or in the manner of its presentation, so that the reader should be able to appreciate something of the individuality of approach which goes to make up the subject of human genetics, and which, indeed, gives it much of its fascination.

HARRY HARRIS
*The Galton Laboratory*
*University College London*

KURT HIRSCHHORN
*Division of Medical Genetics*
*Department of Pediatrics*
*Mount Sinai School of Medicine*

# Contents

*Chapter* 3

## Chapter 4

*Chapter 1*

# Analysis of Pedigree Data*

J. H. Edwards

*Department of Human Genetics*
*University of Birmingham*
*Birmingham, England*

## THE NATURE OF PEDIGREE DATA

A pedigree is defined by a series of individuals connected by the bonds of parentage and possessing various characteristics, either attributes or variates, at one or several times. The unit from which any pedigree may be assembled involves an identity, a pair of parental identities, and a set of one or more characters, of the form of Fig. 1.

Given any set of such units connected by flexible and extensible bonds, a pedigree may be assembled by matching all labels of equal identity. Sets of data may be tabulated in a form which can easily be linked into pedigrees by either man or machine, as shown in Table I.

The bonds of a pedigree relate to gametic paths, and the study of pedigrees is aimed at the study of the genetic determinants of the phenotype

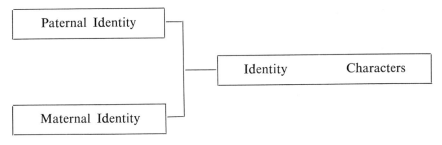

Fig. 1.   Basic unit from which any pedigree may be fabricated.

*Part of this work was done while the author was at the New York Blood Center, and was supported by grant HE 09011 from the National Institutes of Health.

**TABLE I. Basic Data for Medical Research. Basic Units of Pedigree Formation**

| Civic data | | | | | | | Medical data | | | | | | | | | | | | | | | | | | | |
| --- | --- | --- | --- | --- | --- | --- | --- | --- | --- | --- | --- | --- | --- | --- | --- | --- | --- | --- | --- | --- | --- | --- | --- | --- | --- | --- |
| Propositus | | Mother | | Father | | Date | Markers | | | | Variates | | | | States | | | | Events | | | | Environment | | | |
| Iden. | B.D. | Iden. | B.D. | Iden. | B.D. | | I | J | K | L | A | B | C | D | P | Q | R | S | p | q | r | s | w | x | y | z |
| ××× ××× | ××× ××× | ××× ××× | ××× | ××× ××× | ××× ××× | ××× | 0 | — | — | — | — | — | — | — | — | — | — | — | — | — | — | — | — | — | — | — |
| | | | | | | ××× | 1 | 0 | — | — | 107 | — | — | — | — | — | — | — | — | — | — | — | — | 1 | 6 | — |
| | | | | | | ××× | 1 | 0 | 1 | — | — | 51 | — | — | — | — | 1 | 0 | — | — | — | — | — | — | — | 112 |
| ××× ××× | ××× ××× | ××× ××× | ××× | ××× ××× | ××× ××× | ××× | 0 | — | — | — | — | 37 | — | — | — | — | — | — | — | — | — | — | — | — | — | — |
| | | | | | | ××× | 1 | — | — | — | 213 | — | — | — | — | — | — | — | — | — | — | — | 3 | 7 | — | — |
| | | | | | | ××× | 1 | 0 | — | 1 | — | — | — | — | — | — | — | — | — | 1 | — | — | — | — | — | 12 |
| ××× ××× | ××× ××× | ××× ××× | ××× | ××× ××× | ××× ××× | ×××× | — | — | — | — | 112 | — | — | — | 0 | — | — | — | — | — | — | — | — | — | — | — |
| | | | | | | ×××× | 1 | — | 1 | — | — | — | — | — | — | — | — | — | — | — | — | 1 | — | — | — | — |
| | | | | | | ×××× | — | 1 | — | 1 | — | — | — | 11 | — | — | 2 | — | — | — | — | — | — | — | — | — |
| ××× ××× | ××× ××× | ××× ××× | ××× | ××× ××× | ××× ××× | ×××× | — | — | — | — | — | — | — | — | — | — | 0 | — | — | — | — | — | — | — | — | — |
| | | | | | | ×××× | 1 | 0 | — | — | 170 | — | — | — | 3 | — | 1 | — | 1 | — | — | — | — | — | — | — |
| | | | | | | ××× | 1 | 0 | — | — | — | — | 32 | — | — | — | 2 | — | — | — | — | — | 1 | — | — | 67 |
| ××× ××× | ××× ××× | ××× ××× | ××× | ××× ××× | ××× ××× | ×××× | — | — | — | — | — | — | 47 | — | 2 | — | 0 | — | — | — | — | — | — | — | — | — |
| | | | | | | ××× | — | — | — | — | — | — | — | — | — | — | — | — | — | — | — | — | — | — | — | — |
| | | | | | | ××× | — | — | 1 | — | — | — | 44 | — | — | — | 3 | — | — | — | 1 | — | 0 | — | — | — |

and of the way in which they determine the phenotype; pedigree analysis is necessarily indirect, and only necessary because of the technical difficulties in studying both the nature of gametic information, which is not usually expressed in the haploid state, and the manner in which it is expressed. In addition to attempting to resolve the way in which what happens is happening, the analysis of pedigrees can alone throw light on the breeding structure of populations by providing data on inbreeding and on the familial correlation of fertility.

The former problem, the relationship of genetic determinants to phenotypic determination, involves data on characteristics of several individuals in any pedigree. The latter problem, the genetic structure, may be resolved in terms of identity alone if the population is known in sufficient depth. Almost all that is known of human breeding structure is derived from the frequency of matings, such as those between first cousins, with fairly high genetic correlations of the spouses' gametes; as this is straightforward, it will not be discussed further. Attempts to infer gametic correlations from various characteristics of spouses, including birth place, surname, and blood group, have not as yet been applied to sufficiently extensive data to give precise estimates. A detailed discussion on this estimation from blood-group phenotypes is presented by Yasuda.[44]

The characteristics of the individuals in a pedigree may relate to some effectively constant feature, such as sex or blood-group phenotype, in which case time of observation is irrelevant, or of some state or attribute developing during post-natal life, such as most diseases, or to some variate such as weight, in which case observations which do not give age are of little value.

We may conveniently break down observations into *states*, into *events*, or times of change of state, and into *variates*, or indefinitely divisible measurements. States which are permanent within the age range usually encountered, and are explicable on simple genetic hypotheses, such as sex or the ABO blood groups, may be designated *markers*. All these may be recorded in numerical form. Markers can be defined by 0 and 1, or no-response and response to some test; states may be defined by one of several integers relating to stages, and events may be defined by the time relating to the happening of any defined event, that is, to a change in state. This division into states, including markers, events, and variates, covers the complete description available for formal analysis. Other information, such as photographs, X-rays, palmar-patterns, psychiatric reports, etc. may be of greater interest, but such data can only be analyzed formally if drastically simplified by qualifying or quantifying, and the loss of information on numerical translation will often outweigh the ease of manipulation it confers.

The formal analysis of pedigrees reduces to the largely independent problems of single-marker analysis (segregation), multiple-marker analysis (allelism and linkage), state analysis (often termed the study of heritability), and variate analysis.

The units from which pedigrees are assembled are usually presented in vertical array, and the individuals coded by shape and shading, with children below parents, in conformity with the pre-Darwinian convention that progeny descend, each generation being further from grace.

Pedigrees are usually collected and analyzed in order to provide information on the way in which the similarities between relatives are executed. Occasionally pedigrees, particularly very small pedigrees consisting of sibs or twins, are collected to see if relatives are similar: this may now be regarded as self-evident, and I will not discuss the question of whether relatives are more similar than nonrelatives, but assume this, and consider only the evidence which may be shed on the nature and intensity of the determinants underlying this evident similarity.

Since the analysis of conditions expressed fully in the heterozygote, or hemizygote, is obvious, and since in other conditions the complexities exclude analyses without either using electronic computers or segmenting the pedigree into small modules, the advantages of the costly and tedious of large pedigrees showing erratically manifest conditions seem very limited. display

Any pedigree can be compounded from basically simple units which convey information on identity and parentage and on characters. The information on identity can be of any form; truncated lettering and birth date are convenient. The coding of data is more complicated. Variates are readily coded as numbers. Markers which relate to presence or absence of an attribute may be coded in binary form, a particularly appropriate procedure, since computers handle data internally in this form.

Suppose we consider a set of responses − + + − +, etc., to some stimulus such as an antibody, with identity A, B, C,..., etc. (for simplicity writing − as 0 and + as 1, giving the sequence 01101, etc.). If two gameto-types specify any phenotype unequivocally, though not necessarily uniquely, they can be related to the phenotype by the simple dominance relationship usual with qualitative responses in diploid organisms:

| Paternal gametotype | 0 | 0 | 1 | 1 |
| Maternal gametotype | 0 | 1 | 0 | 1 |
| Phenotype | 0 | 1 | 1 | 1 |

Then, if the phenotype is defined by the binary series 01101, etc., this could be related to various pairs of gametotypes under the constraints above.

For example, considering three determinants, we could have

| | | | | |
|---|---|---|---|---|
| Maternal | 011 | 011 | 011 | 011 |
| Paternal | 000 | 001 | 010 | 011 |
| Diploid | 011 | 011 | 011 | 011 |

and three others due to interchanging maternal and paternal. That is, various pairs of four gametotypes of chromosomes are consistent with this phenotype.

Any set of phenotypes may have a set, of between 1 and $2^n$ gametotypes, related to $n$ determinants. These numbers are difficult to communicate without error, either in speech or writing, and also provide difficulty in sorting and cataloging. A simple solution is to divide the series into triplets, starting at the left, and to specify each triplet by a simple number 0–7, any remainder of one or two responses being separated by a comma. The transforming of a triplet into octal numbers is fairly simple following the rule

| 4 | 2 | 1 | |
|---|---|---|---|
| 0 | 0 | 0 | 0 |
| 0 | 0 | 1 | 1 |
| 0 | 1 | 0 | 2 |
| 0 | 1 | 1 | 3 |
| 1 | 0 | 0 | 4 |
| 1 | 0 | 1 | 5 |
| 1 | 1 | 0 | 6 |
| 1 | 1 | 1 | 7 |

So that the series 11001011010101 can be coded into triplets 110,010,110,101,01, and then into octals 6265,01, or, more conveniently, 62652, (14), where the figure in parentheses specifies the number of tests.

The problem of missing data is most readily handled by the use of a "mask," so named because it may be regarded as a piece of paper with holes which can be laid over the array of 0's and 1's from the tests to show only the tests done, and an array we may call "marker," the result of the tests done. The mask may be specified by a series of zero's and ones, one referring to a test done, and both mask and marker may also be specified in octal digits. The order of the tests is not crucial, provided it is specified, since transforming from one order to another is simple.

A coding procedure which makes use of this system for recording data with one locus or other state-system per card is shown in Fig. 2. The results (positive, negative, doubtful, and not done) are presented by mark-sensing,

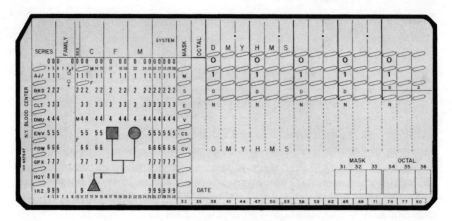

Fig. 2. Card designed to provide full identification of an individual and parentage, and coding of any set of up to 12 binary responses. A batch of cards for each individual is produced and coded, with identity in the left half and identification of the responses in the right half (for example, −A, −B for ABO responses, −M, −N, −S, −Z in the MNSs). The identifiers are allocated up to two columns, the third being used for the response which is graded as 0 (negative), 1 (positive), other (including, particularly, undone (N) and doubtful (0). Quantitative data by date and time may also be coded. The system is indefinitely extensible.

and the computer defines the marker array (0 unless positive, when 1) and the mask array (0 unless positive or negative, when 1). The three hole positions needed for the mark sense are very convenient, as two may be used to label the test (A, $A_1$, B or M, N, S, Z—where Z denotes $\bar{s}$, since there is no lower case available on card punches) in the $A_1$ $A_2$ $B_O$ and MNSs systems, respectively. The left-hand part of the card, defining the relationship, is duplicated on each card so that an indefinite series of cards specifies the phenotype of the individual.

## THE PURPOSE OF PEDIGREE ANALYSIS

Pedigree analysis is concerned with the structure and function of the genetic determinants, and with the statics and dynamics of gene action. I propose to discuss only the former. In pedigree analysis we may assume a general structure of the genetic framework, and, within the restraints of the structure we assume, we may use the data to improve our knowledge of this structure; that is, we attempt to estimate various structural parameters, or, where the mechanism is too complex for the few degrees of freedom available from the data, to summarize the results in some summarizing index, such as a correlation coefficient or a heritability estimate.

This distinction between structural parameters and summarizing indices is of major importance, for the former are, in principle, capable of continuously improved estimates, and of verification by such direct methods as sequential analysis of the products of transcription or translation, or the definition of allelic position by somatic cell hybridization. Eventually the genetic factors and their products will be resolved directly, but, until then, the uncertain inferences from multiple imperfect observations of the phenotypes of relatives are alone possible. In the summarizing indices, on the other hand, there is no obvious way in which more numerous observations will make contact with the results of qualitatively new techniques, since there is no clearly defined basic structure.

The raw materials on which our inferences are based are, firstly, a map of the genetic determinants, a map known to consist essentially of a sequence of almost $10^{10}$ nucleotides, of four varieties, divided into 24 distinct and independently segregating units (the 22 autosomes and the two sex chromosomes). This map, which may consist largely of repeated identical units, is inferred to be in functional units of around 1000 nucleotides, which we may, for simplicity, regard as genes. This map of genetic structure is readily described since it is linear and static and any inferred set of genetic factors may be subdivided into those sharing identity of position by gametic exclusiveness, the alleles, and into linkage groups from evidences of correlated gametic transfer. In both cases structural parameters of physical position have a direct physical sense.

The second map, the metabolic map, is of a different order of complexity. In its simplest form it consists of a large number of points, or pools, the metabolites, between which are the paired metabolic channels through which, under the guidance of the gene products, one from each parent, metabolites are assembled and broken down (Fig. 3).

This is a very complex structure with many thousands of points and far larger numbers of channels. Some channels appear to be major connections whose blockage or perversion will produce serious predictable consequences, like traffic blocks on city bridges. Other unique channels may be inferred if they are near the end of some metabolic peninsular, as in the anomalies of pigmentation. But most channels, like most roads, appear to be in complex networks and only capable of resolution in terms of very numerous parameters. It is in this situation, which appears to underly most normal variation in man (and all normal variations may be regarded as pathological in that any population partitioned on any variate, such as tall and short, might be expected to show differences in morbidity and mortality), which pedigree analysis is now expected to resolve.

Unfortunately, the resolving power of pedigree studies seems inadequate to make much advance, for there are too few degrees of freedom. Many

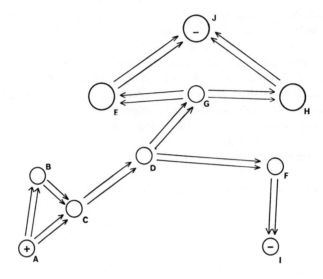

Fig. 3.   Fragment of metabolic map, with metabolites *A* entering
system, and *I* and *J* leaving. Arrows show normal routes.

pedigrees can be summarized in terms of sib-pairs and, where this is possible,
even allowing the luxury of complete ascertainment, there are only two
degrees of freedom (three types of sib-pair constrained to sum to unity), so
that this very complicated network must be summarized in terms which
have no very clear structural meaning in the sense that they do not clearly
relate to physical entities or their relationships.

In view of the difficulties of understanding what is being analyzed in
variance partitioning procedures, it is perhaps worth considering formally
models whose behavior might be expected to simulate that found in man, as
it would seem that it is not possible to determine any structural parameters
of any organism or mechanism without an explicit model of the working
parts. In view of the great advance in the last twenty years, an advance which
includes the first clear understanding of replication, transcription, translation,
and the integration of enzyme pathways, it would seem unlikely that numerical
procedures developed without the restraints of this knowledge would have
a very high resolving power in defining or measuring those structures still
obscured by the receding shadow of the unknown. The assumptions made in
variance partitioning procedures stem from Fisher's classic paper[16] on the
numerical consequences of Mendelism. This paper, which introduced the
terms variance and epistacy, and the concept of indirectly estimating partial
dominance, has been reprinted with extensive annotations by Moran and
Smith.[28] It is not clear from Fisher's text, or from his book of 1930, exactly

what he envisaged as the connecting link between the genotype and the phenotype. It seems likely that he visualized a set of weakly interacting particles, and sought to interpret deviations from the simplest consequences of mixing in the same general way as in the mixing of gases or liquids.

We may consider the evolution of models of increasing complexity relating genetic variability and phenotypic variability. Our first model, which is clearly false in diploid organisms, is to postulate genetic factors $a_1$, $a_2$, $a_3$, etc., each of which exerts an independent effect $w_1$, $w_2$, $w_3$, etc., so that the overall effect is $W = Sw_i$. The model has the advantage of simplicity and the disadvantage of being incompatible with the known mechanisms of chromosomal inheritance in metazoa. It also suffers, though perhaps not fatally, from a paucity of segregational variability. Fisher, in rejecting this possibility on theoretical grounds,[16] appeared to assume that matter is infinitely divisible, so that no variance is maintained by particulate segregation. In practical consequences its implications on direction of inheritance are straightforward, although providing no information on velocity or anticipated goal. It is certainly not obvious that dogs and horses, which are usually bred on the assumption of blending, have changed less rapidly than those species, such as the cow and the chicken, which have been exposed to the more sophisticated models appropriate to diploid inheritance.

We may advance a simple diagrammatic model (Fig. 4) in the form of a series of resistances (or, to overcome the problems of adding reciprocals, of conductances) which we suppose are wired in series to complete a circuit including a battery and a dial measuring the current. Clearly, the response is $W = Sw_i$, where $w_i$ is the conductance of the $i$th element. Further, if a machine is assembled from components derived by random selection from two other machines, the mean response, and the distribution of response, over the complete set of the $(n!/(n/2)!)^2$ hybrids will be determinate.

Fisher's basic 1918 model may be drawn in the same way as a device containing paired elements, with the restraints that hybrids are formed arbitrarily by selection from one component of the unordered pairs (Fig. 5).

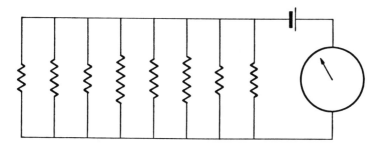

Fig. 4.   Electrical analog of organism with independent units.

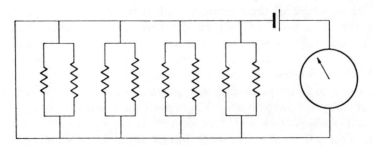

Fig. 5.  Electrical analog of organism with paired units of independent
action, i.e., showing allelism but neither dominance nor epistacy.

Then, the expectation, $W = Sw_i(a_i + b_i + c_i)$, where $a_i$ and $b_i$, each of
which may take values of 0 or 1, refer to alleles which act as though they had
a conductance of $w_i$ or zero, while $c_i$ refers to a further resistance. This
model may be simplified with advantage by excluding $c_i$, giving
$W = Sw_i(a_i + b_i) + C$. The production of further machines by taking
one element from the unordered pairs of two other machines will provide the
same mean distribution as in the preceding model, but has a vastly increased
segregational variability with but $2^{2n}$ possible sets of elements.

Fisher showed that an analagous mathematical model would not quite
fit the expected pattern of heritability of variance on this assumption of
unordered pairs of independent elements, and that a better fit was obtained
by allowing some interaction between pairs at each locus, suggesting the
approximate model shown in Fig. 6. Where the circuit is buffered by some

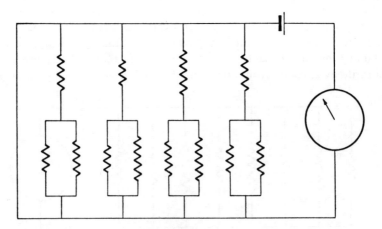

Fig. 6.  Electrical analog of organism with paired units with independent
action of pair, i.e., showing allelism and dominance, but no epistacy.

constant resistances related to each locus and the expectation, as the first approximation, is $W = Sw_i(a_i + b_i)^k$ so that the phenotypic effects of the three genotypes are as 0 to 1 to $2^k$, which ranges from complete dominance when $k = 0$ to complete intermediacy when $k = 1$. This definition of dominance is used purely for typographical convenience and, like other definitions, has no particular biological significance. Dominance as defined statistically is not clearly related to the phenomena at single loci, since no estimate of the variability in dominance is made although, *a priori*, this might be expected to be large and would greatly affect its estimate as well as confounding any estimates of epistacy.

Since this failed to specify adequately the expected phenotype, Fisher introduced the concept of interactions between loci, which he termed epistacy; these may be expressed roughly but simply in the model of Fig. 7, where $W = f[Sw_i(a_i + b_i)^k]$, where $f$ relates to some function which buffers or continuously decreases the rate of change of $W$ with the variable elements $a_i + b_i$. Now that we know the approximate implications of this model (the circuit diagrams are not exactly analogous to the formulae, both being kept as simple as possible both conceptually and typographically), we may ask whether it can be used heuristically. It can clearly be used as a definitive demonstration of the sufficiency of Mendelism as an explanation of graded heritable variation, a demonstration of profound significance, which was first explored on human data. It is of interest that Fisher used this argument almost exclusively demonstratively, reserving the heuristic and pragmatic use of variance partitioning procedures mainly for the selection of optimal environments through fertilizer trials.

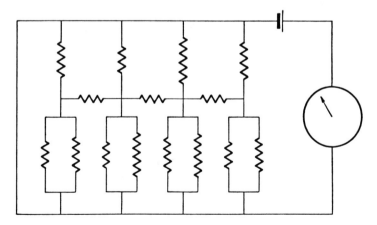

Fig. 7.   Electrical analog of organism with paired elements with full interaction, i.e., allelism, dominance, and epistacy.

Suppose we start from model 4, encase it in a box, and represent each locus by a swith which we code by 1 and 0 for on and off in the simple two-allele case (Fig. 8). A study of the contents of this box by pedigree analysis is equivalent to finding sets of components defined by the rules of parentage, one switch position from each pair being arbitrarily conveyed by each parent, and sibs being defined by common parentage. Ultimately, with an infinite number of families, we would get as much information as could be obtained by throwing various switches and watching the dial. This must be so, since each family will increment the information, but the information cannot exceed that available from direct study. However, even if we could do this, but could not look inside the box, our inferences based on the tabulation of $W$ for each of the $2^{2n}$ settings of $2n$ switches would be far from simple. Suppose the situation were further confused by an arbitrary choice of battery, assumed conveniently Gaussian in its distribution of charge. Clearly the strength of familial likeness will decrease if this is random, but may actually increase if, as will occasionally, be the case in man, this environmental variation, which includes the fetal environment, shows a greatly restricted variation within families.

Even if given the connections between the components and permitted to work the switches rather than having to infer indirectly from pedigree studies, it would be a formidable undertaking to decode the structure. If only pedigree data were available, this would be far more difficult; even the number of switches would be indeterminate in practice. In view of our knowledge of hereditary variations in enzyme structure, and the complex nonlinear interaction of enzymes with substrates, and with one another, any analagous diagram of anything so complex as growth, or intellect, or shape, or disease liability, would be far more complicated than the simple circuits which we have considered. It would also be far more complicated than such devices as television sets or computers, and would wholly lack the constraints on variety and untidiness imposed by industrial practice.

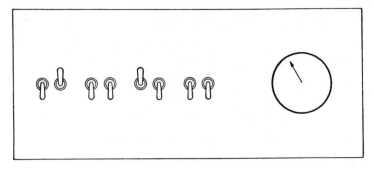

Fig. 8.  Model of system with concealed circuit.

In order to conform to the real world of metabolic pathways we would have to envisage an arbitrarily large number of components connecting various nodes in a vast network, and to replace the simple resistances by structures whose resistance was a function not only of the current they were carrying, but, in some cases, of the current their neighbors were carrying, and could, in some cases, as in the many coupled reactions exchanging energy-rich bonds, take a negative value. It might seem clear from this that there is no realistic chance of making any progress toward the decoding of the composition of the box from observations made from the outside, that is, from observations of the nature of those available in pedigree studies. This is not necessarily a contraindication to studies of heritability, for, if we take the simpler example of physics, accurate and useful information can be obtained on the assumption that the number of components acting is so large that they conform to simple statistical distributions.

Any randomly wired black box will show heritable features provided there is some convention by which the rules of parentage are defined in terms of arbitrary selection of paired components. Even if it is accepted as impossible to decode the wiring from the outside, we may ask what interpretation we can place on estimates of heritability either heuristically, in terms of advancing our knowledge, or administratively, in terms of legislating for alterations in the environment or in attempting to influence the fertility of some phenotypes.

Clearly we could anticipate most of the features which have been found in pedigree studies of the end results of numerous enzymatic activities, including complex disorders. Although the total response is likely to be nonlinear, the effect of any individual switch is likely to be small, and, therefore, to become almost linear over its usual range of activity as the number of switches increases. Further, the extreme ranges due to nearly all the switches being on, or nearly all the switches being off, will be relatively rare, and, for the same reasons, interactions between switches may appear to be small even if physically common on the wiring diagram. That is to say, we would not expect much dominance or epistacy in complex conditions. As there is no particular reason why our dial should read a linear function of whatever it is measuring, this again introduces a further element of nonlinearity, although, where the range of the majority occupies a small part of the possible range, as, for example, in height in man, various transformations may make relatively little difference.

Unfortunately, since variance partitioning in genetics preceded any clear understanding of what was being partitioned, in terms of transcription, translation, and the interaction of primary products with one another and with the environment, it is very difficult to know how its foundations relate to any biologically plausible field of cellular activity. One necessary assumption appears to be the constancy of direction of genetic effects due to one locus notwithstanding variations at other loci, or environmental variations; that is, the assumption that interactions are weak and evenly generalized, and thereby adequately handled by such corrections as epistacy or dominance, and generalized by a linear algebra. Recent knowledge of enzyme action suggests a structural complexity of such bewildering intrinsic variety that interactions can hardly be expected to be either weak or consistent, and even the basic assumption that all the genotypes could be mapped in a linear continuum, and all the environments into another linear continuum, would seem very unlikely and quite incompatible with the essential requirement of stability.

The breakdown of variability into causes peculiar to families, and other causes, may be made on the assumption of additivity, or even multiplicity, of effects, provided it is assumed that these effects are mutually monotonic;

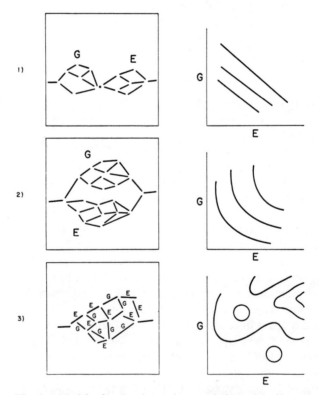

Fig. 9.  Models of interacting pathways relating to heredity and environment. In (1) and (2) heredity and environment are compartmentalized so that the overall effect can be estimated from the effects of both. In (3) they are intimately related and a meaningful summation is not necessarily possible.

that is, that any elemental environment differences, or any interchange at any locus, will always act in the same direction. [Fig. 9(1, 2)]. Where there is interaction [Fig. 9(3)] it may be very difficult or impossible to answer general questions on either genotype or environment.

## THE ANALYSIS OF MARKER DATA AT SINGLE LOCI (ALLELISM AND SEGREGATION)

In general, we assume a pedigree whose members respond to stimuli A, B, C, D, etc. (e.g., sera) with responses $A$, $B$, $C$, $D$, or $a$, $b$, $c$, $d$, to use the simple dichotomy of response or its negation used by both Mendel and Boole, and advocated earlier by de Morgan. They are inappropriate for most computers, but readily expressed as 1 or 0 in a binary sequence of defined order. Such binary arrays are used internally by electronic computers in the same representation, and are particularly easy to program.

The problem of the pedigree analysis of markers is to define which of these responses are consistent with determination by single factors (simple segregation) and thereby may be regarded as markers, which pairs show gametic exclusiveness (allelism), and which others show dependent segregation (linkage). The former problem is now adequately solved with fair precision by simple methods which are usually adequate, and with greater precision by various maximum-likelihood estimation procedures[19,23,31] now integrated by Morton into his segran programs.[27,33]

The detection of allelism, although fairly simple in that gametic exclusiveness implies a partial diploid exclusiveness, so that the distribution of some sets of responses in the diploid will be either proscribed or less common than otherwise expected, the interpretation of an allelic pattern and the elucidation of the minimal allele set have so far escaped any formal solution. The problem is easily specified. Given a set of binary responses in various pedigrees, we may ask what is the minimum set of alleles consistent with the findings. We may form the "OR" set, so called since the two haploids are expressed in the diploid in the OR relationship,

$$0 \quad \text{OR} \quad 0 = 0$$
$$1 \quad \text{OR} \quad 0 = 1$$
$$0 \quad \text{OR} \quad 1 = 1$$
$$1 \quad \text{OR} \quad 1 = 1$$

This gives for a pair of possible responses, the results shown in Table II, where the margins show the two gametes, and the body of the table the consequences of all possible pairs.

**TABLE II.**

|     | 00 | 01 | 10 | 11 |
| --- | --- | --- | --- | --- |
| 00 | 00 | 01 | 10 | 11 |
| 01 | 01 | 01 | 11 | 11 |
| 10 | 10 | 11 | 10 | 11 |
| 11 | 11 | 11 | 11 | 11 |

Where many factors are involved, as in the HL-A system, a similar table can be formed with a square of $2^{12}$ and $2^{24}$ cells, most of which are empty, presenting the problem of what is the smallest set of gametes which would give all the diploids found. While most of the information may be from the pedigree data, this is even more difficult to handle algorithmically. The matter is fully discussed on existing data by Ceppelini et al.[3]

Although segregation analysis may be used to explore the hypotheses of simple segregation expected from simple expressed factors, this is not usually a problem. A more serious problem arises when two different mechanisms are producing the same consequence and it is desired to estimate any two of the three parameters $p = ap_1 + (1 - a)p_2$, where a proportion of sibships $a$ are exposed to an expectation of some effect $p_1$ and the rest an expectation $p_2$. Where sibships of various sizes are present ancillary information on ascertainment may be present. Since in complete ascertainment the results can be reduced to sib-pairs of three varieties (both unaffected, one affected, both affected), the procedure on sibships is limited to estimating two parameters. The major application of this anlysis has been the estimation of the proportion of sporadic cases simulating a recessively determined condition,[32] the estimation of the proportion of autosomal and sex-linked recessives,[4] and the estimation of specific parameters relating to disturbed segregation, as, for example, in heterozygote advantage.[32]

In general, given a set of $n$ observations of a sibship of size $s$, the basic expectation will be a vector defined by the binomial expression $[p+(1-p)]^s n$, where $p = ap_1 + (1 - a)p_2$ and the realized expectation, after ascertainment, is obtained by multiplying the binomial expectation, cell-by-cell, with the relative chance of ascertainment and then multiplying throughout by some factor to maintain the total equal to $n$. The log-likelihood is then found by summing (observed) $\times$ log(expected) cell-by-cell and finding iteratively a solution to $p = ap_1 + (1 - a)p_2$ where one or two of the three variables are fixed.

The simplest ascertainment vectors for sibships with 0, 1,..., $s$ cases affected are ascertainment in the relative proportions

$$1 \quad 1 \quad 1 \quad 1 \quad 1 \quad 1 \qquad 1,$$
$$\text{or } 0 \quad 1 \quad 1 \quad 1 \quad 1 \quad 1 \qquad 1,$$
$$\text{or } 0 \quad 1 \quad 2 \quad 3 \quad 4 \quad 5 \qquad s$$

which relate to complete, truncate, and multiple ascertainment, respectively, but various hybrid forms may be proposed, or, in various ingenious ways, defined by a parameter which is simultaneously estimated.[33]

## THE ANALYSIS OF MARKER DATA OF MULTIPLE LOCI (LINKAGE)

A pedigree may be regarded as a system generated by a set of initial states, the gametes, which, as a result of various events, both fortuitous and due to their internal structure, and, in particular, the constraints of allelism and the proximity of loci, lead to various permutations manifest in various phenotypes. Complete specification, in terms of all possible initial states, is usually impractical, since it involves some $m^{2n}$ states for $m$ types of gametes related to $n$ founder-members, and a modular approach to pedigree study is necessary.

The basic unit of the pedigree is the individual, his or her defining gametes, and the gametic set he or she can produce. Given complete knowledge of the defining of gametes, we could determine the complete set of potential gametes produced, from which information on allelism and linkage could be gained through exclusiveness and association. In the absence of this knowledge we are compelled to define gametes in terms of probabilities. For example, in the ABO systems we replace the known gametes

| A | B | O |   | A | B | O |   | A | B | O |
|---|---|---|---|---|---|---|---|---|---|---|
| 1 | 0 | 0 |   | 0 | 1 | 0 |   | 0 | 0 | 1 |

by a gamete represented by the vector

| $p$ | $q$ | $r$ |
|-----|-----|-----|

$(p + q + r = 1)$ which, in the absence of other information, we assume to be the population allele proportions (more usually termed gene frequencies). A knowledge of the vector of the gametic partner, of the phenotype of the resulting diploid, of the gametic determinants of the phenotypes, and the assumption of some parameters relating to segregation will allow the vector of the resultant gametes to be defined. This can be done successively, working from ancestor to descendent, over any pedigree (Fig. 10).

The comparison of the fit of various parameters is slightly more complicated, since it is constrained by the knowledge that, although the parents of a child or sibship both produce a probability distribution of gametes, they themselves must have been produced from only one gamete of each type, so that an inner loop involving up to $m^4$ steps, where $m$ is the number of gametic types, is needed. This is not very onerous to modern computers.

Given a sufficient body of data, we may generate a set of likelihoods for several recombination frequencies between every pair of loci, and from these define a set of linkage groups equal to not more than the number of chromosomes, and within each linkage group define the order. In practice this is impractical, due to the magnitude of the combinatorial problem, and automatic procedures are likely to be limited to the arbitration between different sets of linkage groupings and optimization of position within specified orderings. The basic procedures for likelihood estimation have been described in detail elsewhere.[26,29,30,42]

A particular case of linkage analysis arises when data are available relating visible abnormalities to data on markers. Unfortunately, the difficulty in clarifying the exact chromosomes in the common translocations, the probable uniqueness of most rare translocations, the small size of deficiencies which are not lethal, and the uncertainty about the proportion of trisomy due to post-zygotic events, which would lead to two of the three chromosomes being isogenic, has made this form of linkage study almost totally unrewarding

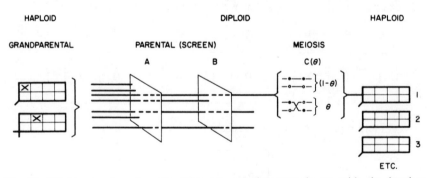

Fig. 10.  Basic procedure for generating an outgoing gametic set with the ingoing possibilities and the phenotypes, if known, at loci $A$ and $B$.

so far, apart from data on the origin of extra and deficient sex chromosomes. The latter are fully discussed by Race and Sanger.[37]

A number of procedures are available for comparing the likelihoods of various recombination fractions, either through tabulated scoring procedures,[26,29] or directly by using electronic computers.[41] These generalized computer programs are at present too elaborate for use without very extensive supervision.

Ascertainment introduces complications, but the bias introduced is usually trivial, although complicated to correct, and, in practice, usually only possible to correct by making unrealistic assumptions.

Due to the ease of clinical recognition of X-linked disease, the presence of common variants which are sex-linked (glucose-6-phosphate-dehydrogenase deficiency and the common forms of color-blindness), and the presence of one X-linked antigen for which antisera are available, most linkage results in man relate to the X chromosome.[1,37]

As a result of any of these scoring or computing procedures a set of likelihoods is derived, relating to a series of values of $\theta$, the recombination fraction, or, in some cases, to various pairs of paternal and maternal recombination fractions. These scores have the great advantage that their logarithms (which are usually given) are additive, allowing a simple addition of scores from different data. The interpretation of likelihoods in more succinct terms can be difficult, but, since they can be expressed graphically, this is unnecessary. So far the paucity of data excludes some of the more serious problems of integrating results of numerous pairs of loci to give a chromosome map. The present position is summarized by Renwick.[39]


## VARIATES

The most precise estimates of similarity of relatives are those in which measurements are made of some characteristic whose biological variability greatly exceeds the variability of measurement. Height, and lengths of various bony parts provided the classical data of Galton[18] and of Lee and Pearson.[22] Similar data may be derived from counting components of complex patterns, such as fingerprints.[20] Given any set of such measurements, we may estimate the genotypic correlation on the assumption of the inheritance of noninteracting particulate determinants, and compare this with the phenotypic correlation found; the ratio of the phenotypic to the genotypic correlation may then be used to summarize the extent of the hereditary determinants, or the heritability.

More complicated partitions of variance, and a comparison of the parental and sib similarities, may provide evidence of dominance or epistacy;[16]

however, as yet, data on man is inadequate for this, due to small numbers and bias from the differing environments in different generations.

## THE ESTIMATION OF PHENOTYPIC CORRELATION

Phenotypic similarities within sets of relatives are fairly easily estimated when the variate studied is directly measurable, and extensive analyses of numerous structural and biochemical, physiological, and psychological variates have now been carried out following the basic regression procedures of Galton[18] and their elaboration by Fisher.[16]

In the study of the familial distribution of attributes it is necessary to postulate either the segregation of small numbers of distinct determining factors, usually two, as in classical Mendelism, or to postulate very large numbers, and to assume that the discontinuity can be interpreted as a result of some underlying continuity, extreme values of which have an increased liability to be classified as a distinct minority. The simplest model, in which this liability is abrupt at a threshold (Fig. 11), arises in classifications which are based on thresholds, as in such terms as tall, premature, or hypertensive. Such models may also be utilized in the study of disorders on the assumption of a sudden threshold and a normally distributed underlying variate. This interpretation of disease was introduced by Hippocrates, under the concept of diathesis, and formally studied by biometric techniques by Pearson and others (see several articles in Volumes I and II of *Biometrica* and the introduction to the first edition of Pearson's "Tables for Statisticians Biometricians"[35]). Pearson clearly appreciated the need to express the relationship of pairs of attributes (Fig. 12) due to arbitrary thresholds, either semantic, as in tallness, or biological, as in susceptibility to smallpox, in terms of the correlation of the underlying variates, and for this purpose an exact solution was proposed by Pearson[34] and, at a prodigious cost in labor, tabulated for values of $r = 0.05$ to $0.95$ in intervals of $0.05$.[12] Little use

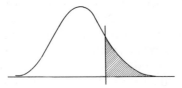

Fig. 11.   Pearson's model of a phenotype which is the result of extreme values of some normally distributed variate.

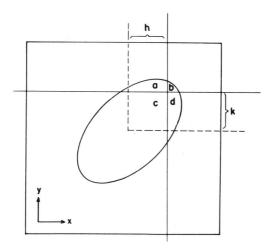

Fig. 12. Pearson's model of phenotypes of pairs of
measurements, such as height of sibs, which provide
a model for the familial concentration of some trait,
such as "tallness."

appears to have been made of this work, largely because of the computational
labor required to reach a solution. Curiously enough, Pearson never extended
the application of these coefficients to the definition of the degree of
resemblance between relatives, and the triviality of many of the examples
demonstrating the value of this procedure must have contributed to its
disuse. He did, however, use the "equiprobable $r$" to estimate the correlation
coefficient for eye color in father and son at $0.53 \pm 0.027$ (Pearson,[35]
p. XXXVIII).

Everitt[12] considered a bivariate normal surface defined by the correlation
coefficient $r$, which is divided into four quadrants (Fig. 12) by dichotomies $x$
and $y$ units of standard deviation from the mean ($h$ and $k$ in his terminology),
and tabulated the integrals whose solution gives the volume of one of the four
quadrants defined by $x$ and $y$. By interpolation $r$ may be obtained, with some
labor, from the volumes of any quadrant.

If we consider the simple case of pairs of observations on, for example,
the heights of father and son, then, following Galton,[18] these may be regarded
as being samples from a universe bounded by a bivariate normal surface. If
some arbitrary threshold is designated to define "tall," then we may dicho-
tomize this normal surface into four quadrants whose volumes would be
equal to the expected numbers, respectively, of: ($a$) tall sons with short fathers,
($b$) tall sons with tall fathers, ($c$) short sons with short fathers and ($d$) short
sons with tall fathers.

This model has been applied to characters, such as some forms of disease manifestation, in which the underlying variate is not available for study.[2,7-9,14,15,24,34,35,38] It is clear from this model that although the distributions of height of all fathers and all sons are both normal, the height distribution of the sons of either short or tall fathers is not normal. This is easily seen, since their sum is normal and the two distributions are asymptotic to different tails of the distribution of their sums. These distributions, which are asymptotic to opposite tails of a normal distribution, and whose sum is a normal distribution, may be referred to as conjugates to the normal curve. Unfortunately, they have so far proved analytically intractable, and may differ so considerably from normality that normal approximations are misleading.

In the case of quantitative inheritance the distributions of the frequencies $a$, $b$, $c$, and $d$ specify the amount of common determination between relatives, and, by estimating $r$ and dividing it by the value expected on a completely inherited variability due to independently acting hereditary units, we may estimate some summarizing index, in the way Falconer has suggested. On the assumption that the common familial environment imposed by the single uterus through which sibs pass and the common nutritional environment imposed on children are trivial, we may relate this ratio to heritability in the sense used by Wright.[42a]

Figure 13 shows the relationship between population incidence, in the relatives of "affected" individuals, and $r$, from which $r$ can be obtained approximately. This is similar to Fig. 3 in Falconer's paper,[14] but the estimates differ slightly, his estimates being about $10\%$ lower in the range of his examples.

Where the incidence of the trait in the population is large, or over $5\%$, an approximate estimate may be made from the approximation $z = (\pi/8) \log_e(bc/ad)$, with variance $(\pi/8)^2[(1/a) + (1/b) + (1/c) + (1/d)]$ (Edwards,[10] where $r \approx z$. When $r$ may be obtained more accurately from $z$ this approximation to its variance may still be of use; the approximation $V_r \approx V_z(r/z)^2$ may also be useful.

Within the limits of precision of human data so far available, linear interpolation from Fig. 13, which shows the inverse of the incidence in relatives against the inverse of the incidence in the population, provides an adequate measure of the underlying phenotypic correlation on the assumption of normality and abrupt truncation of the underlying variate. Once found, this correlation coefficient is difficult to interpret unless the nongenetic familial factors, such as dietary customs, both in quantity and variety, the environment imposed by the single uterus common to sibs, and the medication and diagnostic standards of families, are assumed trivial.

Although, in general, the heritability, as defined in this context by Falconer, will tend to be correlated with the extent of hereditary determina-

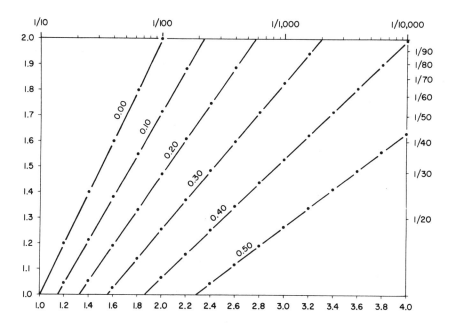

Fig. 13. Incidence in the population (horizontal) and in relatives of affected persons (vertical axis) for relatives with various phenotypic correlations (figures on lines). The scales are the incidence and the logarithm of its reciprocal.

tion, its use in arbitrating about environments is likely to be confusing, since there is no necessary connection between the value of heritability and the opportunity for environmental control. Heritability confounds necessity and sufficiency even when it measures heritable variation, and confounds the genetic and environmental features common to families when it does not. For example, exposure to dairy products is now endemic; if, as is possible, this is the major factor in arterial disease, increasing uniformity of exposure will decrease the environmental variation and necessarily "increase" the heritability. On the other hand, increasing uniformity of exposure increases the opportunity for elimination by legislation or widespread environmental change, as in the case of tuberculosis and rickets and other familial disorders of the past, so that a high heritability may imply ease of elimination.

The simple mathematics implied by the central-limit theorem on the assumption of very large numbers of hereditary particles will allow precise solutions with the aid of simple graphs or tables. However, we should be cautious in applying such models to rare conditions, since, although the number of factors may be very large, the opportunities for indefinite gradation are constrained by the relatively small number of chromosomes by which these factors are conveyed.

Consider the consequences of a set of $n$ loci with equally effective pairs of equally common alleles. Then, if the full range of phenotypic expression is $r$, its standard deviation $s$ may be shown to be $r/\sqrt{2n}$ units, and, as there are $2n + 1$ possible alternative phenotypic values, the interval between the possible phenotypic values will be approximately $r/2n$ units, or $(r/2n)/(r\sqrt{2n})$ units of standard deviation.

The latter reduces to $1/\sqrt{2n}$, so that, if we consider the consequences of 50 loci, the precision of the model cannot exceed 0.1 units of standard deviation; in order to work with a precision of 0.01 units (and the incidences implied by thresholds of 3.0 and 3.1 units are 0.00135 and 0.00097, and differ by a ratio of 1.4 to 1), we must postulate at least 20,000 evenly and independently segregating and equally effective loci. This coarseness in the model seems to impose a lower limit of incidence of disorders which can be approximated with any semblance of realism. Perhaps we should regard between $-2$ and $+2$ standard deviations, or the minority limit of about 3 %, as a reasonable limit to the resolving power of this model. The situation is complicated in practice by the inequality in both the effectiveness and the proportions of different alleles, as well as their interactions, and while it may be reasonable to assume that every allele has some effect on any variate, there are likely to be few variates in which a substantial part, say a tenth, of the variance is not attributable to a very few loci.

The concept of resolving power in this context is difficult. It is not, however, altogether false to consider optical analogies. Light microscopy will resolve protozoa adequately, bacteria to some extent, and viruses hardly at all: variance partitioning and distribution by truncation may be similarly limited to the more frequent attributes. This excludes most diseases in man (although not the causes of most deaths) and, in particular, all congenital malformations. Its use in ranges beyond this seems to be little more than an extremely complicated way of transforming a very small number, such as an incidence, to some number more readily handled, such as the logarithm of its reciprocal. The fact that these transformations are monotonic and that, with a few very rare exceptions, all disorders in man are familial, ensures that any such transformation will lead to a consistent calculus which can, to some extent, be used to grade the degree of hereditary resemblance.

Variance partitioning and allied methods based on truncation appear to give a rough measure of strength of inheritance, or heritability, and allow a rough ranking of disorders in forms of hereditary influence at the times and places studied. However, the heritability so defined is highly specific to the population studied, and is in no sense a feature of the disease considered in isolation.

The hereditary contribution to variance thus appears analogous to other measures of complex situations, such as the concepts of monopoly or utility in economics, or neuroticism in psychiatry. Such concepts can only be expressed quantitatively in relation to situations which are artificially simple, and their great value in determining the quantitative behavior of models should be distinguished from their use as estimates to specify complex structures in terms of a few dimensionless numbers. In particular, we should appreciate that heritability estimates are not a feature of a disease, but a feature of a disease manifest in a specific population, so that we cannot meaningfully talk about the heritability of, for example, diabetes, or spina bifida, but only of the heritability in a specific population on such assumptions as the triviality of familial patterns of diet or of the constrained variability of a single uterus.

## ANALYSIS OF STATES

States which are specified by certain genotypes, such as albinism, haemophilia, or Apert's syndrome, do not normally lead to any difficulties in pedigree analysis, although estimation of their segregation may be complicated due to ascertainment. Where the genotype completely specifies the phenotype, the techniques considered in the discussion of markers may be used. In practice, advances in biochemical and clinical techniques, and in the knowledge of the types of manifestation to be expected, make segregational analysis of decreasing value in the study of specified disease, although of value in resolving mixtures of disorders which cannot yet be specified. In theory, abnormal segregation is an attractive explanation for the maintenance of genes which are harmful in various combinations; in practice, the rather small disturbances which would be an adequate explanation are usually smaller than the effects of bias due to incomplete or inaccurate ascertainment and small compared to the sampling variability of the numbers usually available. Unfortunately, these limitations are inversely correlated, since the diagnostic standards must necessarily always deteriorate as the number of observers increases, or as the intensity of each observation decreases.

States sometimes represent the manifestation of some genetic variant which takes time to express itself, and this leads to serious difficulties due to the pattern of such inheritance closely simulating that expected from multi-factorial inheritance. Basically, we may assume a probability $p$ of carrying a genetic factor manifest in the heterozygote with a probability of $f(t)$, which is a function of age $t$. The expectation of being affected is therefore $pf(t)$, and of being unaffected is $1 - pf(t)$, and the chance of an offspring of age $t'$ also being affected is $(1/2) pf(t) f(t')$, and so on.

Such algebraic formulations quickly get out of hand, since they fail to discriminate between the most likely hypotheses, which cannot even be defined distinctively, since the function $f(t)$ can hardly be uninfluenced by numerous genetic factors. Various procedures have been recommended for the distinction of multifactorial and single-factor inheritance on the assumption that because one locus is of major importance, all others are of trivial influence. Vogel and Kruger[43] advanced several criteria which make this assumption.

This difficulty is more readily appreciated if we consider a set of loci $A$, $B$, $C$, $D$,..., $Z$ which relate to some variate, and assume values beyond some threshold to define an attribute. Then, where the total range of the phenotype is $r$, we may consider a series of cases in which (1) variation due to locus $A = rp$, and (2) variation due to loci $B-Z = r(1 - p)$. As $p$ changes slowly from 1 (complete penetrance) to $1/n$, when $n$ is the number of loci, there will be a steady loss of pattern in the manifestation of the pedigrees examined. Vogel and Kruger's criterion assumes that there is no such spectrum of disproportionate influence of different loci, and implies an intrinsic difference in the biological basis of single-factor and many-factor inheritance, although we have no evidence of two basic mechanisms, and, as Fisher demonstrated,[17] we have both observational and theoretical reasons for expecting evolution by modification of the effects at one locus through other loci.

We will consider four basic models for the expression of states in pedigrees (Fig. 14). Since states are defined by discontinuity, they must be interpreted by a model which has (1) only one factor, or (2) many factors and a single threshold, or (3) many factors and a discontinuity imposed by some function relating a change in state to some function, such as the sum, of many factors. We may consider these models in relation to two factors at a large number of pairs of loci $a$, $b$, $c$, $d$, etc., each of which may take the values 0 or 1 depending on the alleles they contain.

The four models amount to, where $s = a + b + c + d \cdots$ and $t$ is the threshold,

1. If $a = 0$, phenotype is in state 0; if $a = 1$, phenotype is in state 1.

2. If $s < t$, phenotype is in state 0; if $s \geqslant t$, phenotype is in state 1.

3. Phenotype is in state 1 with probability $f(s)$, where $f$ is function of $s$, and is otherwise in state 0.

4. This resembles 3, except that the probability depends on the absolute differences between $s$ and its mean value.

Model 1 adequately covers the transmission of such states as Huntington's chorea or phenylketonuria, in which the phenotype is fairly consistently determined by the genotype, although there is nearly always considerable familial variation in the expression of such disorders, the severity

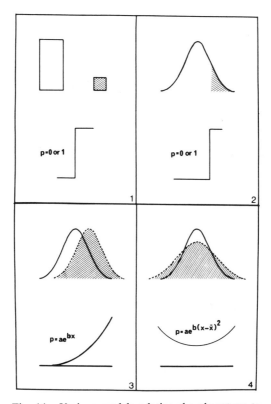

Fig. 14. Various models relating the phenotype to the genotype. In (1) the genotype is discontinuous and divides the population into groups with probabilities of affectation of 0 and 100 %. In (2) the total genotypic effect shows a normal distribution with probabilities of affection of 0 and 1.0 across a threshhold. In (3) the liability increases steadily and experimentally with the genotypic distribution. In (4) the liability increases with the deviation from the mean.

of which varies greatly from family to family. Variation may be due to various forms of mutant alleles, as in haemoglobinopathies due to mutants in any defined chain, or due to modification by a homologous allele, a form of expression only manifest by fairly sophisticated parent–child and child–child comparison,[40] or through the genetic background.

Model 2 has already been discussed as a special case of variate analysis where a variate, overt or inferred, is assumed to distinguish two states determined by a threshold defined only by its partition proportions on the assumption of a normal curve.

Model 3, in which liability increases steadily with incidence,[9] has the intuitive advantage of realism, in that it does not involve an arbitrary threshold, and the considerable analytical advantage that if the risk is specified as $ae^{bx}$, the parameter $b$ has the effect of bodily shifting the derived normal curve (the curve of distribution of the variate in the affected population) along the $X$ axis, and $a$ is purely a scaling parameter which, in collusion with $b$, determines the incidence or proportion of the affected subset. Since the variance is unaffected, the area of this curve (the incidence) is determined by the height at the mean or mode. The theoretical objection that the incidence is not constrained to less than unity is rarely a practical problem, due to the extreme rarity of the population when $x$ exceeds 3 or so.

If as a model we consider hypertension and one of its complications, apoplexy, then we may infer an underlying distribution of blood pressure with unit variance, and suppose that any individual with a blood pressure of $x$ units is exposed to a risk of affliction equal to $ae^{bx}$. The diseased subset will have a distribution of $x$ determined by the distribution

$$ae^{bx}(2\pi)^{-1/2} \exp - \tfrac{1}{2}x^2 = a(2\pi)^{-1/2} \exp - \tfrac{1}{2}(x - b)^2 \exp \tfrac{1}{2}b^2$$

so that the mode, and mean, of the affected population occurs when $x = b$. The incidence is then $a(2\pi)^{-1/2} \exp \tfrac{1}{2}b^2$.

Assuming the underlying population has a genetically determined distribution of $x$, due to numerous factors, then two populations with a genetic correlation $r$ may be shown by similar algebra[10] to have a relative risk $\exp(rb^2)$. This is the ratio of incidence in relatives of affected persons compared to the population incidence. Penrose[36] termed this $k$. It has the particular advantage of simplicity and ease of estimation. If, to follow the terminology used by Falconer,[14] we allow $p$ and $q$ to refer to the incidence in the population and in relatives, then $\log_e k = \log_e (q/p)$, with approximate variance $(1/P) + (1/Q)$, where $P$ and $Q$ are the numbers of cases observed in the two groups. The exact variance includes as further terms the reciprocals of the numbers of unaffected, and can normally be ignored. Normally $P$ is so much greater than $Q$ that it may also be ignored, the variance being $1/Q$.

Estimation of $b$ is simple since

$$\log_e k = b^2 r, \qquad \text{or} \qquad b = [(\log_e k)/r]^{1/2} = [(0.42 \log k)/r]^{1/2},$$

where $r$ is the genotypic correlation. We have $b = (0.82 \log k)^{1/2}$ for first-degree relatives. Since the incidence $p = a \exp \tfrac{1}{2}b^2$, $a$ is also easily estimated.

To a first approximation $b$ may be regarded as a parameter expressing the familial tendency, which may be largely due to genetic determinants, while $a$ is related to the environmental determinants; this formulation has the advantage that it is very obvious that whatever $b$ is, this in no way excludes the prospect of reducing the incidence through environmental modification acting over $a$. Morton[33] has rephrased the formula as $e^{a+bx}$, where his $a$ is the natural logarithm of mine. As these are arbitrary scaling constants, this makes little difference.

This formulation should be regarded as an alternative to the heritability argument.

A modification of the continuous increment model, in which the variance rather than the mean varies, is shown in Fig. 14(1). This model is also considered in detail, from a slightly different standpoint, by Falconer.[15]

In some contexts, such as erratic behavior, it is easy to imagine an inherited tendency with various consequences showing a familial concentration. In terms of specific disorders, it is difficult to imagine that, for example, high and low blood pressure should predispose to identical disorders, although both must impair viability, presumably through different handicaps. Birth weight and gestation show an elegant symmetry in viability, but the causes of death at the extremes are quite different.[21]

Algebraically, the situation is fairly simple. If the population distribution of some variates is $(2\pi)^{-1/2} \exp - \frac{1}{2}x^2$, and the liability is $a \exp bx^2$, the derived population will have the distribution

$$a(\exp bx^2)(2\pi)^{-1/2} \exp - \tfrac{1}{2}x^2 = a(2\pi)^{-1/2} \exp - \tfrac{1}{2}x^2(1 - 2b)$$

which has a variance increased to $1/(1 - 2b)$ compared to the population variance. As the unaffected population will have a reduced variance, the model is particularly attractive, in that it is inheritantly stable.


## HERITABILITY

In conditions which are not adequately explained by single-factor insufficiency, where we must postulate several factors variously confused by differing environments, models relating the genetic determinants to the phenotype are available if it is assumed that (1) the number of factors is very large, (2) that none has any major effect, (3) that the influence of the environment may be regarded in simply additive terms, and (4) the familial correlation of environmental variables is trivial. This approach, the heritability argument, has been discussed with great clarity and several examples by Falconer,[14,15] while its use in experimental genetics and breeding programs is fully explained in his book.[13]

Since there are, in my opinion, difficulties in finding conditions in man in which conditions 1–4 are all likely to be satisfied, and since Falconer's papers are definitive and widely available, I will not discuss this approach further, although the preliminary estimation of phenotypic correlation, on which heritability is based, has been discussed above. It is important to point out once again that "heritability" is not a structural parameter, comparable to the position of a locus, the sequence of amino acids in a protein, or the Menton–Michaelis constant of an enzyme, but a "summarizing index" which is specific to a set of data, and cannot (like the structural parameters considered above) be assumed similar in different environments. Since it does not relate to a specific mechanism, but summarizes very numerous assumed mechanisms, it is difficult to utilize a heritability estimate either at the level of advising a patient or of advising on allocation of resources. Pearson[34] considered that the highly heritable nature of tuberculosis made environmental change unlikely to be effective.

In summary, we have two basic sets of analytical procedures, the single-factor analysis, in which there is a well understood mechanism, explicable in several structural parameters, largely common to all organisms, and the many-factor, often translated as multi factorial or polygenic in Latin and Greek, a translation which confers neither brevity nor clarity, in which the simplicity of the algebra permitted by the assumptions of large numbers of noninteracting or feebly interacting components permits the summarization of a set of observations in terms of a "heritability" varying between zero and unity.

In intelligence or height it appears intuitively reasonable to assume a very large number of loci influencing the phenotype, none of which has any major effect. In other fields, such as metabolic disorders dominated by simple compounds which are handled by small numbers of enzymatic pathways, such as diabetes or gout, we may also make this postulate without fear of contradiction from data, although it would seem unwise to exclude the possibility that variation might be dominated by a few major routes determined by the enzymes produced from a few loci.

It appears to be believed widely that disorders with a high heritability, that is, a pattern of inheritance consistent with Mendelian factors expressing themselves with little disturbance from the environment or from each other, are less amenable to environmental control. In the extreme case where the anticipated heritable variation, on the assumption of trivial environmental effects, is realized, this may be true within the population studied, although it need not be true in other populations. However, where the situation is so complex that the assumption of a very large number of genetic factors has to be made in order to create a simple algebra, and the variation observed exceeds that anticipated from simple genetic variation, there is no reason to suppose any simple connection between the extent of heritability so expressed and the effects of environment changes on the distribution of these variates. Even man's height, the yardstick of biometric certainty fifty years ago, when estimates were made with the precision of a hair's width, is now known to be particularly prone to nutritional influence.

The basic requirement of preventive medicine is the detection of necessary causes and their elimination. Heritability estimates, since they confound sufficiency and necessity, can give little guidance in this field.

## OTHER USES OF PEDIGREE DATA

The interpretation of pedigrees in relation to data on states, events, and variates has been described. Such data are largely irrelevant to the dynamics of gene flow, and the basic genetic structure of the population must be studied. The analysis of population structure requires the linking together of individuals by the bonds of parentage, and the analysis of this structure in terms of various parameters.

The problem of formal structure is simple, since, if each birth is regarded as an event in space and time, then latitude, longitude, and date define a three-dimensional universe of people, and the lines connecting individuals to their parents provide all the data available on relationships. This structure will have some of the properties of a crystal,[9] and can, to some extent, be summarized in terms of the correlation of valencies, or numbers of offspring, between various related individuals, or linked points, and the enumeration of ancestors.[9,10] The former partially defines the correlation of fertility within families, a poorly studied set of parameters which greatly influences the chances of survival of mutants of defined viability. Such parameters may be termed branch parameters, since they partly define the branch structure of the family tree.

Enumeration of ancestors defines the root structure of the family tree, and the extent to which the roots join up to form an ancestral net is most readily summarized in terms of the number of ancestors at any rank, or of its consequence, the inbreeding coefficient, which defines the gametic correlation. Various procedures have been developed for automatic enumeration of ancestors,[25] a task well suited to electronic computers. Enumeration, or root searches of pedigrees, does not in itself solve the problem of gametic correlation, but unbiased estimates of adequate precision can be made by branch searches from randomly designated ancestors using Monte Carlo methods,[5] and these would appear in many ways preferable.

These structural parameters, based on relationship without reference to characterization of individuals other than by sex and fertility, may be supplemented by various estimates derived from the correlation of phenotypes of mating pairs, and the divergence of the phenotype distribution of individuals from that expected if the gametes were uncorrelated. Both these methods are discussed in detail by Yasuda[44]: in practice, on present data, the variances of the estimates are large, and their value at present largely theoretical.

The evaluation of the inbreeding coefficient, or some other more exactly defined parameter of common heritage, is essential for any clear understanding of the dynamics of mutant alleles which are severely disabling when homozygous, and for any evaluation of the contribution, if any, of heterozygote advantage to the origin or maintenance of genetic diversity.

The interpretation to be imposed on the fine structure of pedigree data remains, at present, largely unexplored; in large part this is due to lack of data on which to explore. Until such data are available little information on either the genetic structure of human populations, or on its implications in relation to the fate of mutants of defined relative viability, can be anticipated. Now that the severe analytic problems of stochastic studies can be bypassed by simulation, it will be possible to study very elementary problems of gene flow empirically either on real data, or, where this is insufficient, on simulated data based on structural parameters estimated from the real data. Until this is done the fundamental unknown in population genetics, the probability of distribution of the numbers of a gene of specified, or neutral, relative viability will continue to be unknown. While societies with adequate records may hardly be typical of the past, they are at least preferable to nothing, and may be relevant to the future.

## SUMMARY

An attempt has been made to review the ways in which the study of several related persons can give information on the nature of their genetic determinants. A distinction is drawn between structural parameters, which relate to physical structures such as genes and chromosomes, and summarizing indices, which are related to determinants which cannot be resolved.

## BIBLIOGRAPHY

1. Berg, K., and A. G. Bearn, *Progress in Medicine. Genetics* (1968).
2. Carter, C. O., Inheritance of congenital pyloric stenosis, *Brit. Med. Bull.* **17**(3):251–253 (1961).
3. Ceppelini, R., *et al.*, Genetics of leukocyte antigens: a family study of segregation and linkage, *in* "Histocompatibility Testing" (E. S. Curtoni *et al.*, eds.), pp. 149–187, Williams & Wilkins, Baltimore (1967).
4. Chung, C. S., O. W. Robison, and N. E. Morton, A note on deaf mutism, *Ann. Hum. Genet.* **23**:357–366 (1959).

5. Edwards, A. W. F., *in* "Conference on Computer Application to Genetics," in press.

6. Edwards, J. H., A note on the practical interpretation of $2 \times 2$ tables, *Brit. J. Prev. Soc. Med.* **11**:73 (1957).

7. Edwards, J. H., The Simulation of Mendelism, *Acta Genet. Statist. Med.* **10**:63 (1960).

8. Edwards, J. H., The genetic basis of common disease, *Am. J. Med.* **34**:627 (1963).

9. Edwards, J. H., Linkage studies of whole populations, *in* "Proc. III Int. Congress on Human Genetics," p. 479 (1966).

10. Edwards, J. H., *in* "Record Linkage in Medicine," (E. D. Acheson, ed.), Livingstone, London (1968).

11. Edwards, J. H., The familial predisposition in man, *Brit. Med. Bull.* **25**:58 (1969).

12. Everitt, P. F., Supplementary tables for finding the correlation coefficient from tetrachoric groupings, *Biometrika* **VIII**:385 (1914).

13. Falconer, D. S., "An Introduction to Quantitive Genetics," Oliver & Boyd, London (1960).

14. Falconer, D. S., The inheritance of liability to certain diseases, estimated from the incidence among relatives, *Ann. Hum. Genet.* **29**:51 (1965).

15. Falconer, D. S., The inheritance of liability to diseases with variable age of onset, with particular reference to diabetes mellitus, *Ann. Hum. Genet.* **31**:1 (1967).

16. Fisher, R. A., The correlation between relatives on the supposition of Mendelian inheritance, *Trans. Roy. Soc. Edinburgh* **52**:399 (1918).

17. Fisher, R. A., "The Genetical Theory of Natural Selection" (1930).

18. Galton, F., Co-relations and their measurement, chiefly from anthropometric data, *Proc. Roy. Soc.* **XLV**:135 (1888).

19. Haldane, J. B. S., The estimation of the frequencies of recessive conditions in man, *Ann. Hum. Genet.* **8**:255–262 (1938).

20. Holt, Sarah B., Quantitative genetics of finger-print patterns, *Brit. Med. Bull.* **17**:247–250 (1961).

21. Karn, M. N., and L. S. Penrose, Birthweight and gestation time in relation to maternal age, parity and infant survival, *Ann. Hum. Genet.* **16**:147–164 (1951).

22. Lee, A., and K. Pearson, On the laws of inheritance in man. 1. Inheritance of physical characters, *Biometrika* **2**:357.

23. Lejeune, J., Sur une solution "*a priori*" de la méthode "*a posteriori*" de Haldane, *Biometrics* **14**:513–520 (1958).

24. MacDonell, W. R., A study of the variation and correlation of the human skull, with special reference to English crania, *Biometrika* **3**:191 (1904).

25. McKusick, V. A., and H. E. Cross, *in* "Record Linkage in Medicine," (E. D. Acheson, ed.), Livingstone, London (1968).

26. Maynard-Smith, S., L. S. Penrose, and C. A. B. Smith, "Mathematical Tables for Research Workers in Human Genetics," Churchill, London (1961).

27. Mi, M.-P., Segregation analysis, *Am. J. Hum. Genet.* **19**:313–321 (1967).

28. Moran, P. A. P., and C. A. B. Smith, Commentary on R. A. Fisher's paper on The Correlation between Relatives on the Supposition of Mendelian Inheritance, Eugenics Laboratory Memoirs, Vol. XLI, pp. 1–62.

29. Morton, N. E., Sequential tests for the detection of linkage, *Amer. J. Hum. Genet.* **7**:277–318 (1955).

30. Morton, N. E., Further scoring types in sequential linkage tests with a critical review of autosomal and partial sex linkage in man, *Amer. J. Hum. Genet.* **9**:55–75 (1957).

31. Morton, N. E., Genetic tests under incomplete ascertainment, *Amer. J. Hum. Genet.* **11**:1–17 (1959).

32. Morton, N. E., and C. S. Chung, Are the MN blood groups maintained by selection? *Amer. J. Hum. Genet.* **11**:237–251 (1959).
33. Morton, N. E., *in* "Conference on Computer Application to Genetics, 1968," in press.
34. Pearson, K., On the laws of inheritance in man, II. On the inheritance of the mental and moral characters in man and its comparison with the inheritance of the physical characters, *Biometrika* **3**:131 (1904).
35. Pearson, K., "Tables for Statisticians and Biometricians," C.U.P. (1914).
36. Penrose, L. S., The genetical background of common diseases, *Acta Genet. (Basel)* **4**:257 (1953).
37. Race, R. R., and R. Sanger, "Blood Groups in Man," Blackwell, Oxford (1968).
38. Record, R. G., and J. H. Edwards, Environmental influences related to the aetiology of congenital dislocation of the hip, *Brit. J. Prev. Soc. Med.* **12**:8 (1958).
39. Renwick, J. H., Progress in mapping human autosomes, *Brit. Med. Bull.* **25**:65 (1969).
40. Renwick, J. H., Nail-patella syndrome; evidence for modification by alleles at the main locus, *Ann. Hum. Genet.* **21**:159 (1956).
41. Renwick, J. H., and D. Bolling, A program-complex for encoding, analyzing and storing human linkage data, *Amer. J. Hum. Genet.* **19**:360–367 (1962).
42. Renwick, J. H., and S. D. Lawler, Genetical linkage between the ABO and nail-patella loci, *Ann. Hum. Genet.* **19**:312 (1955).
42a. Wright, S., Coefficients of inbreeding and relationship, *Amer. Naturalist* **56**:330 (1922).
43. Vogel, F., and J. Krüger, Multifactorial determination of genetic affections, *in* "Proc. of the III International Congress on Human Genetics," p. 437 (1966).
44. Yasuda, N., An extension of Wahlund's principle to evaluate mating type frequency, *Amer. J. Hum. Genet.* **20**:1–23 (1968).

*Chapter 2*

# Autoradiography in Human Cytogenetics

## Orlando J. Miller*

*Department of Obstetrics and Gynecology*
*and*
*Human Genetics and Developmental Biology*
*College of Physicians and Surgeons*
*Columbia University*

## INTRODUCTION

Autoradiography, or radioautography, is a technique for studying the location or amount of a substance by tagging it with a radioactive isotope and recording the location and number of as large a proportion of the resultant disintegrations as possible in a photographic emulsion. Autoradiography has been applied to numerous problems in human cytogenetics, including the accurate identification of specific chromosomes and their genic content, the organization and segregation of the genetic material, the control of gene duplication, transcription, and the role of chromosomes in development and evolution.

Monographs dealing with autoradiographic studies of protein synthesis,[150] cell biology, and molecular genetics[47,77] have recently been published, and the methods of autoradiography have been extensively reviewed.[11,40,234,238,261] Consequently, these areas will not be extensively reviewed here. On the other hand, many of the investigators applying these techniques in human cytogenetics have paid little attention to the quantitative and, particularly, the statistical aspects of autoradiography, and these will therefore be presented in somewhat more detail.

* Career Scientist of the Health Research Council of the City of New York. This work was supported in part by a grant from the National Institute of Child Health and Human Development of the U.S. Public Health Service under grant HD 00516.

## TECHNICAL ASPECTS

### Radioactive Isotopes

### Types Useful in Autoradiography

Radioisotopes spontaneously decay into a different isotope, with the released energy in the form of $\alpha$-, $\beta$-, or $\gamma$-rays. Only the first two are important in autoradiography, the second especially so. The main source of $\alpha$-particles is the heavy metals, whose rarity in living tissues limits their usefulness. An unusual application was the recent demonstration of a total switch from production of tadpole hemoglobin chains to frog hemoglobin chains after metamorphosis, using $^{203}$Hg *in vitro*.[262]

Most of the isotopes useful in biological work are $\beta$-emitters. These include $^3$H, $^{14}$C, $^{32}$P, $^{35}$S, $^{59}$Fe, and $^{125}$I. The first four of these atoms are almost universally present in biological material, and their radioactive isotopes make very useful markers. A $\beta$-particle, or electron, is so light and easily deflected by orbital electrons that it tends to follow a highly irregular path, whose length is related to its initial energy. Sometimes the choice of isotope is dictated by the problem under study, e.g., to study genetic abnormalities in the synthesis of a cysteine-containing mucopolysaccharide, one might choose an isotope such as $^{35}$S.[161a] In light-microscope autoradiography tritium ($^3$H) is usually the isotope of choice because its $\beta$-particles have the shortest path distance and therefore permit the highest resolution. Their average range in deoxyribonucleic acid (DNA) or protein (density 1.3) is only 0.7 $\mu$. In photographic emulsion (density 3.5) 99 % of tritium $\beta$-particles will penetrate no further than 0.8 $\mu$ and rarely penetrate beyond the first layer of silver bromide crystals in AR-10 stripping film.[210] However, the ultra-thin tissue sections and monolayer emulsions used in electron-microscope autoradiography permit almost equally high resolution with other $\beta$-emitters.[41]

### Rate of Radioactive Decay

Decay of radioisotopes occurs at a fixed rate characteristic of each isotope. The number of disintegrations is measured in curies (Ci), or microcuries ($\mu$Ci). One microcurie is the amount of a radioactive substance necessary to produce $3.7 \times 10^4$ disintegrations per second (dps). The time required for half the atoms to decay is called the half-life of that isotope. Tritium, with a half-life of 12.26 years, disintegrates at the rate of about 0.112 % per week, while $^{14}$C, with its much longer half-life, 5600 years, disintegrates at only 0.000238 % per week. The rate of disintegration of radioactively labeled compounds, measured in curies per mole, is called the specific activity of the compound. Since one mole of any substance contains

$6.025 \times 10^{23}$ molecules, the substitution of one tritium atom for hydrogen in each molecule would yield $6.025 \times 10^{23}$ atoms of tritium per mole, which would produce $1.20 \times 10^{15}$ dps, equal to $3.2 \times 10^4$ Ci. Thus, the specific activity of the substance would be $3.2 \times 10^4$ Ci/mole, or 32 Ci/mM. With isotopes of short half-life, such as tritium, high specific activities are attainable, and this is essential if one is to detect small structures or those containing relatively few molecules of a specific kind. These problems are magnified in electron-microscope autoradiography, where ultra-thin sections are used.[238,261]

## Photographic Emulsions

### Types of Emulsions

Photographic emulsions consist of a suspension of silver bromide crystals in gelatin. The characteristics of photographic emulsions that are important in autoradiography have been reviewed extensively.[11,40,77,234] Nuclear emulsions differ from those used in regular photography by their smaller and more uniform size of silver bromide crystals (ranging from $0.03–0.4$ $\mu$ in different nuclear emulsions to $0.5–3.0$ $\mu$ in standard film). Nuclear emulsions are of two main types: stripping film and sol-gel dipping emulsions. The most commonly used stripping film is Kodak AR-10, which has a $5$-$\mu$ layer of emulsion supported by a $10$-$\mu$ layer of gelatin. The best method of handling stripping film appears to be that of Schmid and Carnes,[244] in which the photographic plates are soaked in alcohol prior to cutting and stripping the film from the glass. This greatly reduces sparking and the resultant formation of latent images, without requiring the careful control of humidity otherwise necessary during the stripping process. The result is an easier, more rapid technique and a lower background of silver grains in the final autoradiograph. Stripping film plates can be stored for a relatively long time, and are thus ideally suited for the usually small-scale operations of human cytogenetics. Liquid emulsions are quite satisfactory for qualitative and quantitative autoradiography both at the level of the light microscope[139] and the electron microscope.[238] They are relatively easy to use, many slides can be coated quickly, and the thickness of the emulsion can be controlled, most simply by diluting the emulsion to a variable degree.[76] One drawback of the liquid emulsions is that they develop a high background rather quickly, so that the shelf life may be only one to two months.

The sensitivity of an emulsion, i.e., the likelihood that an electron striking the emulsion will produce a silver grain, depends upon the rate of energy loss by the radiation striking it. At the low energies characteristic of tritium the rate of energy loss is very high, and a relatively insensitive emulsion will record tritium almost as well as a highly sensitized one, and usually with a lower background. One can therefore use Kodak NTB-2 instead of NTB-3 emulsion or Ilford K2 instead of K5.[234] Sensitivity can be increased by gold latensification, a process by which metallic gold is deposited onto latent images.[11] The sensitivity may be greatly reduced by latent-image fading due to oxidation of the reduced silver by air or by contact with some biological specimens. These sources of error can be prevented by exposing the emulsion in an inert gas atmosphere and by coating the specimen with a thin layer of carbon, about 50 Å thick[11,231]

## Removal of Silver Grains or Emulsion

The presence of abundant silver grains tends to obscure the underlying labeled specimen, making it difficult to correlate the grains with specific biological structures, such as chromosomes. This problem can be resolved by photographing specific regions of the specimen prior to autoradiography, to obtain the highest-quality view of the structures under study, relocating the same cells after autoradiography, and using the photograph as a guide to the specific location of grains.[4,14,89] This method has the disadvantage that a large proportion of the cells photographed may be unlabeled. An alternative approach is to photograph the labeled specimen after autoradiography, then to remove the silver grains by bleaching with potassium ferricyanide solution. Better resolution of the underlying specimen is obtained if the emulsion is also removed by trypsin digestion.[20] If the specimen is coated by a very thin layer of some water-impermeable substance, such as polyvinyl chloride or Formvar, the entire emulsion can be easily removed, thus facilitating examination of the labeled portions of the specimen[22] and also permitting repeated filming in order to obtain more-quantitative analyses of labeling intensities.[264]

## Two-Emulsion Technique

Various double-labeling techniques involving the application of two separate layers of nuclear emulsion have been worked out[61,78] to enable the investigator to study two processes simultaneously. These techniques take advantage of the short path distance of tritium $\beta$-particles. Most of these will not penetrate even 1 $\mu$ of nuclear emulsion overlying the tritium-labeled specimen, and virtually none will penetrate a layer of stripping film, whereas the $\beta$-particles produced by $^{14}C$ decay have an average path distance of 12 $\mu$ in emulsion and are thus easily picked up in a second layer of stripping film, though with lower resolution.

## Autoradiographic Efficiency

The efficiency of an autoradiographic procedure is defined as the ratio of the number of radioactive decays recorded to the number that occurred in a labeled source, and can be calculated by comparing grain counts with disintegrations per unit time scored in a scintillating counter.[234] Dewey *et al.*[69] found that the efficiency of AR-10 stripping film was the same for tritium $\beta$-particles originating in interphase nuclei as in metaphase cells, being $10.8 \pm 0.5\%$ for exposure times from 4 to 200 hr. This means that self-absorption of the $\beta$-particles in the metaphase cells was roughly the same as that in the interphase cells, a finding seemingly at variance with the observations of Maurer and Primbsch,[165] who found complete absorption of tritium-produced $\beta$-rays in no more than 3 $\mu$ of nucleoplasm, 2 $\mu$ of cytoplasm, and 0.6 $\mu$ of nucleolus. Others have reported film efficiencies of 5 and 7 % for smears of mammalian cells (reviewed by Dewey *et al.*[69]), while Falk and King[76] found an efficiency of 16 % for 0.5-$\mu$ thick sections and progressively lower efficiencies as section thickness was increased. Small variations in thickness and differing densities of cellular organelles can thus reduce the accuracy of quantitative evaluation of disintegration rates.

## Resolution

The error in localizing the site of a radioactive decay, i.e., the resolving power of an autoradiographic technique, can be defined in several ways.[210] In human cytogenetics we are usually concerned with resolution as the distance that must separate two labeled sources before they can be distinguished from each other. When one observes distinct silver grains rather than heavily labeled objects with continuous densities, resolving power has only statistical validity, although the results will be the same, *given adequate sample size.*[264]

The photographic process limits resolution in two ways. First, the latent image need not be at the exact spot where the silver bromide crystal was hit, and second, the resultant silver grain need not form symmetrically around the latent image. Consequently, both the size of the silver bromide crystal and the size of the developed silver grain affect the resolution of the autoradiographic technique. The best resolution of autoradiograms is less than the resolving power of the light microscope by a factor of about five (1 $\mu$ *vs.* 0.2 $\mu$)[113] and of the electron microscope by a factor of at least 100 (500 Å *vs.* 5 Å). With the electron microscope a resolution of 1500–2000 Å (0.15–0.2 $\mu$) is relatively easy to attain, even with tissue sections as thick as 1000 Å.[238] For higher resolution much thinner sections and more cumbersome techniques are necessary.

## Special Considerations in the Study of DNA

### Types of Labeled Precursor

Thymidine is an almost specific precursor of DNA, i.e., it is virtually not incorporated into any other molecules except water-soluble intermediates, which are removed from the specimen during the processes of fixation, washing, and autoradiography. Bryant[30] has detected a slight incorporation of tritium into cytoplasmic and nuclear protein after administration of ³H-thymidine (³H-TdR), but this amounts to no more than about 2.5 % of the tritium (see Figs. 12 and 13).

Adenine, cytosine, and guanine are present in both DNA and RNA. Uridine is present only in RNA, but is partially converted to cytidine within cells, and can therefore be incorporated in both DNA and RNA. However, ³H-5-uridine (³H-5-UdR) is a specific precursor of RNA, since tritium in the 5 position will be removed by the methylation reaction leading to cytidine. Labeled thymidine is the precursor of choice in studies involving DNA synthesis, but most of the labeled nucleoside bases mentioned above can be used in such studies, simply by removing RNA from the specimen with RNAase prior to autoradiography. Information of several types should be obtainable in this way. By using cytosine, guanine, or 5-methyl-cytosine, a base present in very low proportions in human DNA, it should be possible to find out whether any chromosome or relatively large chromosome segment has a base composition that differs significantly from that of other chromosomal regions. Sigman and Gartler[254] found a late-replicating X chromosome less frequently with ³H-cytidine labeling than with ³H-TdR, suggesting that the late-replicating portions of the X have a higher proportion of thymine than of cytosine.

### Availability of Labeled Precursors

Under the usual conditions of culture and dose ³H-TdR is very rarely exhausted from the medium.[14,147,203] On the other hand, it is possible to add so little ³H-TdR that it can be exhausted in a matter of minutes.[144] Lang et al.[147] determined the relative amount of labeled thymidine in the media in HeLa cell cultures over a 50-hr period. It fell to half the original value in approximately 8 hr. In vivo, labeled precursors are removed from the circulation much more quickly, so that single injections are comparable to pulse-labeling unless the intracellular precursor pool is large.[146,277]

### Tritium Effect

Incubation of human leukocytes with tritium-labeled nucleosides can lead to chromosome breaks,[17] although about 1700 tritium disintegrations (from incorporated $^3$H-TdR) are required to produce one visible chromosome aberration.[69] Either a single tritium disintegration is relatively ineffective, or the damage is readily repaired. In support of the latter is the finding that isotopically labeled DNA ($^{14}$C or $^3$H) is more susceptible to enzymatic degradation with deoxyribonuclease.[233]

The incorporation of $^3$H-TdR has a number of effects on cellular systems similar to those of radiation.[142,253] One of these effects, a lengthening of $G_2$, must be taken into consideration when designing some experiments.

## Quantitative Aspects

Thymidine is now available labeled with tritium in the 5-methyl group (which is stable in aqueous solution) at specific activities from 0.36 to about 15 Ci/mM. The specific activity to use depends on several considerations: the size of the object to be labeled, the time during which this is to be carried out, possible harmful effects of high-specific-activity thymidine, and so on. In calculating the dose required to give a certain range of disintegrations per week per cell, one must take into consideration the overall efficiency of the detection system, i.e., what proportion of disintegrations will produce silver grains. In one study with a film efficiency of about 5 % Lajtha and Oliver[144] estimated that to obtain 10 grains over a cell in a smear preparation using a 25-day exposure time, about $6 \times 10^4$ tritium atoms must be in the cell.

Conversely, the amount of $^3$H-TdR that has been incorporated into cells can be estimated from the grain count. Dewey et al.[69] used this method to determine the maximum rate of incorporation of thymidine into cells. This was $2.5 \times 10^8$ molecules, or 0.10 $\mu\mu$g per labeled cell per hour. The same result was obtained whether the specific activity was 1.9 or 6.6 Ci/mM, i.e. the maximum rate of incorporation occurred at a concentration of thymidine of 0.25 $\mu$g/ml.

## *Statistical Aspects of Autoradiography*

The probability that a given atom of a radioactive element will disintegrate within a time interval that is much shorter than the half-life of the element is very small. Consequently, the fluctuation in the number of disintegrations in a labeled source per unit time follows a Poisson distribution. Overman and Clark[202] give a general treatment of this problem which holds for any type of nuclear radiation entering any type of detector.

One characteristic of the Poisson distribution is that the mean and variance are equal. Thus, any observed value, say, the grain count of a chromosome, can serve as an estimate both of the mean and the variance; the standard deviation of a single measured value is given by the square root of that value. If a chromosome has nine grains over it, there is a 5 % chance that another chromosome in the same cell with an equal number of tritium atoms will have less than three or more than 15 grains. This means that even in the absence of any other source of variation, one does *not* expect an equal number of grains over two chromosomes that are synchronously synthesizing DNA. These purely random fluctuations of radioactive decay limit the accuracy with which grain counts estimate the amount of label incorporated by an object as small as a metaphase chromosome, especially one of the smaller ones. Stubblefield[264] has devised a method of replicate autoradiography by which it is possible to increase the number of observable grains over a chromosome to almost any desired level, thus reducing these chance fluctuations in grain counts to a minimum. Alternatively, one can do grain counts on a larger sample of chromosomes.

The variance in grain count between synchronously replicating chromosomes can be further increased over that of a Poisson distribution by: chance variation in the proportion of labeled molecules incorporated, variation in the closeness of apposition of emulsion to specimen, variable interaction between emulsion and biologic specimen, variations in the density of silver bromide crystals in the emulsion, or shifts in their position during development. The effect of any of these factors (except the first) will be to alter the probability that a disintegration will be recorded, and this will increase the variance of the count distribution.

Another possible source of variation is that several grains may be produced by a single disintegration. This is not a problem in track autoradiography, since the number of tracks shows a Poisson distribution even though the number of grains does not.[211] In most tritium autoradiography tracks are not produced, because of the short path distance of even the most energetic beta rays from tritium decay, and it is questionable whether a significant proportion of tritium decays produce more than one grain. A simple way to test this is to apply stripping film repeatedly to the same labeled cell. After exposing each film for the same length of time one would expect, if there is no more than a single grain per disintegration, a Poisson distribution of grains. In Stubblefield's data[264] on grain counts over individual chromosomes after 10 repeated filmings of a single cell the mean and variance were approximately equal.

Another way to test this point would be to prepare uniformly labeled DNA by allowing incorporation of labeled precursor for a period of time longer than the generation time, and studying grain counts in stripping films over such DNA. A Poisson distribution of grains has been observed over uniformly labeled bacteria,[40,204] mammalian chromosomes,[69] and dissociated chromosomal fibers.[119] Consequently, it appears that in AR-10 stripping film a single disintegration rarely activates more than one silver grain.

When labeled precursor is available to asynchronously dividing cells for only a relatively short portion of the S period of any cell, uneven rates of DNA synthesis and cellular asynchrony will increase the variability in grain counts of specific chromosomes. The failure of Gilbert et al.[99] to observe a Poisson distribution in grain counts over human chromosomes is probably due to this factor, rather than the one they suggest, variation in the number of grains produced by individual tritium disintegrations.

Since so many studies of human chromosomes are carried out in a manner similar to that used by Gilbert and his associates, increased variances are often encountered. Painter and his associates[204] observed a variance in grain counts over HeLa nuclei that was more than 10 times the mean after pulse-labeling with $^3$H-thymidine for 30 min, but only 3.3 times the mean after 24 hr incubation with labeled thymidine. They concluded that the high variance of grain counts after short tracer incubations is due to variation in the rate of DNA synthesis throughout the cell cycle (complete absence in $G_1$ and $G_2$, with lesser variations during S), a possibility also suggested by Lajtha et al.,[145] who used the analysis of grain-count distribution to evaluate the nature of synthetic processes at the cellular level.

The value of such statistical approaches is also illustrated by a study of ultraviolet-light-induced DNA synthesis. Rasmussen and Painter[225] found increased incorporation of $^3$H-TdR into the DNA of HeLa cells after u.v. exposure, even into cells presumably in $G_1$ or $G_2$ rather than the S phase. The variance of the grain counts was much lower after u.v. treatment, supporting the hypothesis that repair DNA synthesis is taking place, since the rate of DNA synthesis was similar in all cells, in contrast to the usual finding in asynchronously growing cultures. Similar results were observed after exposure of HeLa cells to X-rays.[226]

DuPraw[71] has pointed out that autoradiographic analysis can be misleading under conditions where only relatively heavily labeled segments reach optimal grain densities. His folded-fiber model of the chromosome shows clearly how the presence of label can easily go undetected at certain levels along a chromatid, and provides an explanation of Stubblefield's observation[264] that regions of high labeling intensity are often connected by intermediate areas of lower specific activity.

## DNA SYNTHESIS AND THE CELL CYCLE

### The Timing of DNA Synthesis

### The Cell Cycle and the S Period of DNA Synthesis

When somatic cells are exposed to a labeled precursor of DNA for a short time, say, 10 min, only a proportion of the interphase cells, and none of the mitotic cells, incorporate the label into DNA. In the germ line a small amount of DNA synthesis, perhaps 2% of the total, occurs during meiotic prophase, a finding which may have implications for the mechanism of crossing over.[284] The period during which DNA synthesis occurs in a cell is called its S period. In most cell types it is preceded and followed by intervals in which DNA synthesis is normally absent although RNA and protein synthesis occur. The cycle of chromosome duplication and cell division can be visualized as a clock face, divided into segments proportional to the duration of each phase: the $G_1$, or presynthetic period, the S, or synthetic period, the $G_2$ or postsynthetic period, and M, or mitosis. Methods for determing the duration of the phases of the cell cycle by autoradiography have been reviewed by Cleaver.[47] In brief, one can use a pulse-chase technique, continuous labeling with or without a colchicine block, pulse labeling combined with spectrophotometry, or pulse labeling combined with time-lapse cinemicrography.

## Pulse Labeling: The Pulse-Chase Technique

The standard method for studying the cell cycle *in vitro* is to expose cells for a short period of time to labeled thymidine, then to replace the medium containing the "hot" thymidine with one containing an excess of unlabeled thymidine, and continue incubation of the cells for various periods of time before terminating the culture and preparing autoradiographs. The purpose of the "cold" thymidine is to dilute the intracellular pool of DNA precursors to ensure that no further label will be incorporated after the pulse. By plotting the percentage of labeled metaphases against elapsed time since the pulse (Fig. 1), it is possible to determine the length of $G_2$, S, the generation time, and (by subtraction) $G_1$. After the pulse no labeled metaphases are seen for about 2 hr, which is therefore the shortest period of time required for cells labeled in their late S phase to pass through $G_2$ and prophase in order to reach metaphase. If every cell spent the same amount of time in $G_2$, the curve of labeled metaphases would rise almost vertically from 0 to 100%. Instead, the increase in labeled metaphases is slow, requiring several hours. The slope of the curve serves as a measure of variation in $G_2$. The average length of $G_2$ is given by the time required to obtain 50% labeled metaphases.

As the cohort of labeled cells moves on through the cell cycle, unlabeled cells begin to reach metaphase and the percentage of labeled metaphases falls. The time required for the transit from 50% labeled metaphases on the ascending slope of the curve to the 50% point on the descending curve serves as an estimate of the average duration of the S period, and the lesser slope of the descending curve serves as a rough indication of the variability in the duration of the S period from cell to cell.

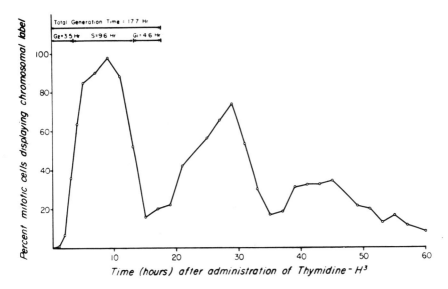

Fig. 1.   Cell cycle times estimated by the standard pulse-chase method. Three successive cycles are detectable, indicating a relatively high degree of synchrony in cell growth in phytohemagglutin-stimulated human leukocytes. (From Cave.[43])

The percentage of labeled metaphases continues to decline with time after the pulse label, but instead of reaching zero, it begins to rise again as a result of a second wave of mitosis in labeled cells. The time interval between successive comparable precentages on the ascending slopes of the curve of labeled metaphases gives an estimate of the cell cycle or generation time. Similarly, an estimate of the duration of the $G_1$ period is obtained by subtracting the length of $G_2$ ($+$ prophase) $+$ S from the cell cycle time.

The duration of $G_2$ $+$ prophase, usually referred to as $G_2$, varies from about 2 to 7 hr for individual cells. This varies with cell type and conditions of growth, but is usually 3–6 hr is diploid human leucocytes,[43,44,88,134,220] adult skin,[8] or embryonic cell strains,[179] and in heteroploid HeLa cells.[224] The same studies have shown that the average duration of the S period usually ranges from 6 to 12 hr. German[88] obtained a much longer value for the length of S, nearly 24 hr, in cultured leukocytes, but Takagi and Sandberg[270] have suggested this might be due to scoring numbers of second division figures. They observed a very short generation time in cultured leukocytes from two human males, and in one the cells labeled 13.5 hr before their examination at metaphase showed labeling of only one of their chromatids, indicating an intervening round of DNA synthesis in the absence of tritiated thymidine.

The $G_1$ period is the most variable portion of metaphase, for reasons that need not concern us here. However, variations in generation time are usually accompanied by similar and nearly proportional changes in all phases of the cell cycle. Sisken and Marasca[255] used a combination of autoradiography and time-lapse cinemicrography to study the kinetics of proliferation of a heteroploid line of cultured human amnion cells. They found that $G_1$ and the generation time were quite variable, whereas $S + G_2 +$ prophase $+$ metaphase was nearly constant. They concluded that compensating mechanisms help regulate the length of successive phases of the mitotic cycle in individual cells. By the hypothesis of an inverse relationship between length of successive parts of the cycle, it would be expected that cells inhibited from beginning DNA replication by fluorodeoxyuridine (FUdR) would upon release from the inhibition be able to complete the S period more rapidly than unblocked cells, and this appears to be the case.

An understanding of the elementary principles of cell kinetics is necessary in order to interpret the results of many autoradiographic studies. Cleaver[47] and Lajtha and Gilbert[143] have recently reviewed the methods, models, and problems involved in such studies. Variations in the length of specific phases of the cell cycle between cells of the germ line and of the soma have been described.[276a] However, such variations are common between cells within most tissues, both *in vivo* and *in vitro*. These variations in length of individual phases of the cell cycle contribute to the overall asynchrony in the growth of cells. They also make it impossible to predict when in its S phase a pulse-labeled metaphase cell was incorporating label. Thus, while it can be used to determine general rates of synthesis[270,271] or grossly different labeling patterns,[180] pulse labeling is not as suitable for detailed analysis of the sequence of DNA synthesis at the end of the S period as continuous labeling.

## Continuous Labeling Technique

The use of continuous labeling of chromosomes has greatly simplified the interpretation of terminal labeling patterns of metaphase chromosomes and made possible more-exact qualitative and quantitative studies of the end-of-S DNA synthesis. When tritiated thymidine is added in sufficient concentration to be available throughout a given incubation period the end of the S period can be used as a point of reference because every labeled metaphase cell will have incorporated ³H-thymidine from some unknown point in the cycle until the end of its S period. If nuclear emulsion is exposed to labeled metaphases of high enough specific activity and for sufficient time to rule out gross chance fluctuations in grain density, an unlabeled chromosome or chromosome segment can be presumed to have completed its DNA replication prior to the addition of ³H-TdR. Furthermore, the number of labeled metaphase chromosomes[187] and their grain density, or intensity of labeling,[98,99] are indications of how close the cell was to the end of its S period at the time $^3$H-TdR became available for incorporation into its DNA. Thus, labeled metaphase cells with equal grain counts will have incorporated $^3$H-TdR for about the same portion of their terminal S periods, a relation not generally found with pulse labeling.

Another feature of continuous or terminal labeling is that colchicine or similar mitotic spindle inhibitors can be used to accumulate cells in metaphase without altering the general validity of the results. This makes it possible to determine the average time scale of events near the end of the S phase. This has been done both in synchronized cultures and in asynchronously growing cells. In synchronized cultures it is much easier to determine the rate of DNA synthesis in relatively specific intervals of the S period. Using an autoradiographic technique and the CMP line of human epithelial adenocarcinoma cells that had been synchronized by a double blockage with excess thymidine, which inhibits DNA synthesis, Kasten and Strasser[129] demonstrated a rather rapid increase and slower decrease in the rate of DNA synthesis (using a qualitative scale rather than exact grain counts) at the beginning and end of the S period. An unexpected finding was the abrupt cessation in nucleolar DNA synthesis and marked decline in other DNA synthesis for at least 1 hr in the middle of the approximately 9-hr S period of these cells. Stubblefield et al.[265] confirmed the occurrence of intermittent cessation of DNA synthesis during the S period in synchronized Chinese hamster cells, and presented scintillation counting data on the rate of RNA synthesis (to be described later) that may shed light on the significance of this distinctive pattern of DNA synthesis.

While studies in synchronized cells have many advantages, there are also several disadvantages; the method used to bring about synchrony may interfere with incorporation of labeled precursor (e.g., excess thymidine leads to a large pool of unlabeled precursors), may disturb the pattern of replication, and is usually more difficult, requiring additional processing or handling of the cultures, with the possibility of introducing further complications. Much information can be obtained by working with asynchronously growing cells, such as those usually found both *in vivo* and *in vitro*.

### The Rate of DNA Synthesis

The relative rate of DNA synthesis in labeled cells can be estimated from their grain counts after a short exposure to $^3$H-TdR. In asynchronously growing cells, as usually found both *in vivo* and *in vitro*, there is a wide range of grain counts over the nuclei, indicating variation in the rate of DNA synthesis throughout the S period. Takagi and Sandberg[270] related this variation in rate of synthesis to the stage of the S period by pulse-labeling cultured leukocytes for 10 min at various times prior to termination of each culture. They processed all preparations simultaneously to minimize technical sources of variation, and counted the number of silver grains over each chromosome in the labeled metaphase cells as an index of their rate of DNA synthesis. Earlier, Dendy and Cleaver[68] had shown that under such conditions the grain count over each interphase nucleus correlates well with its DNA content measured spectrophotometrically by the two-wavelength method. Takagi and Sandberg[270] found a gradual increase in the rate of DNA synthesis (as indicated by the number of grains per cell) to a peak level more than halfway through the S period, with a more rapid decrease in the rate of DNA synthesis toward the end of S. They carried out the same kind of analysis for individual chromosome pairs, and found their patterns to be characteristic. For example, chromosomes 17 and 18 show marked differences from each other at almost every point in the S period. Chromosome 17 initiated DNA synthesis at a higher level and maintained a higher rate of synthesis for the first half of the S period, while chromosome 18 had a higher rate in the last third of the S period (Fig. 2). The Y chromosome and late-replicating X chromosomes had very low rates of DNA synthesis in early S and very high rates of synthesis in the late S period.[271] While studies of this kind, using pulse-labeling, can provide a great deal of information about the average behavior of cells in a culture, they cannot delineate the morphologic sequence and rate of DNA synthesis with the same degree of accuracy as continuous (terminal) labeling.

Gilbert et al.[98] devised a method of determining the rate of DNA synthesis in the final 15–30 min of the S period by arranging terminally labeled metaphase cells in a cumulative distribution based on grain counts. They established an absolute time scale by assuming complete asynchrony of the cultured leukocytes and multiplying the total time during which tritiated thymidine was available by the proportion of labeled metaphases. This came out as 2.49 cells per minute in their particular culture. Their method enabled them to demonstrate a much higher rate of DNA synthesis in the late-replicating X chromosome than in the other chromosomes of the complement. They did not attempt to determine relative rates of DNA synthesis in different autosomes, although their technique could be used for this.

The most detailed quantitative analysis of the terminal replication sequence of a single chromosome has been that of Gavosto et al.[86] They added tritiated thymidine to lymphocytes cultured from a healthy woman for 3 hr and 45 min before termination of the three-day cultures, and colcemide 1 hr and 45 min before fixation. In a random sample of 264 mitotic figures thus obtained 66 (25%) were labeled and 198 unlabeled. On the assumption

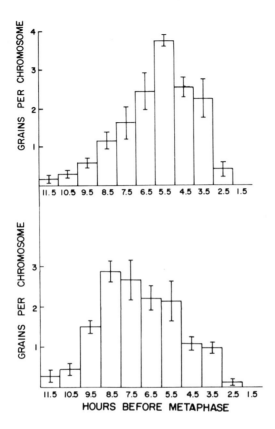

Fig. 2. Grain counts resulting from 10 min pulse-labeling at various times before metaphase. Above, chromosome 18; below, chromosome 17. The average grain counts over these two pairs of chromosomes are different from each other at almost every interval throughout the S period, and it is therefore relatively easy to distinguish them from each other. (From Takagi and Sandberg.[270])

that the culture was replicating asynchronously, i.e., that the number of cells in any stage of the cell cycle is proportional to the relative length of that stage, Gavosto and his associates concluded that the S period occupied 25 % of the 1 hr and 45 min during which metaphase cells were being collected, or 26 min, while the $G_2$ period was estimated as 75 % of the total time of incubation with $^3H$-thymidine, or 3 hr and 19 min. Gavosto and co-workers arranged the labeled metaphase cells in a cumulative distribution by the method of Gilbert et al.,[98] pressing the assumption of a completely

A

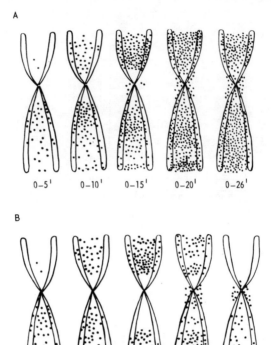

0–5'        0–10'      0–15'      0–20'       0–26'

B

0–5'      5⊥10'     10⊥15'     15⊥20'     20⊥26'

Fig. 3. Sequence in which labeling bands appear in five successive subperiods of the final 26 min of the S period. A. Grains present over the late-replicating X chromosome of cells labeled between 0 and 5 min, 0 and 10 min, or longer. B. In each sketch the grains actually formed in the corresponding subperiods. (From Gavosto et al.[86])

asynchronous culture still further, and subdivided the cells into groups representing 5-min intervals of the S period. The grains over all the late-replicating X chromosomes in each group were transferred to a diagram (Fig. 3). Consequently, by subtracting from each diagram the grains present in the diagram representing the periods closer to the end of S, a good estimate of the location and intensity of DNA synthesis in each time interval, *relative to the end of S*, was obtained.

Still other information can be gained from such quantitative approaches, e.g., Gilbert et al.[98] compared the position of an individual cell in the two cumulative distributions, one based on autosomal, the other on late-replicating X-chromosomal grain count in a series of terminally labeled cells.

They found a mean ranking difference of 10.8, which they equated with a $10.8/2.49 = 4.4$-min internal timing variation between the state of the late-replicating X and of the autosomal DNA synthesis within a single cell. This may be a misleading designation, since the variation may be purely statistical due to chance variations in the incorporation of labeled thymidine and the random nature of radioactive decay, rather than indicating fluctuation in the sequence of DNA synthesis within a cell. On the other hand, if such fluctuations do occur, the hypothesis that the pattern of DNA replication is extremely highly ordered, with virtually no variation, is untenable. Except for this ambiguous evidence, one of the most firmly established principles arrived at by labeling studies of DNA replication is that there is a consistent sequence or pattern of synthesis.

## The Order of DNA Synthesis

DNA synthesis occurs in a definite, orderly sequence. Mueller and Kajiwara[184] labeled the DNA that replicated early in one S period in synchronized HeLa cells with ³H-TdR, allowed several generations of random growth, and then labeled the DNA with bromodeoxyuridine (BUdR) at various points in the S period of the newly synchronized cells. The ³H label was found in the BUdR-containing heavy hybrid DNA that replicated early in the second synchronized cycle, indicating that the DNA molecules that replicated during the initial part of one S period are replicating in the same temporal relation to the other DNA molecules in subsequent S periods in daughter cells.

A similar orderly sequence is observable at the level of whole chromosomes. The pattern is not discernible in every cell, presumably because of chance fluctuations in incorporation of label or grain density of labeled chromosome segments, or, in pulse-labeled cells, because of their asynchronous growth. The order is most easily observed in terminally labeled cells, and somewhat less easily in initially labeled cells, i.e., those labeled at the initiation of the S period. It seems probable that in each species each chromosome has an invariant and characteristic replication pattern.

## CHROMOSOME IDENTIFICATION AND CHARACTERIZATION

Characterization of chromosomes by their labeling patterns can be useful in resolving several types of problems. The first of these is the distinction between morphologically similar whole chromosomes. Increased accuracy of identification of chromosomes is essential to determine the nature of some chromosomal defects, and to distinguish heterogeneity in the clinical effects of a given chromosomal abnormality from heterogeneity in chromosome aberrations. The relevance of this application will be particularly evident in the sections on chromosomes of the B, D, and G groups.

A second type of problem is the identification of chromosomes involved in translocations, inversions, or other structural changes. This is best illustrated in the section on D/D and D/G translocations, where auto-radiographic identification has led to recognition of the nonrandom involve-ment of D-group chromosomes. A third type of problem is the distinction between arms of metacentric chromosomes. While the first two types of problem can sometimes be solved simply by analysis of the labeling patterns of whole chromosomes, the third type requires distinguishing between the labeling patterns of portions of chromosomes, a technique that has a wider variety of uses.

The generally accepted nomenclature for the human chromosomes and their abnormalities is the Denver system as modified at the London and Chicago Conferences. This system[46] is based primarily on chromosome length and secondarily on the position of the centromere, i.e., the length of each arm relative to the other. The chromosome involved in the first auto-somal abnormality discovered, that associated with mongolism, was incorrectly identified as one of the larger G-group chromosomes, i.e., a   21, and this designation is so well established that it seems wiser to modify the system of nomenclature, which is in any case arbitrary, rather than attempt to convince everyone to call it 22-trisomy. Such errors should be much less frequent now, because of the greater accuracy of identification possible with autoradiography.

### Terminal Labeling Characteristics of Specific Chromosomes

Chromosomal labeling patterns have been studied in cultured cells, usually leucocytes, from more than 50 XX and 25 XY individuals. Late-replicating regions have been observed in many chromosomes.[5,88,179] Their location in the autosomes corelates well with the position of secondary con-strictions,[242] but the latter are not present consistently enough to be useful in chromosome identification. The late-S period (terminal) labeling patterns of individual chromosomes, on the other hand, appear to be much more consistent, and have proven quite useful in the identification of chromosomes 4, 5, 13, 14, 15, 16, 17, 18, 21, 22, the late-replicating X, and the Y. To date no satisfactory evidence exists that any C- or F-group autosome can be identified, and there is some doubt regarding the identification of the early-labeling X chromosome.

The ease of chromosome identification by replication pattern depends upon the magnitude of the difference between morphologically similar non-homologous chromosomes in relation to that between homologues. These differences are of two sorts: (1) the number of silver grains, and (2) their location along the chromosome. Most of the earlier studies on human chromosome identification were based on rough approximations of these two parameters, with the exception of the detailed study of Gilbert et al.[99] Only the more obvious differences between chromosomal replication patterns were delineated in such studies, but these have been adequate to differentiate between chromosomes with in B, D, and E groups, where the difference between homologues is much smaller than that between nonhomologues, and less well between chromosomes 21 and 22. As seen in Table I, chromosomes in the B, D, and G groups usually fall into distinguishable pairs (two chromosomes with similar patterns being called labeling homologues) in more than 50 % of terminally labeled cells. In B and G groups, each with two chromosome pairs, it cannot be proven that the same two chromosomes always have the same labeling pattern. In fact, in view of the small difference in silver grains involved, this seems unlikely. The conclusion that labeling homologues are true homologues thus involves a degree of circular reasoning. In the D group, with three pairs of chromosomes and the most common pattern the presence of three labeling patterns, each represented by two chromosomes, it is easier to conclude that labeling homologues are true homologues, but this is still based on the unproved assumption of homologue synchrony in these groups. When there are only five chromosomes in the group, or seven, due to a specific alteration in the karyotype, it is possible to test the consistency of the labeling pattern by comparing the frequency of the most common pattern ($C$) with that of alternate patterns ($A$). The ratio, $C/A$ is 7–12 in the D group, but only 1.6–3.4 in the G group (Table I), indicating how difficult identification of a G-group chromosome is by labeling pattern.

The consistency of the replication pattern of a specific chromosome can best be studied by using a cytologic marker so that the chromosome can be identified morphologically in every cell. In a series of cases in which this has been done a highly consistent replication pattern has been observed for a marker chromosome 4, 5, 13, and 18 (Table II). This has confirmed the accuracy of characterization of these chromosomes by determination of the most common pairs of replication patterns within the groups, and supports the hypothesis that homologues generally replicate fairly synchronously. This hypothesis, however, does not appear to be true except in a very general sense, since evidence of a slight but consistent degree of homologue asynchrony has been obtained in quantitative studies using a series of marker chromosomes.[62,174]

Replication patterns can be determined more accurately by performing grain counts at the microscope and plotting the location of grains along measured chromosomes.[86,95,171,197] A further refinement is the use of marker chromosomes; examples of their use will be given.

TABLE I. Consistency of Identification by Terminal Labeling Pattern

| Chromosome or group | Type of case | No. of chromosomes in group | No. cells scorable | Identification by pairing | | | | Ref. |
|---|---|---|---|---|---|---|---|---|
| | | | | Most common pattern (C) (%) | Alternate patterns (A) (%) | Ambiguous labeling (%) | Ratio C/A | |
| 4, 5 | Control | 4 | 95 | 68 | — | — | — | 92 |
| 4, 5 | t(5p+, 14q) | 3 | 41 | 56 | 0 | 44 | — | 287 |
| 13, 14, 15 | Control | 6 | 84 | 39 | — | — | — | 95 |
| 13, 15 | t(13q15q) | 4 | 30 | 57 | — | — | — | 112 |
| 13, 14 | t(13q15q) | 4 | 76 | 59 | — | — | — | 95 |
| 13 | 13-Trisomy | 7 | 74 | 62 | — | — | — | 294 |
| 13 | 13-Trisomy | 7 | 22 | 86 | — | 14 | — | 94 |
| 14 | t(5p+, 14q) | 5 | 41 | 42 | — | — | — | 287 |
| 14 | t(14qGq) | 5 | 50 | 80 | — | — | — | 295 |
| 14 | t(14qGq) | 5 | 38 | 58 | — | — | — | 112 |
| 14 | t(14qGq) | 5 | 132 | 61 | 9 | 30 | 6.8 | 63 |
| 14 | 14-Trisomy | 7 | 125 | 48 | 7 | 45 | 7.5 | 1 |
| 15 | t(15qGq) | 5 | 40 | 60 | 5 | 35 | 12.0 | 63 |
| 21, 22 | Control | 4 | 113 | 55 | — | — | — | 92 |
| 21, 22 | t(21qGq) | 2 | 40 | 55 | — | — | — | 295 |
| 21, 22 | t(21qGq) | 2 | 23 | 78 | — | — | — | 112 |
| 21 | t(14q21q) | 3 | 50 | 74 | — | — | — | 295 |
| 21 | t(14q21q) | 3 | 38 | 58 | — | — | — | 112 |
| 21 | 21-Trisomy | 5 | 103* | 63 | 18 | 18 | 3.4 | 295 |
| 21 | 21-Trisomy | 5 | 216 | 24 | 14 | 62 | 1.6 | 12 |
| 21 | 21-Trisomy | 5 | 61 | 52 | 21 | 26 | 2.5 | 92 |
| 21 | 21-Trisomy | 5 | 48 | 50 | 21 | 29 | 2.4 | 79 |

* Only moderately to heavily labeled cells were used.

TABLE II. Consistency of Terminal Labeling Pattern of Marker Chromosomes

| Type of marker | No. of chromo-somes in group | No. cells scorable | Labeling pattern Consis-tent (C) (%) | Inconsis-tent (I) (%) | Ambig-uous (%) | Ratio (C/I) | Ref. |
|---|---|---|---|---|---|---|---|
| 4p− | 4 | 209 | 66 | 1 | 32 | 69 | 170, 279 |
| 4p− | 4 | 40 | 98 | — | — | ⩾49 | 213 |
| 5p− | 4 | 209 | 70 | 1.4 | 28 | 49 | 279 |
| 13p− | 6 | 38 | 68 | 3 | 29 | 26 | 62 |
| 15p− | 6 | 17 | 76* | 0 | 24 | — | 62 |
| 18p− | 4 | 22 | 96 | 0 | 4 | — | 62 |
| t(Cq−; 18q+) | 3 | 42 or 72 | 100 | 0 | 0 | — | 34 |

*Probably overestimated because the missing portion labels relatively late.

## The A Group

The chromosomes of the A group appear to undergo relatively synchronous DNA replication.[19,89,99,134,179,256,257,266] In fact, Gilbert et al.[97] found that these pairs of homologues had, on the average, a smaller difference in grain count than would be expected from the observed variances from cell to cell in the "end-of-S" cohort of 226 cells they studied. This could be due to a more constant rate of synthesis for these three pairs of chromosomes than for the entire complement during the end-of-S interval being studied, or to the (probably unconscious) use of labeling pattern as well as morphology in pairing chromosomes 1 and 3. This difficulty does not arise when pairing is made from unlabeled photographs.

One of the dangers of working with this kind of pooled data is that the heterogeneity between cells may swamp real but small differences in the parameter being studied. This difficulty can be overcome in either of two ways. First, one can study a much narrower cohort of terminally labeled cells (on one slide, or on slides simultaneously processed to reduce variation due to technical factors) in which the total grain count is nearly the same, indicating that these cells began incorporating label at approximately the same point in their S period. The use of synchronized cultures would accomplish the same goal, but less effectively with the inefficient methods presently available for maintaining cell synchrony. Second, one could make cell-by-cell (i.e., within-cell) comparisons of grain count over homologous chromosomes. This method has been much abused in the past, usually by those of us who failed to take into account the statistical nature of the relationship between grain density and rate of DNA synthesis and used samples of too limited size.

Thus, in a number of reports one reads that a specific cell shows asynchrony for certain pairs of homologues, when all that has been observed is unequal numbers of silver grains over the presumptive homologous segments. Analysis of large numbers of cells is essential in this method of analysis. Using this method, Takagi and Sandberg[270] found no evidence of asynchronous duplication of homologous regions of chromosomes 1, 2, or 3 in one individual, and concluded that these homologues generally replicate synchronously.

**Chromosome 1.**   The two chromosomes terminate relatively early. DNA synthesis stops earliest near the distal ends of both arms, with late replication persisting in the centromeric region, particularly in the adjacent secondary constriction region.[8,33]

The problem of distinguishing between the two arms of a chromosome as metacentric as numbers 1 and 3 is usually very great. However, when a secondary constriction is visible near the centromere of chromosome 1 it becomes possible to distinguish between the two arms of this chromosome. In such cases it is possible to compare the labeling patterns of the two arms in order to find out if there are characteristic differences. Sofuni and Sandberg[258] carried out such a study. They were unable to demonstrate significant differences between the labeling of the two arms other than in the secondary constriction region, but their analysis of terminal labeling was based on only nine cells. A more-detailed study might demonstrate a difference, which, though small, might be useful in distinguishing a structural change.

**Chromosome 2.**   This chromosome shows very little segmental differentiation in timing of synthesis.[19,89,97,99,134,179,256,257,266] DNA synthesis ends relatively early. The centromeric region is not late-replicating, and the distal end of the long arm is first no terminate DNA synthesis. Castilla *et al.*[42] used the persistence of this feature to rule out a terminal deletion in two cases of mentally retarded males with a peculiar facies, a cleft palate, inguinal hernias, simian crease, talipes equinovarus, and a chromosome 2 whose long arm was approximately 20% shorter than normal.

**Chromosome 3.**   The pattern of replication of chromosome 3 is generally similar to that of chromosome 1. The two arms, which are morphologically indistinguishable, also have generally similar labeling patterns. Fine distinctions could not be recognized without some means of identifying each arm. The centromeric region is relatively late-replicating, though perhaps not so much so as chromosome 1.[19,89,97,99,134,179,242,256,257,266] Buchner *et al.*[33] found a slightly different pattern, which may be related to the relatively small samples that have generally been studied.

A problem which has been generally overlooked is the occasional inability to distinguish between chromosomes 1 and 3 in a particular cell. Since there is still no independent method of evaluating the accuracy of identification of these chromosomes by morphologic criteria, the degree of confusion between them is unknown. Such misclassification would tend to blur the distinctions between the labeling patterns of specific chromosomes. This problem could be resolved by using a marker chromosome 3, or perhaps by comparing the labeling patterns of presumptive chromosomes 1 and 3 in cells where both chromosomes 1 have a visible secondary constriction, assuming, of course, that it is always chromosome 1 which shows such a constriction; this is a reasonable assumption, since no more than two A-group chromosomes have such a constriction in any cell, and these chromosomes appear longer.

Despite these limitations, the terminal labeling patterns of chromosomes 1 and 3 are clearly different from those of X-isochromosomes and the common types of D/D translocations, $t(13q14q)$ and $t(13q13q)$, the structural variants that commonly resemble chromosome 3. Consequently, one can identify these abnormal chromosomes by autoradiography and characterize them in more detail, as will be described shortly.

## The B Group

The long arms of two of the four morphologically indistinguishable chromosomes of the B group terminate DNA synthesis later in the S period, and are thus more heavily labeled than the other two in terminal-labeling studies.[90,99,242] The reverse pattern is found for the short arms.[33] On the assumption that homologues in this group replicate synchronously, it has been generally concluded that the labeling pattern can be used to distinguish between chromosomes 4 and 5. This conclusion has been supported by numerous studies with B-group marker chromosomes. German et al.[91] found consistently early termination of replication of the long arm of the deleted chromosome in cells from two individuals with a deletion of part of the short arm of a B-group chromosome, and the cri du chat (cat-cry) syndrome. Miller et al.[171] and Warburton et al.[279] confirmed this in 13 more cases. Wolf et al.[288] found consistently late termination of replication of a deleted B-group chromosome in cells from a child with an apparently different clinical syndrome but a similar deletion of the short arm. Miller et al.[171] found consistent late replication of a similarly deleted chromosome in an individual who was ascertained in a search for older patients with clinical features of the cri du chat syndrome. As Table III indicates, additional cases of both types have now been described, and in each case the labeling pattern is quite consistent (Fig. 4 and 5).

**TABLE III. Chromosome Identification by Labeling Pattern in Autosomal Abnormalities**

| Clinical picture | No. of unrelated cases | No. identified by labeling pattern | Chromosomal abnormality | Ref. |
|---|---|---|---|---|
| 13-Trisomy syndrome | 8 | 8 | 13+ (trisomy) | 26, 31, 94, 95, 162, 294 |
| 18-Trisomy syndrome | 2 | 2 | 18+ | 89, 293 |
| Spontaneous abortion | 1 | 1 | 18+ | 73 |
| 21-Trisomy syndrome | 13 | 13 | 21+ | 13, 92, 242, 295 |
| Multiple malformations | 2 | 0 (but not an x) | $C+$ | 74, 229 |
| Malformations + cat cry | 1 | 1 | 14+ | 87 |
| $4p-$ Syndrome | 9 | 9 | $4p-$ | 39, 170, 171, 213, 288 |
| Multiple malformations | 1 | 1 | $t(4q+?, C)$ | 197 |
| $5p-$ (cat cry) syndrome | 20 | 20 | $5p-$ | 18, 90, 99, 171, 207, 242, 247 |
| $5p-$ (cat cry) syndrome | 1 | 1 | $t(5p-, 14)$ | 287 |
| Primary amenorrhea | 1 | 1 | $t(5q, C)$ | 161 |
| $13q-$ Syndrome | 3 | 3 | $13r$ (ring) | 1, 27 |
| $13q-$ Syndrome | 1 | 1 | $13q-$ | 115 |
| $13q-$ Syndrome + absent thumbs | 1 | 1 | $13q-$ | 1 |
| $13q-$ Syndrome + absent thumbs | 1 | 1 | $14r$ | 259 |
| Normal carriers | 3 | 3 | $13p-$ | 21, 151, 207 |
| 13-Trisomy syndrome | 2 | 2 | $t(13q13q)$ | 94, 207 |
| Carriers or affected | 6 | 6 | $t(13q14q)$ | 26, 66, 95, 237 |
| Carriers or affected | 1 | 1 | $t(13q15q)$ | 112 |
| Carriers or affected | 14 | 13 | $t(14qGq)$ | 26, 63, 112, 168 |
| Carriers or affected | 4 | 3 | $t(15qGq)$ | 26, 63, 168 |
| Carriers or affected | 1 | 1 | $t(14, 15)$ | 26 |
| Carriers or affected | 1 | 1 | $t(C, 15)$ | 63 |
| Multiple malformations | 1 | 1 | $t(14-, ?)$ | 62 |
| Normal | 1 | 1 | $15p-$ | 62 |
| Mental retardation | 1 | 1 | $17r$ | 96 |
| Multiple malformations | 1 | 1 | $18r$ | 206 |
| $18p-$ Syndrome | 3 | 3 | $18p-$ | 96, 167, 228 |
| $18q-$ Syndrome | 1 | 1 | $18q-$ | 227 |
| Normal carrier | 1 | 1 | $t(18q, Cq)$ | 34 |
| Chronic myelogenous leukemia | 6 | 3 | $21q-$ | 104, 153, 242 |
| Carrier or affected | 3 | 3 | $t(Dq21q)$ | 112, 295 |
| Carrier or affected | 3 | 2 | $t(21q21q)$ | 64, 607 |

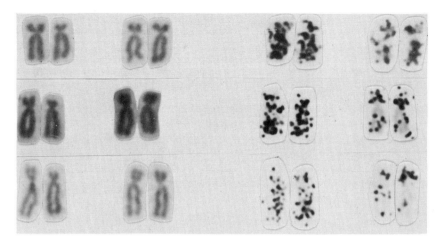

Fig. 4. Partial double karyotypes of terminally labeled B group chromosomes in three cells from an individual with a partial deletion of the short arm of a chromosome 4 (4p−). The deleted chromosome is consistently one of the late-replicating pair, and its long arm is usually more heavily labeled than that of its homologue. (Courtesy of W. R. Breg.)

The studies of Miller et al.[171] and Warburton et al.[279] have confirmed the hypothesis that homologues replicate synchronously in the B group by demonstrating a correlation between length of long arm (and of short arm) and replication pattern. They found the length of the long arm of the 4p− chromosome to be 0.252 ± 0.001 the total length of the four long arms in 247 cells from five cases, while the relative length of the long arm of the 5p− chromosome was 0.243 ± 0.001 in 258 cells from 12 cases. The long arm and the short arm of the late-replicating chromosomes were on the average about 5 % longer than the corresponding arm of the early-replicating chromosomes in 14 cases with a short-arm deletion, in a control group with normal B-group chromosomes, and in a 4/5 translocation carrier. The mean arm ratio of the late-replicating chromosomes was not different from that of the early-replicating chromosomes in samples of 9, 18, 26, and 39 cells, a result at variance with the findings of Ockey et al.,[197] who found arm ratio more useful than length in distinguishing between chromosomes 4 and 5 in a sample of seven cells. Sampling error probably accounts for this discrepancy, although differential contraction is also a possibility.

The quantitative data reported by Warburton et al.[279] brought to light an interesting discrepancy. The long arm of the early-replicating deleted chromosome in 12 cases was shorter than the mean of the early-replicating chromosomes in controls (0.243 ± 0.001 vs. 0.246 ± 0.001), and in suitably labeled cells, shorter on the average than its normal early-replicating homo-

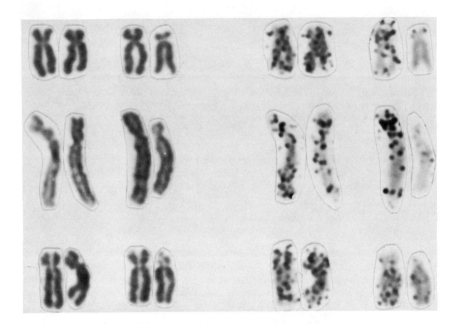

Fig. 5. Partial double karyotypes of terminally labeled B group chromosomes in three cells from an individual with a partial deletion of the short arm of a chromosome 5 (5p−). The deleted chromosome is consistently early in terminating replication; in fact, even its long arm is usually more lightly labeled than that of its homologue. (From Miller et al.[171])

logue. The long arm of late-replicating deleted chromosomes in two cases also were slightly shorter than the long arm of nondeleted late-replicating chromosomes, a finding now confirmed in three more cases (Table IV).

Miller et al.[174] confirmed these differences in length, and showed that they are accompanied by differences in grain counts over the long arms in

TABLE IV.  Relative Lengths of Long Arms of B-group Chromosomes in Labeled Cells

| Type of case | No. of cases | No. of cells | Early replicators Deleted | Early replicators Nondeleted | Late replicators Deleted | Late replicators Nondeleted |
|---|---|---|---|---|---|---|
| 5p− (early repl.) | 12 | 74 | 0.243 | 0.246 | — | 0.256 |
| 4p− (late repl.)* | 5 | 79 | — | 0.246 | 0.252 | 0.256 |
| Controls | >10 | 47 | — | 0.245 | — | 0.255 |
| 4/5 Translocation | 1 | 42 | — | 0.490 | — | 0.510 |

* Including unpublished data on three more cases.

terminally labeled cells. A $4p-$ chromosome has slightly but significantly more silver grains than its labeling homologue, while a $5p-$ chromosome has slightly fewer grains than its labeling homologue (Fig. 5). One explanation of these discrepancies in length and grain count is that a deletion influences both chromosome condensation and replication pattern. It is unclear why the effect on replication should be in opposing directions depending on which chromosome has the deletion. An alternative explanation is that both chromosomes 4 and 5 (and perhaps other autosomes[62]) exist in two functional states, just as the X chromosome does, so that homologous chromosomes undergo asynchronous DNA replication and chromosome condensation.[174]

The differences in labeling between homologues which have been demonstrated are very small and do not affect correct identification of pairs of similarly labeled chromosomes in this group. While the measurement data and the consistent labeling pattern of marker chromosomes support strongly the idea that the homologues in this group replicate synchronously, they do not constitute proof. When there is a structurally altered X chromosome it is preferentially the late replicator, and it is possible that a similar process occurs in the B group. It is thus logically possible that both chromosome 4 and chromosome 5 replicate markedly asynchronously, so that each has an early- and a late-replicating homologue. If so, we do not have a means of identifying either chromosome. Furthermore, all B-group deletions observed so far could involve the same chromosome. Wolf et al.[288] and Carneiro Leao et al.[39] regard the differences between their patients with a deletion of a late-replicating B-group chromosome and individuals with the cri du chat syndrome, who have an early-replicating deleted chromosome, as so striking they have no doubt that a deletion of a different chromosome is involved. Miller et al.,[171] on the other hand, have commented on the marked overlap in clinical features seen in these patients. Since virtually nothing is known of the way chromosomal abnormalities lead to developmental abnormalities, it is perhaps unwise to be overly dogmatic about any of the conclusions based on the very limited amount of information yet available.

The B-group chromosomes are often involved in translocations. Analysis of the labeling pattern permits a distinction between those involving chromosome 4 and those involving chromosome 5. De Capoa et al.[65] described three families in which a translocation carried in a clinically normal individual was responsible for five cases of the cri du chat syndrome. In each case the affected individual had an apparent deletion of part of the short or early-replicating chromosome. Wolf et al.[287] observed the cri du chat syndrome in a 13-year-old female with a presumptive 5/14 translocation between the short arm of an early-replicating B-group chromosome and the long arm of a D-group chromosome having an intermediate labeling pattern, with loss of the centromere region of the D-group chromosome and the distal portion of the short arm of the early-replicating B-group chromosome.

Ockey et al.[197] described an elongated long arm of a B-group chromosome in a patient with phocomelia-like limb abnormalities. The labeling patterns of the other B-group chromosomes indicated that the abnormal chromosome was derived from a late-replicating B-group chromosome, but gave no information about the origin of the extra chromosomal material presumably carried by this chromosome. Mann et al.[161] described a similar elongation of early-replicating B-group chromosome in a chromatin-positive female with a missing C-group chromosome, indicating the presence of a B/C translocation.

## The C Group

Despite numerous attempts to study the labeling patterns of chromosomes in the C group,[19,89,99,134,242] no one has yet succeeded in identifying a single autosome within this group. Even when an extra chromosome or a structurally abnormal chromosome is present in this group, the only discrimination that has been possible is whether the chromosome involved is or is not derived from a late-replicating X.[74,125,229] Secondary constrictions occur somewhat too commonly and inconsistently in this group to be used as markers, although Schmid[242] has emphasized the generally later replication of these regions. The use of distinctive marker C-group chromosomes will probably be essential for determination of the labeling patterns of specific autosomes within this group, but no such study has yet been reported.

## The X Chromosome

Replication Pattern.   In cultured cells from normal females one chromosome in the C group is still actively synthesizing DNA after most of the other chromosomes in the complement have already ceased, or nearly ceased, DNA synthesis.[88,99,180] No such late-replicating C-group chromosome is seen in normal XY males or in chromatin-negative females with gonadal dysgenesis.[180] Consequently, it has been concluded that the late-replicating C-group chromosome in normal chromatin-positive females is one of the two X chromosomes. Chromatin-positive males, whether XX,[82,282a] XXY,[4,5,35,49,82] or XXYY,[28,280] also have one late-replicating C-group chromosome.

Further evidence that this chromosome is an X comes from studies of individuals with more than two X chromosomes or females with one structurally abnormal X chromosome. When there are more than two X chromosomes in the diploid complement the additional X chromosomes are

TABLE V.  Sex-Chromosome Identification by Labeling Pattern

| Karyotype | Number studied | Late-replicating sex chromosomes | Ref. |
|---|---|---|---|
| 45,X | 1 | O | 103 |
| 47,XYY | 6 | YY | 15, 28, 42, 80, 131 |
| 47,XYY | 3 | Y | 35, 141 |
| 47,XXY | 13 | X | 5, 5a, 35, 49, 82, 195a |
| 69,XXY | 1 | O | 246 |
| 48,XXYY | 2 | XYY | 28, 280 |
| 47,XXX | 6 | XX | 35, 93, 103, 180, 187 |
| 48,XXXY | 2 | XX | 82, 103 |
| 49,XXXXY | 6 | XXX | 4, 82, 118a, 187, 235, 296 |
| 49,XXXXX | 1 | XXXX | 103 |
| 45,X/46,XX/47,XXX | 1 | O/X/XX | 103 |
| 46,XY/47,XXY/48,XXXY | 1 | O/X/XX | 117 |
| 46,XXp− | 4 | Xp− | 9, 96, 260 |
| 46,XXr | 4 | Xr | 23, 50a, 236 |
| 46,XXr | 3 | O | 216 |
| 46,XXi | 10 | Xi | 7, 93, 103, 172, 192, 269 |
| 46,XXq+ | 1 | Xq+ | 122 |
| 46,Xt(Xq+,Cq−) | 1 | Xq+* | 193 |

* The presumptive translocated segment is *not* late-replicating.

late-replicating. This has been shown for XXX,[93,103,187,192] XXXY,[82,103] XXXXY (Fig. 6a),[7,82,187,235,296] and XXXXX[103] individuals and mosaics, as shown in Table V. In every case the maximum number of sex chromatin bodies or late-replicating C-group chromosomes is one less than the number of X chromosomes, thus supporting the hypothesis that these late-replicating C-group chromosomes are indeed X chromosomes. The three late-replicating C-chromosomes in XXXXY cells replicate synchronously, i.e., they show no more variation in grain count among themselves than expected by chance.[235]

The labeling pattern of structurally abnormal X chromosomes identified on the basis of their phenotypic effect has provided still further confirmation of this idea. With few exceptions, in females with one normal X and one abnormal X it is the structurally abnormal chromosome which is late-replicating, not the normal X. This has been shown in the case of deletions involving the long arm,[96] the short arm,[9,260] or a ring chromosome,[23,236] as well as for duplicated or X-isochromosomes,[7,67,103,172,192,198,269] an enlarged X chromosome of undetermined nature (Fig. 6b),[122] or an X-autosomal translocation (Fig. 6c).[193] The only possible exceptions have been three early-replicating ring-X chromosomes described by Pfeiffer *et al.*,[215,216] and these may have another explanation.

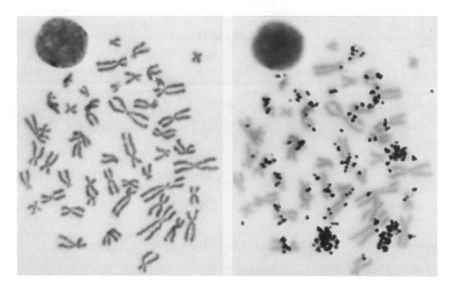

Fig. 6a. Terminal labeling of an XXXXY cell, showing three late-replicating X chromosomes in nearly-peripheral locations. Kodak NTB 3 emulsion. (Courtesy W. R. Breg.)

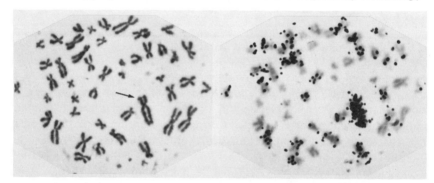

Fig. 6b. Terminal labeling of an enlarged X (Xq+) chromosome, showing the uniformly late replication of the entire chromosome. (From Hugh-Jones et al.[122])

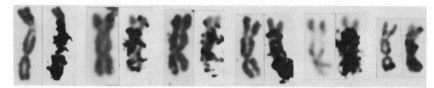

Fig. 6c. Presumptive X-autosome translocation chromosome from six cells. This chromosome has a late-replicating portion about the size of a normal X, and, in these terminally labeled cells, a lightly labeled segment presumably derived from an autosome. (From Neuhäuser and Back.[193])

An important feature of the cases with structurally abnormal X chromosomes is that the size of the sex-chromatin body parallels the size of the late-replicating X chromosome. Furthermore, in a proportion of cells the sex-chromatin body appears to synthesize DNA out of step with the rest of the nuclear chromatin (Fig. 7).[10] These findings, in addition to the one-to-one correspondence between the maximum number of late-replicating X chromosomes and the maximum number of sex-chromatin bodies, strongly support the hypothesis that the late-replicating C-group chromosome is an X chromosome, and that the sex-chromatin body is formed by this late-replicating X chromosome. It is not yet clear, however, whether each cell contains a late-replicating X but only some of these form a sex-chromatin body, or whether every late-replicating X forms a sex-chromatin body. Mittwoch favors the latter idea on the basis of evidence that the proportion of XX cells with a late-replicating X is about the same as the percentage of chromatin-positive cells. Not all published reports support this idea, although German[88] reported a variable proportion of cells with a heavily labeled X in three normal females, and Jacobs et al.[125] found that only about a third of the terminally labeled metaphase cells in their female controls have a heavily labeled C-group (X) chromosome. Rowley et al.[235] reported three late-replicating X chromosomes in virtually every "suitably labeled" (whatever that means) XXXXY cell, and so did Mukherjee et al. [187] in cultured leukocytes from an XXXXY male who had three peripheral sex-chromatin bodies in only 7% of his buccal mucosal cells. Mukherjee et al.[187] also

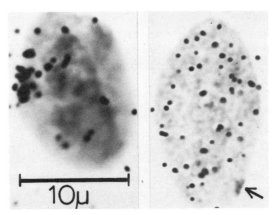

Fig. 7. Asynchronous DNA synthesis in sex chromatin, contrasted to the rest of the interphase nucleus. One nucleus shows general labeling except over the sex chromatin; in the other nucleus there is a dense cluster of grains, presumably over a sex-chromatin body. (From Atkins et al.[10])

consistently found two late-replicating X chromosomes in cells from an XXX female, although only 2% of her buccal mucosal cells contained two sex-chromatin bodies. While the tissues studied were different, the marked discrepancy between these frequencies suggests that variations in the number of sex-chromatin bodies are not due simply to variations in the number of late-replicating X chromosomes. The apparent discrepancies between laboratories cannot yet be evaluated, nor the underlying problems solved, because of the almost universal failure to report results in sufficient detail.

The late-replicating X chromosome is most easily identified by auto-radiographic terminal-labeling pattern of any chromosome in the entire complement. The other (early-replicating) X chromosome has never been clearly identified because it cannot be distinguished from the other C-group chromosomes. Schmid[242] suggested that the early-replicating X chromosome had certain distinctive labeling characteristics (Fig. 11), and this appears to have been confirmed by Lubs[157] by use of a marker X chromosome.

Morphologic Characteristics.    Several attempts have been made to characterize late-replicating X chromosomes. When karyotypes are prepared without knowledge of the labeling pattern the late-replicating X is shorter than the generally accepted values for the X (e.g., those included in the reports of the Denver and London Conferences) and varies in length in individual cells from the longest to the shortest in the C group.[4,14,88,187] Measurements confirmed the extreme variability in length of this chromosome relative to other members of the C group, and the shorter mean length, between that of chromosome 8 and 9.[24]

Chandra and Hungerford[45a] found a 75% correspondence in 57 cells between the chromosome selected by morthology as belonging to the group of four "6 or X" chromosomes (internally indistinguishable) and the heavily labeled C-group chromosome, thus supporting their contention that this chromosome can be placed in a group with three morphologically similar chromosomes with some success, but also indicating the limited accuracy of morphologic identification of this chromosome.

When more than one late-replicating X is present in diploid cells it is possible to compare their morphology in the same cell. Mukherjee et al.[187] suggested there might be a consistent difference between the morphology of one of the two late replicating X's in an XXX female or of the three late-replicating X's in an XXXXY male, but their sample was too small to be convincing, especially since the apparent difference in morphology was not based on measurements. A similar qualitative difference in the arm ratio and size of the late-replicating C-group chromosome was observed by Hsu et al.,[117] who interpreted their results as indicating a deleted X chromosome, but presented no quantitative data (relative grain counts or measurements) in support of this hypothesis. Reitalu[230] has suggested that the shortness of the X in Hsu et al.'s case may be due partly to its strong state of contraction, and he compares it with an observation of Jacobs and her co-workers in the case of an XX/XXX mosaic in which the extra presumptive X chromosome had the same morphology as a number 10.

The importance of quantitative data on length and arm ratio of the late-replicating X chromosome can be illustrated by reference to a case of Mukherjee and Burdette.[191] They reported an elongation of the short arm of the late-replicating C-group chromosome in a female with a ring chromosome 3, and concluded that the tip of one arm of a number 3 was translocated to the X. Their figures do not support this claim, nor does their comparison with "the other X chromosome," since there is no way this chromosome can be identified. Comparison of the late-replicating X with the longest or most metacentric C-group chromosome in a series of cells from this case or with the late-replicating X in other individuals might have confirmed the presence of an altered morphology, although such a change in morphology need not have arisen by the postulated translocation, but might be a simple polymorphism.

X-Autosome Translocation.   The peculiar behavior of X chromosomes, resulting from the existence of two functional states with alternative replication patterns, creates a special problem in recognizing a translocation between an X chromosome and an autosome. Even if the structural change itself does not modify the replication pattern, a number of different labeling patterns are theoretically possible. The structurally normal X chromosome may be preferentially inactivated and thus consistently late-replicating. In that case it would not be possible to distinguish an X-autosome translocation from a translocation involving two autosomes. Mann et al.[161] reported a case of this type.

On the other hand, X-chromosome inactivation may occur randomly, so that in some cells the structurally normal X chromosome will be late-replicating, while in other cells the X-chromosome portion of the two translocation chromosomes will be late replicating. This has been observed in mice[159] as well as in man. A variable proportion of the attached autosomal material may also be inactivated by a kind of "spreading effect," which has been described in X-autosome translocations in mice, though not in man.

Thirdly, the structurally normal X may always be active, with the translocated bits of X preferentially inactivated. This has been observed in mice, where the effect of an excess of autosomal material is apparently minimized by inactivation of the X to which this autosome segment is attached.

Neuhäuser and Back[193] have presented strong evidence for the presence of an X-autosome translocation in a female child with multiple malformations. The chromosome number was 45, with two missing C-group chromosomes and an additional submetacentric chromosome similar to, but distinguishable from, chromosome 2. The marker chromosome was generally late-replicating except for the distal portion of its long arm (Fig. 6c). Normal-appearing sex-chromatin bodies were seen in 50 of 300 buccal mucosal cells and drumsticks in 11 of 400 neutrophils. The authors concluded that an unidentified portion of a C-group autosome was translocated to the tip of the long arm of an X chromosome, which is preferentially late-replicating, but the replication of the autosomal segment has remained independent of that of the X. Other reports of possible X-autosome translocations have also appeared,[161] but without the necessary crucial evidence for proving their nature.

Marker X.   Lubs[157] has recently observed a marker C-group chromosome in three generations of a family. The four carrier males were mentally retarded, while the carrier females were normal. Autoradiographic analysis showed that the marker chromosome was an X. It was late-replicating in six of 20 informative cells, whereas another C-group chromosome was late-replicating in the other 14 cells. Thus, the presence of a secondary constriction near the end of the long arm, forming a satellite, was not associated with preferential inactivation of the marker X. The labeling pattern of this chromosome was studied in 18 cells from two carrier males. The long arm was later-replicating than the short arm and the satellite. No comparison with the labeling pattern of the C-group autosomes was given, although Lubs claimed that chromosome 6, i.e., one of the longest C-group chromosomes, sometimes has a similar pattern.

**Ring-C Chromosome.**   Any ring chromosome is a rather unsatisfactory object for autoradiographic analysis because the chromatids are virtually always overlapping, and the labeling of the underlying chromatid will therefore not be quantitatively reflected in the resulting autoradiogram. However, the asynchronous duplication of the X chromosomes is sufficiently marked that even relatively small ring-X chromosomes can sometimes be identified, since they are preferentially late-replicating.[50a,236] On the other hand, Pfeiffer et al.[215] failed to observe late replication of a ring-C chromosome in a very thorough study of a 12-year-old girl whose clinical features strongly supported the identification of the ring as an X. They suggested that the ring consisted mainly of the early-replicating chromosomal material found in the centromeric region and that no change in replication pattern was involved. A similar explanation has been given to account for the absence of late replication in two small centric fragments possibly of X-chromosome origin.[50a] For both these reasons the conclusion that two small ring-C chromosomes which are not late-replicating are therefore of autosomal origin[6] is not compelling.

## The D Group

The six chromosomes in the D group can be divided into three pairs on the basis of their terminal labeling patterns. One pair is quite late-replicating in the distal and sometimes the middle third of the long arm. The second pair terminates DNA synthesis only slightly earlier in the S period, but has a different labeling pattern with late replication in the centromeric region. The third pair terminates DNA synthesis earlier with the late-replicating segment also in the centromeric region (Figs. 8 and 11). Yunis et al.[294] have referred to these three labeling patterns as $D_1$, $D_2$, and $D_3$ respectively ($D_1$ because it occurs in three D-group chromosomes in $D_1$-trisomic cells), while Giannelli and Howlett[95] call them A, B, and C patterns. The relative lengths of chromosomes with the various labeling patterns have been determined;[90,95] these support the hypothesis that the longest chromosome pair, number 13, has a $D_1$ or A pattern, chromosome 14 a $D_2$ or B pattern, and the shortest chromosome pair, number 15, a $D_3$ or C pattern. These differences in labeling intensity and grain location are not always clear-cut in a particular culture, and it may be necessary to vary the

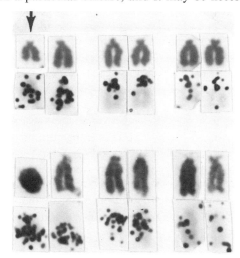

Fig. 8. Partial double karyotypes of terminally labeled D-group chromosomes from cases with 46,XY,13q− (above) and 46,XY,13r karyotypes (below). The arrow indicates the 13q− and ring chromosomes. Kodak AR-10 stripping film, one-week exposure. (Courtesy of P. W. Allderdice.)

time for incorporation of label before suitable labeled cells are obtained. Even then, analysis of a reasonably large sample of cells, perhaps 30 or more, may be necessary to determine the labeling pattern of the D-group chromosomes. No confidence can be placed in the pattern observed in a single cell because of the statistical considerations discussed earlier. A good quantitative study is that of Buchner *et al.*[33]

In the eight cases of the $D_1$-trisomy syndrome tested thus far an additional chromosome with a $D_1$ (or A) labeling pattern has always been present.[26,31,94,162,293] Giannelli and Howlett[95] were unable to assign the chromosome responsible for the $D_1$-trisomy syndrome to a size class even though they presented convincing evidence that the chromosomes with the A pattern were the longest D-group chromosomes in cells from a normal individual and from a presumptive 13/14 translocation heterozygote, and that the longest pair of D-group chromosomes were the last to terminate DNA synthesis. Identification of the chromosome involved thus rests only on the labeling pattern and the phenotypic correlation. In D-trisomic cells from a 46,XX/47,XX,D+ individual who did *not* have the clinical findings of the $D_1$-trisomy syndrome the extra chromosome had a $D_2$ or B pattern of labeling rather than a $D_1$ pattern.[87] The consistent correlation of labeling pattern of the extra chromosome with the phenotype strengthens the case for identifying the $D_1$, $D_2$, and $D_3$ labeling patterns with specific chromosomes.

Another approach to the identification of chromosomes in the D-group has been the study of D/D translocation chromosomes of the centric fusion type. Two types of rearrangement are informative: (1) a translocation between nonhomologous chromosomes, as shown by the absence of the translocation chromosome in at least one child, and (2) an isochromosome for the long arm of a D-group chromosome, as shown by the presence of only translocation-trisomic offspring. Information on seven cases of the first type indicates that when the two arms are derived from different chromosomes they have different labeling patterns. In six cases the translocation chromosome has had a $D_1/D_2$ (13/14) pattern,[26,66,95,237,291] while one has had a $D_1/D_3$ (13/15) pattern.[112] Information on two D-group isochromosomes, each associated with $D_1$-trisomy syndrome, indicates that each had a $D_1/D_1$ labeling pattern.[94,207] This supports the identification of chromosome 13 as the one with a $D_1$ pattern and strengthens the interpretation of the above translocations as 13/14 and 13/15 in type.

Sometimes a structurally altered chromosome is present in association with such a characteristic clinical picture that one is assured the same chromosome is responsible for the abnormality in each case. Such markers are ideal for studies on chromosome identification. Patau[207] emphasized that use of a marker chromosome may turn an exceedingly difficult statistical problem into an almost trivial one. He used a telocentric $D_1$ chromosome to show the consistent labeling pattern of a specific chromosome, and to show that on the average the $D_1$ chromosomes terminate DNA synthesis later than the other two pairs in the D-group. Bias and Migeon[21] observed a $D_1$ labeling pattern in a virtually telocentric D-group chromosome which was present in 13 phenotypically normal individuals in three generations of one family. Lieber *et al.*[151] also observed a $D_1$ pattern in a telocentric chromosome in 14 normal people in four generations of another family. In the latter family the index case was a child with multiple malformations who also had the telocentric chromosome 13. The presence of a quadrivalent in cells from a testis biopsy from a carrier male relative indicates that the normal carriers of the telocentric 13 have a reciprocal translocation.

Allderdice and her associates[1] observed a $D_1$ pattern in a D-group ring chromosome in a patient with characteristic clinical features, and in a second D-group chromosome with a deletion of 20 % of its long arm (Fig. 8) in a clinically similar patient with, in addition, absent thumbs and associated anomalies. They were unable to rule out a terminal deletion by labeling pattern. It was difficult to separate the other five D-group chromosomes into matching pairs and a singleton in a consistent fashion by total grain count alone, although the pattern of labeling was more informative. This method of identification of a "missing pattern" has been widely used in the case of D/G, G/G, and other translocations,[63,168,214] and appears to be a useful technique which gives consistent results (Table I), although its reliability has not been adequately tested.

Some of the interpretations which have been made by the "missing pattern" technique may have to be revised. A recent case with absent thumbs, associated anomalies, and a ring-D chromosome may serve as an example. Because a ring chromosome has overlapping chromatids, autoradiography does not give an accurate estimate of the intensity or location of its labeling. Consequently, one must rely principally on the "missing pattern" method of identification of the source of the ring. In one study[259] the missing pattern was clearly not a $D_3$ or 15, and appeared likely to be a $D_2$ or 14. In view of the close phenotypic similarity between this case and the one of Allderdice *et al.*,[1] it seems likely that inadequacy of the "missing pattern" technique, especially when used with a relatively small sample of cells, has led to an erroneous conclusion. Alternatively, one could conclude that a deletion of similar portions of two different chromosomes in the D-group can produce very similar phenotypes. Hollowell *et al.*[115] have described somewhat different clinical findings in a three-year-old girl with a ring chromosome 13, and thus raised the question of the specificity of phenotype with a deletion of chromosome 13.

It is questionable just how far one should press this point of clinical similarity or dissimilarity between cases. Yunis and Hook[292] have interpreted two unique structurally abnormal chromosomes as partial $D_1$ chromosomes because of a few phenotypic features shared with $D_1$-trisomic individuals. The karyotypes in the two cases were 46,XX,G—,C+ and 47,XY,G ? (with satellites on each arm). It is doubtful whether the clinical or the auto-radiographic studies in either of these cases provide an adequate basis for the conclusion that each has partial $D_1$-trisomy.

A potentially more promising approach to chromosome identification is the use of genetic markers. Bloom et al.[27] reported anomalous inheritance at the haptoglobin locus in two unrelated individuals with a ring chromosome identified as a number 13 by autoradiography. They concluded that the haptoglobin locus might be near the tip of either arm of chromosome 13. Hollowell et al.[115] found an Hp 2—1 heterozygous individual with a ring chromosome 13, identified autoradiographically, indicating that the locus is either not on this chromosome, or is very close to the tip of one arm, so that it can be present or absent in a ring chromosome. Bias and Migeon[21] found several individuals with a telocentric chromosome 13, identified autoradio-graphically, who were heterozygous at the haptoglobin locus, and concluded that this locus was not on the short arm of 13, unless extremely close to the centromere. Their conclusion appears to be unjustified, since the related individuals in question may be balanced translocation carriers, as in the family described by Lieber et al.[151]

Terminal labeling studies have been informative as regards chromosome identification in D/G translocations of the centric fusion type, despite the necessity of depending upon the "missing pattern" method (Table I). Of 17 unrelated cases studied, 13 were reported to be of the $D_2G(14/G)$ type,[26,63,112,168,242,291] three were the $D_3G(15/G)$ type, and one was either a $D_1/G$ or a $D_2/G$ type. Not a single case has yet been found that is clearly of the $D_1/G$ type, even though the $D_1$ chromosome is frequently involved in the D/D centric fusion type of interchange. This finding probably accounts for the absence of $D_1$-trisomic individuals in the numerous families with D/G translocations that have been published.

Jacobsen and Mikkelsen[126] have studied a familial reciprocal transloca-tion involving two D-group chromosomes. The mother of the proband has karyotype 46,XX,2D—,t(Dq+,Dq—). The larger translocation chromosome terminates DNA synthesis late, and appears to have a $D_1$ labeling pattern, although the distal portion, nearly half of this chromosome, is lightly labeled. The labeling pattern of the four normal D-group chromosomes does not permit pairing and recognition of the two missing patterns. The identity of the small translocation is obscure; its size and labeling pattern fail to distinguish it from the G-group chromosomes. The authors suggest that this smaller chromosome, which is present in addition to a full set of normal D-group chromosomes in the proband, carries that portion of the $D_1$ chromosome which is responsible for some of the clinical abnormalities in $D_1$-trisomy, because the propositus has coloboma, cataract, epicanthus, transverse palmar crease, and seizures.

Bloom and Gerald[26] found a presumptive $D_2/D_3$ labeling pattern in a reciprocal D/D translocation chromosome. They found a $D_1$ labeling pattern in the presumptive D portion of A/D, B/D, and C/D translocation chromosomes. De Capoa et al.[63] found a presumptive $D_3$ pattern in a C/D translocation chromosome. The direct identification of this pattern was supported by finding only one normal D-group chromosome with a $D_3$ pattern. Pitt et al.[217] studied a familial D/D translocation in which the labeling pattern of the reciprocal translocation chromosomes was clearly not a $D_1$.

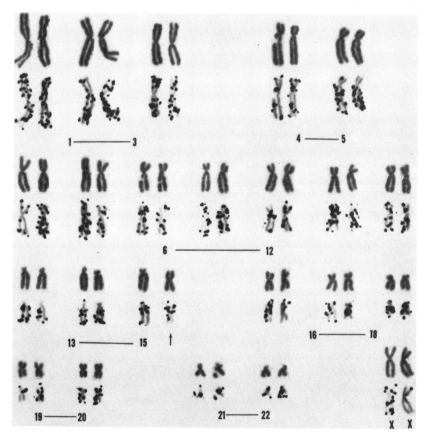

Fig. 9.   Double karyotype of a cell, labeled at the initiation of its S period with ³H-TdR, from a patient with an inversion of a chromosome in the D group, identified as number 13 by both initial and terminal labeling. The initial-labeling pattern shown here is the reverse of that seen in terminally labeled cells. (From Cohen et al.[50])

Autoradiography was used by Cohen *et al.*[50] to support their hypothesis that an amenorrheic woman whose karyotype appeared to be 46,XX,D−,E ?+ (Fig. 9) had an inversion of chromosome $D_1$, with a karyotype 46,XX,inv(13 ?$p + q-$).

## The E Group

The pattern of DNA synthesis in the E group can be very helpful in chromosome identification. Chromosome 16 has a late-replicating region in the proximal part of one arm (generally considered the long arm) corresponding to the secondary constriction sometimes seen there.[7,89,187,242] Chromosome 17 appears to be the first pair in this group to terminate DNA synthesis.[14,89,99,134,180,242] Chromosome 18 is generally late-replicating, especially for such a small chromosome.

Giannelli and Howlett[96] combined autoradiography with measurements in an attempt to validate the accuracy of morphologic and autoradiographic identification of E-group chromosomes. They found that in one case all the chromosomes could be identified by morphology alone, in one case only pair number 16 could be so identified, and in two cases none could be identified in this way. Labeling studies permitted more accurate identification, particularly in combination with morphologic indices.

In view of these findings, it is unfortunate that relatively adequate labeling studies have been reported for only one case of the $E_1$ (presumptive 18)-trisomy syndrome.[293] In this case there was an additional late-replicating chromosome in the E group, supporting the general impression that the clinical syndrome is due to 18-trisomy. Further confirmation would be highly desirable, since the possibility that 17-trisomy occurs has not been ruled out, and no other clue exists to the phenotype it might produce. El-Alfi *et al.*[73] identified a presumptive 18-trisomy by labeling pattern in a 25-week aborted hydrocephalic fetus. At such early stages of fetal life the phenotype is still of little value as a clue to identification, making autoradiography just that much more important.

Autoradiography has been somewhat more widely used to identify deleted or otherwise structurally abnormal E-group chromosomes. Migeon[167] observed late replication in a virtually telocentric chromosome whose long arm was comparable in length to that of a chromosome 17 or 18. She concluded that it was a number 18 with a partial deletion of its long arm. Giannelli and Howlett[96] studied the labeling pattern of the E-group chromosomes in two girls with Ullrich's syndrome. Each had a short-arm deletion of chromosome 18, judged by combined autoradiography and measurement. The clinical findings in these 18$p-$ cases were somewhat different from those usually reported in patients with an E-group short-arm deletion, and this raises the question of the degree of confidence with which one can identify chromosomes by the clinical effects associated with a deletion or other change.

Reinwein et al.[227] identified a chromosome 18 with a partial deletion of its long arm by its persistent late replication. Giannelli and Howlett[96] identified a ring chromosome in a mentally retarded girl as a number 17 because of its light terminal labeling and the clear morphologic distinction of the remaining E-group chromosomes. One other ring-E chromosome has been studied: Palmer et al.[206] identified a ring-18 in a child with multiple malformations by its heavy labeling.

Jacobsen and Mikkelsen[126] identified chromosomes 18 and 21 autoradiographically in individuals with a familial $t(18p-,21p+)$ translocation. Buhler et al.[34] used labeling studies in a C/E translocation heterozygote to show that chromosome 18 was involved in the translocation. The proband, a son of this heterozygote, had a partial C-trisomy. Because of the small size of the C-group chromosome presumed missing as a result of this translocation, the authors concluded they were dealing with a 12/18 translocation. It is unfortunate that labeling studies are still of no use in distinguishing between the various C-group autosomes, since morphologic characterization of a missing chromosome in this group is of notoriously questionable accuracy.

## The F Group

Chromosomes 19 and 20 are indistinguishable by their labeling patterns. Both pairs terminate DNA synthesis relatively early in the S period[89,134,242] and almost synchronously.[99] However, one commonly sees one of the four chromosomes labeled at a time when the other three are unlabeled, or, conversely, three labeled and one unlabeled.[153,187] This is not evidence of asynchronous DNA synthesis, despite the claims of these investigators, because of the high probability of getting just such a result by chance with completely synchronous DNA synthesis. Judging from the published figures, many of the labeled F-group chromosomes had only one or two silver grains, and the mean grain count over the F group must have been very small. Consequently, a fairly high proportion of F-group chromosomes with equal tritium content would be expected to show no silver grains in a given short exposure to film. The assumption that unlabeled chromosomes have already terminated DNA synthesis is not really valid under these conditions, especially with the relatively short exposure of film to the specimen usually used in autoradiographic studies.

Despite these limitations, the distinctive early termination of DNA synthesis of F-group chromosomes can be helpful in identifying structurally modified chromosomes that are morphologically similar, e.g., 21/22 or 22/22 translocation chromosomes.

## The G Group

The chromosomes of the G group are so small and their termination of DNA synthesis so nearly synchronous that it is difficult to obtain grain densities high enough to permit distinction between chromosomes in this group. Nevertheless, some consistent results have been obtained (Table II). Schmid[242] found three heavy and two lightly labeled G-group chromosomes on terminal labeling in 21-trisomic mongols of each sex, but he gave no quantitative data on the number of cells or the number of individuals studied. Yunis et al.[295] presented data on terminal labeling of cells in four 21-trisomic mongoloid females. In each case he found 10–25 cells with three heavy and two lightly labeled G-group chromosomes, and only about one-third as many cells with the reverse pattern, two heavy and three lightly labeled G-group chromosomes. Despite the lack of grain counts, these data support the author's conclusion that the mongolism chromosome is the G-group chromosome that terminates DNA synthesis relatively late. Similar results have been obtained in four male and eight female mongols.[13,79,92] They support the conclusion that either the terminal phases of DNA synthesis of chromosomes 21 and 22 lie close together, or there is asynchrony of the homologues. Cave and Levitsky[45] were unable to demonstrate any consistent pattern of DNA synthesis in the G group in 92 cells from 17 females with Down's syndrome. However, they used a pulse-labeling technique rather then terminal labeling, and pooled cells labeled at various points in the S period. Their results are thus not comparable to those obtained with the generally more useful terminal-labeling technique.

Studies on D/G and G/G translations in mongols or their parents have tended to confirm the late replication of the mongolism chromosome (Table I). Yunis et al. [295] found one heavy and two lightly labeled G-group chromosomes in each of two D/G (presumptive 14/21) translocation carriers. They also observed one heavy and one lightly labeled G-group chromosome in each of two G/G (one a presumptive, one a proven 21/22) translocation carriers. Higurashi et al.[112] reported similar observations: 18 of 23 labeled cells had one heavy and one lightly labeled G-group chromosome, with the presumptive translocation chromosome heavily labeled in only one arm. Two cases with a presumptive 21/21 isochromosome have shown two lightly labeled G-group chromosomes and a more heavily labeled isochromosome,[63,207] as expected if the mongolism chromosome is later-replicating than the other G-group chromosome.

German[90] showed by measurement that the later-replicating pair of G-group chromosomes are shorter than the other two. This has also been claimed by Schmid,[242] Yunis et al.,[294] and Patau.[207] Since the mongolism chromosome is so firmly established as number 21, it would probably be wiser to continue to refer to it as number 21, despite the slight inconsistency this introduces into the Denver classification. There is, in any case, still no proof that mongolism is only produced by partial or complete trisomy of this chromosome 21, even though this seems intuitively likely.

The labeling pattern of at least six different Ph[1] chromosomes has been studied. In three cases the Ph[1] chromosome was late-replicating;[153,242] in three more the Ph[1] chromosome had an indeterminate pattern, i.e., it was not clearly late-replicating.[104] Differences in the size of the deletion, or small sample size, could be responsible for this difference.

## The Y Chromosome

Usually, the Y chromosome terminates DNA synthesis later than chromosomes 21 and 22, i.e., it can be distinguished from them by its heavier terminal labeling.[89,134,135,242] This is not always so, however; in some cases no late-replicating Y has been observed.[44] Only a few quantitative studies have been carried out, notably by Kikuchi and Sandberg,[135] who found the Y to be among the last chromosomes in the complement to terminate DNA synthesis.

A number of presumptive XYY individuals have been described in whom labeling studies were carried out. The results have been somewhat inconsistent. In some cases the two presumably genetically and morphologically identical Y chromosomes have had identical grain densities and labeling patterns,[15,28,42,80] while in other cases markedly asynchronous duplication has been observed.[135,141] No consistent difference in morphology between these has been observed, although in one case of similar labeling both Y's were very small,[42] while in one of the opposite type of case the Y chromosomes were much larger.[135] In one case with asynchronous duplication of the two presumptive Y chromosomes these two chromosomes were of different sizes,[141] an observation that casts real doubt on the identification of one of them.

### Initial Labeling Patterns

Kikuchi and Sandberg[134] and Bianchi and Bianchi[19] reported asynchrony in the initiation of DNA synthesis in different chromosomes in pulse-labeled cultured human leukocytes. This did not appear to be as marked as that found near the end of the S period, nor as easy to study. Consequently, the pattern of initiation of DNA synthesis has not been as much used as an aid in chromosome identification. Two methods of study have been used. First, pulse-labeling cells in asynchronously growing cultures at various times before fixing the cells, and second, blocking DNA synthesis with FUdR in order to pile up a very large proportion of cells in late $G_1$, and relieving the block in the now synchronized cells with tritiated thymidine. For the readily identifiable chromosomes, 1, 2, and 3, the initial labeling patterns appear to be the reverse of the terminal labeling patterns (Fig. 10), i.e., a segment of chromosomes that is terminally labeled is initially unlabeled, and *vice versa*.[198,256-258,270,271] The same is true for the X and Y chromosomes, and the initial labeling patterns of chromosomes in the B, D, and E groups are also compatible with this general rule, although only one suitable marker chromosome has yet been studied and found to conform to this rule (Fig. 9).[50]

It has been claimed that the heteropycnotic, late-replicating X chromosomes also begin DNA synthesis late,[44,118a,198,222,223] although this has not been generally observed in asynchronously growing cultures.[19,134,189] On the other hand, Takagi and Sandberg[271] have observed delayed initiation of DNA synthesis in one C-group (presumptive X) chromosome in XX cells and in the Y chromosomes in XY cells.

The evidence of late initiation of DNA synthesis in heteropycnotic X chromosomes in synchronized cultures is unequivocal. Petersen[212] and Hsu and Lockhart[118a] observed three unlabeled C-group chromosomes in

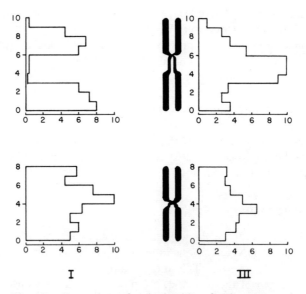

I                                                III

Fig. 10.  Comparison of grain densities of a chromosome 1 having an elongated secondary constriction region with that of its normal homologue: I, initial labeling; III, terminal labeling. Note the late replication of the elongated segment, and the inverse relationship between grain densities at the two ends of the S period. (From Sofuni and Sandberg.[258])

cultured XXXXY cells when ³H-thymidine was added at the beginning of the S period in FUdR-blocked cultures. Priest et al.[223] found 0, 1, and 2 unlabeled presumptive X chromosomes per diploid cell in XY, XX, and XXX cell lines, respectively, and determined that these chromosomes began DNA synthesis more than 2 hr after the other chromosomes, which corresponds to nearly half of the 6-hr S period in such synchronized cultures. The unlabeled hetero-pycnotic X chromosome showed the same variability in length, ranging in rank from second to fifteenth in the C-group,[223] as it does as a heavily labeled late-replicating chromosome.

Ockey et al.[198] found an isochromosome for the long arm of the X chromosome consistently unlabeled with ³H-thymidine during the initiation of the S period in FUdR-synchronized cultures. On the other hand, Mukherjee et al.[185] found a similar isochromosome X lightly labeled very early in S in nonsynchronized cultures. It is possible that their method did not give true initial labeling, since they left ³H-TdR in the culture for several hours and did not chase with cold thymidine. Continued incorporation of label into DNA from an intracellular pool would serve to blur the initial labeling patterns. However, similar experiments in bovine cell cultures with good pulse labeling gave similar results, with simultaneous onset of DNA synthesis in the two X chromosomes and later appearance of markedly asynchronous duplication.[190] Since the S period is shorter in synchronized cultures than is asynchronously growing cultures,[222] it is possible that different rates of synthesis at the beginning of S under the two conditions of culture are responsible for the different labeling patterns observed. This is in keeping with the light initial labeling Stubblefield[264] observed over X and Y chromosomes in the Chinese hamster in FUdR-synchronized cultures.

### Comparison of DNA Content of Chromosomes

Autoradiography can be used as a means of comparing the DNA content of specific chromosomes. Wennstrom and de la Chapelle[282] used this approach to evaluate the nature of a long Y chromosome in two cases. Unfortunately, they did not allow sufficient time for incorporation of ³H-TdR, and thus could not rule out the effect of asynchronous DNA synthesis. Their observation that a long Y chromosome had no more silver grains than a normal-sized Y is therefore not conclusive evidence that the two Y chromosomes being compared had no difference in DNA content.

Methodologically, the study by Crippa and German[57] is better. These workers allowed tissue-cultured fibroblasts to grow in the presence of ³H-thymidine throughout their S period in order to label all the DNA synthesized in one cycle. They found no difference between the number of grains over a morphologically variant chromosome 16 (16q+) and its normal homologue in a series of 20 cells, and concluded that the greater length of the marker chromosome was not the result of an increase in DNA content in its long arm. By increasing the number of cells examined or the grain count over this small number of cells by repeated filmings, any desired level of confidence could be reached. This method might be particularly helpful in characterizing structurally modified chromosomes; e.g., in the case of a chromosome 1 with an elongated secondary constriction region (Fig. 10),[258] is there an insertion of additional genetic material ? To date no attempt has been made to use this approach to estimate the relative DNA content of specific chromosomes or to correlate these values with measured lengths or cytophotometric estimates of DNA content. A better method might be that of Ebstein.[72] She found that ³H-actinomycin-D can be used to label small quantities of DNA cyto-chemically with greater sensitivity than that obtained with the Feulgen reaction.

## THE FUNCTIONAL SIGNIFICANCE OF DNA REPLICATION PATTERNS

### Late Replication and Heterochromatin

The existence of two physical states of chromosomal material has been known for many years. Euchromatin is an extended state, heterochromatin a more condensed or contracted state of the genetic material. Heterochromatin is visible in interphase nuclei, while euchromatin is not. With the electron microscope euchromatin is seen to consist of fibers 50–75 Å thick, while heterchromatin contains thicker fibers, 300–400 Å thick.[108]

Lima-de-Faria[152] discovered that heterochromatin terminates DNA synthesis later than euchromatin. He found this to be so for the heteropyc-notic X chromosome of the grasshopper, *Melanoplus*, during meiosis, and for the clumped autosomal heterochromatin in the rye plant, *Secale*. Sex chromatin is also late-replicating,[10,103] and so are the heteropycnotic X chromosomes which form the sex-chromatin bodies. Further studies by many workers have confirmed the generally late replication of heterochromatin, both autosomal and that in the sex chromosomes.

### Can Condensed Chromatin Replicate without Any Change of State?

Hay and Revel (Fig. 11)[108] and Moses and Coleman (Fig. 12)[182] showed by electron-microscope autoradiography that tritiated thymidine was incorporated only into extended chromatin, with no silver grains seen over condensed chromatin. Consequently, one might expect that sex chromatin,

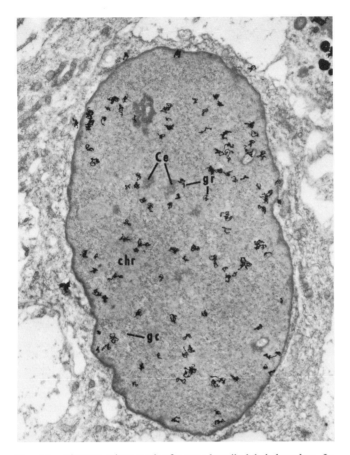

Fig. 11. Electron micrograph of a very heavily labeled nucleus. In areas where the chromatin (chr) forms small clumps it is clear that the silver grains are associated only with the finely textured component. In some regions the central portion of a chromatin clump (Ce) may be denser than the periphery. Similar areas of dense chromatin (heterochromatin) occur commonly along the nuclear membrane. Silver grains (gr) are found over the less-dense chromatin surrounding the centers, but the dense chromatin itself is unlabeled. A few grains are seen over the cytoplasm close to the nucleus. The specimen was fixed after 1 hr of ³H-TdR. gc, granular component. Magnification approximately 5400×. (From Hay and Revel.[108])

and other chromatin masses, would disappear during duplication of the allocyclic X chromosome, but this is apparently not the case. Atkins et al.[10] found labeled sex-chromatin bodies after short exposures of cultured XX cells to tritiated thymidine (Fig. 7), and others have confirmed this. Klinger et al.[138]

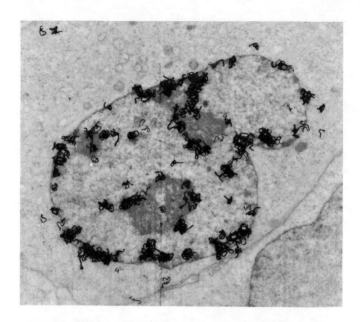

Fig. 12. Electron-microscope autoradiograph of nucleus from HeLa cell exposed to ³H-thymidine for 30 min. Areas of very active DNA synthesis around the nuclear periphery are indicated by dense clusters of grains. Such areas are also associated with the periphery of the nucleolus. There are a few grains that are not associated with one or the other of these areas. The grain over the clear region in the center of the nucleolus indicates that DNA replication is occurring in this area also. Note also the cytoplasmic incorporation. Section coated with Ilford L-4 emulsion and exposed two months. Magnification approximately $7200 \times$. (From Moses and Coleman.[182])

used a combined autoradiographic–photometric determination on the same nuclei to show that labeled cells in the S phase have the same frequency of chromatin-positive cells as cells in the $G_1$ phase. Cells in the $G_2$ phase, with a doubled amount of DNA, had slightly higher percentages of chromatin-positive cells. Comings[52] obtained quite similar results with only 3 min incubation with ³H-TdR. Both groups concluded that heterochromatin could undergo DNA replication while in the condensed state, although Comings pointed out that one could not rule out some segmental uncoiling on a scale that might be detectable only by electron microscopy. Since complete DNA replication of the heteropycnotic X chromosome takes approximately the last 5 hr of the 7.5-hr S period in the cultured cells studied by Comings,[52] a 3-min exposure to ³H-TdR could label no more than

0.05 hr/7.5 hr $= 0.66\%$ of the DNA of this chromosome. Light-microscope autoradiography does not have the resolution necessary to distinguish lateral loops of even much larger size than could be made from this amount of DNA.

The possible effects of the methods used to study sex chromatin have received inadequate attention, i.e., the presence of a sex-chromatin body in a fixed cell is not sufficient evidence that the allocyclic X was in such a condensed state in the living cell. Schwarzacher[250] found a higher frequency of sex-chromatin bodies in cultured cells after fixation and staining than were visible by phase-contrast microscopy of living cells, and concluded that not all sex-chromatin bodies were in equal states of condensation. If such a study were combined with autoradiographic analysis, it might be possible to show whether in living cells sex chromatin is visible only in those cells that are not in the S phase, indicating an obligatory large-scale uncoiling for replication. If not, then the higher resolution of electron-microscope autoradiography will be necessary for solution of this problem.

### Control of Heterochromatin and Replication Sequence

The pattern of DNA replication, which reflects the amount and location of heterochromatin in each chromosome, is coordinated with that of all the other chromosomes in the normal diploid complement. Consequently, the pattern of synthesis of each chromosome cannot be totally autochthonous; there must be some external controlling agency, such as the genome itself[242] or the nuclear membrane.[56] The role of genetic factors can be investigated by studies of aneuploid, triploid, or polyploid cells.

**Aneuploid Cells.** Schmid[242] suggested that an additional chromosome in the complement might be late-replicating, whatever its normal pattern of DNA replication, because the extra chromosome was in some way recognized by the cell and rendered supernumerary. While the observations in 13-, 18-, and 21-trisomic individuals, and those with additional X chromosomes, are consistent with this hypothesis, they are equally consistent with the alternative hypothesis that such degrees of aneuploidy do not influence the pattern of DNA synthesis of individual chromosomes. Furthermore, there is evidence that an additional C-group[74,229] or D-group[87] chromosome need not be late-replicating, nor are both Y chromosomes in XYY individuals always late-replicating.[135]

In general, numerical and structural changes seem to have little or no effect on DNA replication sequences, although structurally abnormal X chromosomes are preferentially late-replicating and long Y chromosomes are sometimes quite late-replicating.[61a,135] The remaining few possible exceptions are explicable in terms of inadequate identification of structurally modified chromosomes,[62] or the existence of two functional states for some of the autosomes, with preferential inactivation of a partially deleted homologue.[62,171]

**Triploid and Tetraploid Cells.** Studies of diploid and tetraploid cells have shown that in general a diploid set of autosomes can maintain one X chromosome in the active state, or, alternatively, can suppress the activity of all but one X chromosome in each diploid complement. Thus, tetraploid XXXX cells generally show two heteropycnotic X chromosomes, whereas the diploid XX cells generally show one. Triploid cells may have either one or two active X chromosomes.[175] This is indicated by the number of sex-chromatin bodies, and also by the number of late-replicating X chromosomes, which can be either one or two less than the number of X chromosomes. Atkins et al.[5] described a diploid/triploid mosaic in which the triploid cells had a 70,XXY karyotype with no late-replicating X and no sex chromatin.

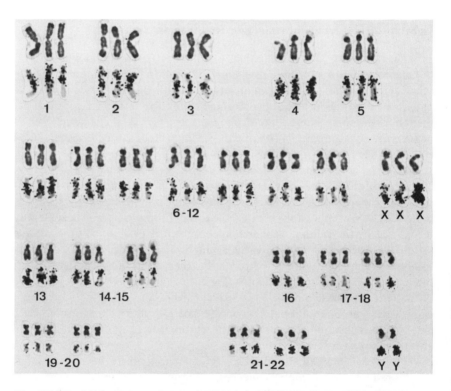

Fig. 13.  Double karyotype of a terminally labeled triploid cell. Note the single heavily labeled X and the characteristic labeling patterns of many other chromosomes, especially those of the A, B, D, and E groups. (From Schmid and Vischer.[246])

Schmid and Vischer[246] described another diploid/triploid mosaic, a malformed male with 48,XXYY/71,XXXYY constitution. Only one late-replicating X chromosome (Fig. 13) and one sex-chromatin body was present in any cell, again indicating that in triploid cells two X chromosomes may be active. It would be interesting to know whether a higher G6PD enzyme level was present in these triploid cells, indicating a breakdown of the usual dosage-compensation mechanism for X-linked genes.

## The Function of Heterochromatin

## General Studies

The significance of late replication has been assessed both directly and indirectly. The results clearly indicate that late-replicating chromosomal segments are genetically inactive, and support the hypothesis that the control of gene action is mediated, at least in part, by the state of chromosomal condensation.

Further evidence that gene action requires extended chromatin comes from studies on protein synthesis. Schultze *et al.*[249] studied incorporation of labeled amino acids into nuclear protein, using grain counts over the nucleus. They found the rate of protein synthesis proportional to nuclear volume, with a constant rate of nuclear protein synthesis per unit volume for each organism tested: mouse, rat, rabbit, guinea pig, and pigeon. The rate of cytoplasmic protein synthesis was proportional to the rate of nuclear protein synthesis, suggesting that all protein synthesis is controlled by nuclear volume, that is, the state of chromosome condensation.

The principle that the heteropycnotic X chromosome is genetically inert,[158] i.e., does not serve as a template for mRNA synthesis, will be discussed in the next section. The corresponding principle that the late-replicating autosomal regions are also genetically inert rests on studies of heterochromatin to be described, on studies of the role of RNA synthesis, and on studies by Kajiwara and Mueller[128] on the incorporation of 5-bromodeoxyuridine (BUdR) into HeLa cells in synchronized cultures. Such incorporation during the last half of the S period had almost no effect on cloning efficiency, while such incorporation during the first half of the S period markedly reduced cloning efficiency. Since DNA which contains BUdR does not synthesize RNA, these results indicate that genes which are duplicated in the last half of the S period are not essential for the synthesis of macromolecules required in clonal growth, and supports the hypothesis that these genes may be inactive.

Kasten and Strasser[129] used a qualitative estimate of grain density over labeled interphase nuclei in synchronized cultures after incubation with

[3]H-UdR as an index of the rate of RNA synthesis. They noted a profound fall in this rate about 3 hr after the beginning of the S period, lasting about 1 hr and coinciding with the maximal rate of the first wave of DNA synthesis. They concluded that DNA could not serve as a template for both RNA and DNA synthesis at the same time. Stubblefield et al.[265] using a more-quantitative method, found an abrupt increase in the rate of RNA synthesis after the first 30% of DNA had been replicated in synchronously growing cells. Both groups of investigators interpreted their results as indicating that most of the DNA involved in transcription (gene action) is replicated in the first third or so of the S period, i.e., represents euchromatin.

Hsu[118] found a much lower rate of RNA synthesis by heterochromatin than by euchromatin, as judged by grain count over the respective areas of mouse L cells. Comings[52] showed that after a 3-min incubation with tritiated uridine only 0.37 times as many silver grains were present over the sex-chromatin body in cultured human XX cells as over comparable areas of euchromatin. He concluded that the sex-chromatin body had only 0–18% as much RNA synthesis in the short time interval tested, but the poor resolution of light-microscope autoradiography seriously limits the accuracy of studies of this kind.

Another approach was used, with great success, by Gall and Callan.[84] They injected [3]H-uridine or [3]H-phenylalanine into adult female newts and removed pieces of ovary at various times afterward in order to study incorporation of label into the lampbrush chromosomes in the oocytes. They found that RNA synthesis in these vertebrate oocytes occurred in extended lateral loops of DNA rather than in the highly condensed chromomeres of the lampbrush chromosomes. Gall and Callan found that the incorporation of [3]H-uridine followed a sequential pattern best explained in terms of a dynamic model, with the loop being continuously unwound at its thin insertion and wound up at the thick, with a constant polarization. The rate of this process was speeded up by prior gonadotrophic hormone treatment. Gene activity thus appears to be associated only with extended chromosome segments; inactive loci appear to be highly condensed. This has been confirmed by electron-microscope autoradiography in calf thymus nuclei.[155] Metaphase chromosomes in both mitosis[219] and meiosis[177] also fail to synthesize RNA, supporting the concept that highly contracted chromosomes cannot act as a template for RNA synthesis. A corollary of this principle is that many agents may regulate RNA (and protein) synthesis by influencing the state of condensation of DNA.[81] Monesi[177] also found that the heteropycnotic XY bivalent in the testes of the mouse was invariably unlabeled throughout the meiotic cycle, while the autosomes incoporated [3]H-uridine into RNA from mid-pachytene through diplotene and diakinesis before ceasing such incorporation completely in metaphase and throughout anaphase of meiosis.

### The Lyon Hypothesis: Two Functional States of the X Chromosome

The Lyon hypothesis, which was put forward to explain the cytologic observations on sex (hetero)chromatin and the behavior of X-linked genes, provides an explanation of this correlation in the case of the mammalian X chromosome. According to this hypothesis,[158] mammalian X chromosomes have two functional states: active and inactive. One X chromosome in each diploid cell is genetically active, i.e., serves as a template for messenger RNA synthesis. Any additional X chromosomes are inactivated at an early stage of embryogenesis, become condensed and capable of forming sex-chromatin bodies. Thus, the maximum number of sex-chromatin bodies is one less than the number of X chromosomes.

In view of Lima-de-Faria's discovery that heterochromatin is late-replicating, it is not surprising that the heteropycnotic X chromosomes which form the sex-chromatin bodies are also late-replicating.[103,180] In fact, this finding is a major support of the hypothesis that these chromosomes are inactive. Several direct tests of this hypothesis have been carried out by exposing cultured cells to $^3$H-uridine for only a few minutes and terminating the cultures immediately. By both electron-microscope autoradiography[155] and light-microscope autoradiography[118] it has been shown that little, if any, RNA synthesis occurs in heterochromatin or in the region of the sex-chromatin body.[52] Similar studies in which cultured cells were pulse-labeled with $^3$H-uridine and metaphases scored several hours later have usually failed to demonstrate this, presumably because of nonspecific absorption of RNA onto all chromosomes.[12,52,209] However, Fujita et al.[83] reported an absence of RNA synthesis by one of the two X chromosomes in XX cells using a similar technique. If confirmed, this would be perhaps the clearest cytologic demonstration of the genetic inactivity of one X in XX cells. Abundant genetic evidence in support of the Lyon hypothesis is available, but will not be reviewed here.

**Random Inactivation of X Chromosomes**   Mukherjee and Sinha[188] provided cytologic proof of the random inactivation of X chromosomes postulated by Lyon by showing approximately equal frequencies of occurrence of a late-replicating horse X chromosome and a late-replicating donkey X chromosome in cells from an interspecific hybrid, the mule. To date there has been no similar demonstration within any species, although the recent study by Lubs[157] may qualify as a direct demonstration of random inactivation in man. On the other hand, there is evidence in man that when the two X chromosomes are structurally different the abnormal X is preferentially inactivated, becoming late-replicating. This is seen in 46,XXp−, 46,XXq−, and 46,XXr cases, and has also been reported in all long-arm isochromosomes X and in cases of 46,XXp+ (Table V).

The Lyon hypothesis provides a ready explanation for the consistent occurrence of a late-replicating structurally abnormal X in these cases, since in cells where the normal X is inactivated functional genes will be completely absent at some loci (in the case of a deletion or isochromosome), and such cells are very likely to be inviable. It is difficult to imagine why a small duplication or perhaps some very small deletions should be lethal on this basis. Consequently, one is left with three possibilities:

1. Small deletions or duplications can occur on an X chromosome without leading to preferential inactivation.

2. Such deletions or duplications very rarely occur.

3. Small deletions or duplications always lead to preferential inactivation, not because the cell would be inviable if such a chromosome were the only "active" one, but because of preferential inactivation by an active process (e.g., Grumbach et al.[103] postulated an episomal factor).

**Inactivation during Embryogenesis.** Kinsey[136] and Hill and Yunis[114] have found direct evidence of X-chromosome differentiation during mammalian embryogenesis, as predicted by the Lyon hypothesis. Kinsey found no late-replicating X in 2–3-day rabbit embryos, while a distinctively late-replicating X was visible in cells from 11–12-day female embryos and adults. Hill and Yunis observed only one arm of each X chromosome in XX eight-cell preimplantation embryos of the Syrian hamster replicating late in the S period, while in mid-gestation embryos and adult skin fibroblast cultures both arms of one X and one arm of its homologue are late-replicating.

### Lack of Inactivation in the Germ Line

Since all X chromosomes appear to be undifferentiated in the zygote, it would not be surprising if inactivation failed to occur in the germ line. Evidence of this has been reported by Utakoji and Hsu[277] for the Chinese hamster and by Mukherjee and Ghosal[186] for the golden hamster.

### Do Autosomes Have Alternate States?

The markedly different patterns of DNA synthesis shown by the two X chromosomes, and their correlation with alternate functional states of the genes carried by these chromosomes, leads directly to the question of whether similar differences between homologues exist for the autosomes. While markedly asynchronous duplication of homologous autosomes does not occur, slight degrees of asynchrony cannot be ruled out on the basis of present evidence. Such asynchronous duplication of homologous autosomes could have the same significance as the more markedly asynchronous duplication of X chromosomes, indicating a functional difference between the two homologues due to inactivation by facultative heterochromatization of loci on one of the homologues. At present no genetic evidence, e.g., dosage compensation, exists in support of this hypothesis, but some cytologic evidence exists.

The level of resolution possible with light-microscope autoradiography is inadequate to show whether homologous gene loci replicate simultaneously or at different times. On the other hand, if the control of gene action is mediated by changes in the state of chromosome condensation, it is possible that relatively large blocks of genes are controlled as units, in which case it may not be unrealistic to expect this to be reflected by the presence of differences between homologues in the distribution of late-replicating chromosomal material. Such differences have not usually been found, as described earlier in this review. However, minor differences might well be missed unless one of the homologues carried a morphologic marker. Using such a marker, Sofuni and Sandberg[258] and Buchner et al.[33] reported correlated differences between homologues of chromosome 1. They found a lower initiation of S and higher end of S grain count over the elongated secondary constriction region than over the corresponding region of the normal homologue in a case of familial elongation of this region (Fig. 10). Since Ockey and de la Chapelle[196] observed fewer grains over the secondary constriction region of chromosome 1 when it is elongated than when it is short, or even invisible in cells from one individual, the differences observed by Sofuni and Sandberg are probably not due simply to greater autoradiographic efficiency over the elongated region. Either they reflect an increment in total DNA content of the region, or indicate a small degree of homologue asynchrony, with the structurally modified chromosome preferentially later-replicating.

Ockey and his associates have suggested that homologous autosomes may replicate slightly out of phase with one another on the basis of correlated differences in length, labeling, and location.[195,198] Further evidence of asynchronous duplication of homologous autosomes has come from the use of morphologic markers. Miller and his associates[171] have found a correlated difference between homologues in both length and replication pattern of the long arm of a B-group chromosome with a partial deletion of the short arm. In five unrelated individuals the long arm of a $4p-$ chromosome was shorter and more heavily terminally labeled than its homologue, while in another five individuals with a $5p-$ chromosome the long arm of the deleted chromosome was shorter and probably more lightly terminally labeled than its homologue (Fig. 5). Similar differences between homologues in labeling and length have also been observed for chromosomes 13, 15, and 18 by de Capoa et al.,[62] who found an even greater difference between homologues for chromosome 14. These investigators found 50 % more grains over a presumptive $14p-$ chromosome than over its labeling homologue. Since the maximum difference in grain counts over the two chromosomes 14 in controls is only 20 %, the findings in this case are perhaps best explained as the result of a translocation between chromosome 14 and a later-replicating chromosome. It seems unlikely that a deletion involving the short arm is responsible for the changes in length and replication pattern of the long arm in all five cases, although this remains a logical possibility.

### DNA Replication Patterns and Differentiation

If tissue differentiation is associated with differences in activity of gene loci, then the chromosomes in cells from different tissues might have different replication patterns. There is evidence (discussed elsewhere) that X-chromosome inactivation takes place early in embryogenesis, with associated appearance of sex chromatin, and, in two mammals, late replication of the facultatively heteropycnotic portion of the X.[114,136] It seems likely that changes in the X chromosome ("differentiation") are responsible not only for the alteration in replication pattern and heteropycnosis, but also for the genetic inertness of the late-replicating X chromosome.

The majority of studies of DNA replication in the human complement have involved leukocytes. However, a number of studies of diploid fibroblast cultures have appeared.[4,5,8,9,179] There are no obvious differences in the time sequence of DNA synthesis between leukocytes and fibroblast-like cells (minor differences would probably not have been noticed in the largely qualitative studies carried out so far in autoradiographic studies of human chromosomes). Similar results have been obtained in animal studies; e.g., Martin[164] found no differences in the gross patterns of autosomal DNA replication in four tissues of the Chinese hamster. However, Utakoji and Hsu[277] observed a striking difference in the replication pattern of the sex chromosomes between somatic cells and cells of the germ line in the Chinese hamster. Furthermore, they found correlated differences in length and replication pattern of the sex chromosomes between different tissues. The long arms of both X and Y chromosomes were shorter in the bone-marrow mitoses than in spermatogonial mitoses. The X and Y chromosomes from lung cells grown *in vitro* appeared to be even shorter than the corresponding chromosomes from bone-marrow cells *in vivo*. This difference, however, was not correlated with any obvious differences in replication pattern. The authors also noted a much longer $G_2$ period in spermatogonia. Their technique, a single intraperitoneal injection of ³H-TdR, gave a peak blood level after 1 hr, with a rapid fall thereafter. Since counts above background were still detectable after 3 hr, they concluded that this *in vivo* technique, while equivalent to pulse labeling *in vitro*, was really equivalent to continuous labeling as far as cells in late S phase are concerned. This seems somewhat doubtful, except for the very end of S, in view of the short duration of peak level and the failure to show that the persistent label in the blood was in the form of tritiated thymidine.

Despite these methodological problems, and the difficulty of working with spermatogonial metaphases, Utakoji and Hsu obtained reasonably convincing evidence that in spermatogonia the long arm of the X and the entire Y are not labeled in late S phase, in marked contrast to their intense labeling in late S in bone marrow. They concluded that since heteropycnosis, late DNA replication, and genetic inactivation appear closely related, the sex chromosomes in spermatogonia are metabolically active, at least in some stages of germ cell development.

## RNA SYNTHESIS AND THE REGULATION OF GENE ACTION

A structural gene acts by serving as a template for the transcription of the genetic message, which is coded in the sequence of bases in DNA, into RNA molecules, which serve as templates for translation of the message into a sequence of amino acids in polypeptide chains.[281] In addition to the structural genes, there are a large number of controlling genes, whose mechanism of action is largely unknown.

Gene action and its control can be studied by using labeled precursors of RNA or protein. In mammalian cells RNA synthesis occurs in the nucleus. While some of the newly synthesized RNA appears to be transferred fairly rapidly to the cytoplasm,[3] there is evidence that a large proportion of the rapidly labeled nuclear RNA is short-lived and is broken down in the nucleus rather than being transferred to the cytoplasm.[105] The nature of this RNA is still uncertain, but it may play a role in the regulation of gene action.

### Nuclear Control

The physical state of DNA is very important in the control of RNA synthesis. Hay and Revel[108] and Littau *et al.*[155] have shown by electron-microscope autoradiography that RNA synthesis takes place in euchromatic areas of the nucleus, not in the heterochromatic areas of condensed chromatin. The rates of nuclear and cytoplasmic protein synthesis, which parallel rates of RNA synthesis, are proportional to nuclear volume.[249] Furthermore, when cells with repressed nuclei are hybridized with cells that are active in RNA synthesis, the repressed nuclei undergo morphological changes, enlarging and becoming less condensed, as they become capable of RNA synthesis.[107] It seems likely that many agents which influence the rate of RNA synthesis act by bringing about configurational changes in DNA.

Frenster[81] has reviewed the evidence that a variety of substances which inhibit or stimulate RNA synthesis act by means of a reversible binding to DNA. Each substance binds preferentially to either single-stranded or double-stranded DNA, and in every case the effect of the ligand on RNA synthesis at preselected gene loci is strongly correlated with the form of DNA preferred. Thus, histones, polylysine, actinomycin D, acridine orange, and chloroquine bind preferentially to double-stranded DNA, and all are inhibitors of RNA synthesis. Testosterone, estradiol, methylcholanthrene, RNA polymerase, and complementary RNA bind with single-stranded DNA, and stimulate RNA synthesis. Most of these agents are rather nonselective, whereas complementary RNA is capable of a selective binding, permitting specific derepression of RNA synthesis.

Certain cations may also stimulate RNA synthesis.[218] In nuclei isolated from both normal and regenerating rat liver only ribosomal RNA synthesis occurs to any extent, and this is reflected by the incorporation of tritiated uridine only into the nucleolus. Treatment of the isolated nuclei with $Mn^{++}$ leads to increased synthesis of a new type of RNA with a correlated shift in the location of silver grains. The selective activation of nonnucleolar RNA-synthesizing sites is indicated by the altered base ratios of the newly synthesized RNA and by the altered location of silver grains on electron-microscope autoradiography.[218]

### Cytoplasmic Control of Gene Action and Replication

The extent of cytoplasmic control of gene action and replication can be investigated by cell hybridization[106,107] or nuclear transplantation.[100,221] Harris and his co-workers produced hybrid cells by taking advantage of the ability of certain viruses, e.g., u.v.-inactivated Sendai virus, to induce the fusion of single into multinucleate cells. In an early study Harris and Watkins[106] showed that cells of human and murine origin could be fused together into artificial heterokaryons, multinucleate cells with nuclei of diverse origins. They proved the different origin of the nuclei within single heterokaryons by autoradiography after labeling one cell type by growing the HeLa cells (or, in some experiments, the Erlich mouse ascites tumor cells) in the presence of tritiated thymidine for about one cell cycle prior to mixing the cells in the presence of u.v.-inactivated Sendai virus (Fig. 14).

Harris and Watkins[106] also used autoradiography to demonstrate the ability of both types of nuclei in the artificial heterokaryons to synthesize RNA, and the ability of the hybrid cells to synthesize protein. Because both

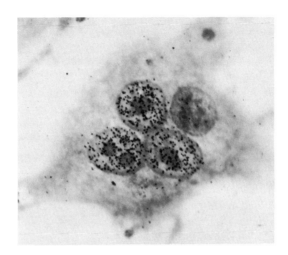

Fig. 14. Autoradiography of a tetranucleate cell containing three HeLa nuclei and one Ehrlich nucleus. The HeLa cells had been grown in tritiated thymidine before the heterokaryons were produced. (From Harris et al.[107])

these functions are carried on, these heterokaryons are very useful for the analysis of nucleo-cytoplasmic relationships. A further application is based on the common observation that mammalian cells, unlike fungi or yeast, use thymidine as a specific precursor of DNA, and the more recent finding that DNA synthesis occurs in some nuclei in heterokaryons. Consequently, mammalian-cell heterokaryons are extremely useful in studies on the regulation of DNA synthesis.

Harris et al.[107] have shown by autoradiography that RNA and DNA synthesis, which normally do not occur in the nuclei of chicken erythrocytes, mouse macrophages, or other repressed cells, can occur in these nuclei when they are in heterokaryons with a cell type in which RNA or DNA synthesis can normally occur, e.g., HeLa cells. In general, in heterokaryons the more-repressed nucleus gains the functional capabilities of the less-repressed nucleus, and undergoes associated morphological changes, becoming less condensed. Thus, in a heterokaryon of chicken erythrocytes and mouse macrophages the erythrocyte nuclei become capable of RNA synthesis, which the macrophage nuclei normally carry out, but neither type of nucleus becomes capable of DNA synthesis. Studies such as these have shown that cytoplasmic factors play a large role in the regulation of both RNA and DNA synthesis.

The effect of small doses of actinomycin D on DNA synthesis can be interpreted in terms of the action of a cytoplasmic initiator of DNA synthesis. Baserga et al.[16] found that a small dose of actinomycin D sufficient to give prompt 50 % inhibition of RNA synthesis has a much slower effect on DNA synthesis, with maximal inhibition only after 4.5 hr. Autoradiographic analysis of this effect showed that the actinomycin has no effect on DNA synthesis once it is initiated, but prevents the initiation of DNA synthesis, presumably because it inhibits a metabolic step essential for initiation of DNA synthesis in $G_1$ cells.

Stubblefield and Mueller[266] and others have shown that protein synthesis is essential for the initiation of DNA synthesis, and possibly for continued DNA synthesis. Bloch and his co-workers[25] found that continuation of DNA synthesis is dependent upon concurrent protein synthesis. Puromycin, which inhibits the synthesis of protein, including histones, also inhibits DNA synthesis. Thus, DNA synthesis may be tied to protein synthesis in higher organisms in which the chromosomes contain both DNA and protein. Histone synthesis, on the other hand, can proceed at a normal rate even when DNA synthesis is inhibited, as with 5-fluorodeoxyuridine (FUdR). Robbins and Borun[232] showed in synchronized HeLa cells that most, if not all, histones are synthesized in the cytoplasm on small polysomes. Two inhibitors of DNA synthesis, cytosine arabinoside and FUdR, caused the selective disruption of these polysomes when added during the S period, but not in $G_1$.

The effect of other exogenous agents, e.g., phytohemagglutinin, can also be interpreted in terms of the action of cytoplasmic initiators of RNA, and eventually DNA, synthesis, i.e., in terms of derepression[285] of functions in a specialized cell. This is somewhat at variance with the stem cell model Moss and Ingram[183] have proposed, unless stem cells are generally repressed unless triggered by a specific stimulus.

Harris and Watkins[106] found that whether or not a mammalian cell nucleus synthesizes DNA cannot be solely determined by events in the cytoplasm. In a single heterokaryon DNA synthesis may be taking place in some nuclei and not in others, and there may be differences in the rate of DNA synthesis in nuclei of different species of origin. Cell hybridization would seem to be a useful technique for analyzing this problem.

### The Timing of Gene Action

The role of chromosomal organization in the timing of gene action is largely unknown except for the apparent genetic inertness of heterochromatin and tissue differences in heterochromatin. Tauro et al.[272] have presented evidence that in one eukaryotic (with true chromosomes) organism, a yeast, the genome appears to be only periodically available for transcription. Gene position along the chromosome controls the order of enzyme synthesis, and there may be only one period of enzyme synthesis per structural gene per generation. In this yeast, which has about 18 tiny chromosomes, the timing of enzyme synthesis is related to the distance of its structural gene from the end of the chromosome; linked genes are expressed in order of their position along the chromosome, allelic genes are always expressed at exactly the same time, and unlinked genes are expressed at different times.

Whether a unicellular eukaryote can serve as a model for all eukaryotes, including man, seems doubtful. Gall and Callan[84] found evidence for an orderly linear meiotic sequence of RNA synthesis along individual loops of the lampbrush chromosomes of newt oocytes, but many of the lateral loops along each chromosome appeared to be actively synthesizing RNA at the same time, indicating either a more complex organization of the chromosomes of vertebrates than of yeast, or a different mode of control of gene action. The chromosomes in higher organisms appear to contain many units of transcription. Gall and Callan estimated the size of one of these in the newt as 1000–2000 $\mu$, which is equivalent to 500–1000 average-sized genes. This is larger by one or two orders of magnitude than the operon postulated by Jacob and Monod.[124] This discrepancy could be accounted for by (1) the type of ordered transcription of adjacent different gene loci found in yeast, or (2) by genetic redundancy, as postulated by Callan[38] on the basis primarily of his findings in the germ line of vertebrates.

Attempts to study the progression of RNA synthesis along mitotic chromosomes have been almost totally unsuccessful. The chromosomes are only individually recognizable at metaphase, a time when no RNA synthesis occurs.[58] On the other hand, when a labeled precursor of RNA is added earlier one usually finds equal labeling of all chromosomes, including both X chromosomes in the female and the Y in the male.[51,209] Fujita et al.[83] reported no RNA synthesis along one of the two X chromosomes in cells from a female, but this has yet to be confirmed. His technique included extensive washing, which might have removed RNA loosely absorbed onto the metaphase chromosomes.

Some information has been obtained by studying stages of the cycle other than metaphase, despite the difficulty in identification of specific chromosomes. Back and Dormer[12] observed labeling along all chromosomes, including therefore the heteropycnotic X chromosome, in prophase after incubation of cells with [3]H-UdR. In similarly treated cells Comings[51] found as many silver grains over early prophase nuclei as over interphase nuclei, which suggests that the suppression of RNA synthesis which occurs during mitosis has not yet begun at prophase. He reported that the partially despiralized heteropycnotic X seen in prophase and the sex chromatin in interphase nuclei showed a lower number of silver grains than were seen over adjacent areas.

While no direct relationship has been found between position along a chromosome and the time of action of the genes located there, some evidence of a functional relationship has been established. For example, Stubblefield et al.,[265] using synchronized cells, found an abrupt increase in the rate of RNA synthesis after 30% of DNA (the euchromatin) has been replicated in the first third of the S period. Kasten and Strasser[129] also observed such an increase in RNA synthesis in synchronized cell cultures, but they were more impressed by a sharp fall in RNA synthesis beginning about 4–5 hr after the beginning of the S phase and coinciding with the maximum rate for the first of the two waves of DNA synthesis. They concluded that the fall in RNA synthesis occurred because RNA cannot serve as a template for both DNA and RNA synthesis at the same time. If this is correct, then clearly the late-replicating DNA is not active in transcription, nor is the very-early-replicating DNA. More quantitative studies would help to clarify these points.

## ORGANIZATION AND REPLICATION OF THE GENETIC MATERIAL

### DNA Replication at the Molecular Level

According to the Watson–Crick model, DNA is made up of two very long polynucleotide chains held together by hydrogen bonds between purine and pyrimidine bases which are attached at regular intervals to the backbone of each chain. Each backbone is made up of repeated deoxyribose phosphate moieties which are held together by phosphodiester bonds between the 3' and 5' positions of the deoxyribose portion of each nucleoside.

DNA synthesis requires primer, or template, DNA.[140] DNA replication is thought to involve separation of the two polynucleotide strands, with each serving as a template for synthesis of a new complementary strand. The two strands of DNA are antiparallel, in the sense that the 3' and 5' positions of the deoxyribose moieties of the two strands have opposite polarities. Consequently, if DNA replication proceeds in linear fashion from one end of the molecule to the other, nucleoside 5'-triphosphate would be added to the 3' hydroxyl end of one polynucleotide chain, while the other chain would be synthesized from the 5' hydroxyl end. DNA polymerase can catalyze the synthesis in the 5' to 3' direction,[140] but no enzymatic mechanism for the synthesis of deoxypolynucleotide in the 3' to 5' direction is known.

Okazaki *et al.*[200] have presented evidence that DNA synthesis may only take place in the 5′ to 3′ direction. They found that DNA synthesis takes place in short stretches along both chains, i.e., that DNA replication is discontinuous. The "units" of synthesis, about 1000–2000 nucleotides long, are then joined together in the cell by a ligase reaction. Autoradiography with labeled thymidine cannot be used to study these units of replication because they contain too few nucleotides. In studies to be described shortly a much larger unit of replication, sometimes called the replicon,[123] has been investigated, usually by light-microscope autoradiography. It is clearly impossible to speak with complete assurance of what is going on at the molecular level from studies with a resolution of only 1 $\mu$. For example, such questions as whether replication, once started, is continuous or discontinuous, and whether replication can occur in both 5′ to 3′ and 3′ to 5′ directions, can hardly be resolved by such studies, nor can the question of whether each DNA molecule replicates only from one end or at many sites along the molecule. Nevertheless, several fundamental questions regarding the organization and replication of the genetic material in microorganisms and in higher organisms, including man, have been answered.

Cairns[35] showed by light-microscope autoradiography that the replication of bacteriophage DNA involves separation of the polynucleotide strands as predicted by the Watson–Crick model. He labeled lambda phage DNA throughout a full cycle of replication in order to render it visible as an autoradiographic track of silver grains. The length of such tracks was 23 $\mu$. Since the molecular weight of lambda phage DNA is $46 \times 10^6$, the weight per micron was $2 \times 10^6$, which fits well with that expected if each track is made by a single DNA double-helix.

Cairns[36] also used autoradiography to show that the replication of bacterial DNA proceeds in much the same way, and that the genetic material of *E. coli* consists of a single circle of DNA 700–900 $\mu$ long. The DNA forms a fork presumably by separation of the two polynucleotide chains, and DNA synthesis proceeds in apparently continuous fashion along both limbs of the fork until replication has progressed all the way along the circular DNA molecule.

In 1963 Jacob *et al.*[123] proposed a model for DNA replication in bacteria and bacterial viruses. They postulated a basic unit of genetic material, the replicon, capable of independent replication. Each replicon carries two specific sites: (1) a structural gene controlling the synthesis of a specific initiator, and (2) a controlling gene or replicator which is activated by the intiator. According to this hypothesis, replication of the bacterial DNA is initiated at the replicator site in response to a signal provided by the initiator, and proceeds until the entire replicon is copied. They postulated that the

initiator locus is attached to a specific site on the bacterial surface, adjacent
to an F antigenic site, and pointed out that the idea of a relationship between
specific surface antigens and DNA replication in bacteria has many implications for the analysis of different types of cellular systems, e.g., the triggering
effect of antigens or phytohemagglutinins on small lymphocytes. The attachment of the bacterial "chromosome" to the surface membrane, which has
been confirmed by electron microscopy, provides a mechanism for the
segregation of daughter "chromosomes" to the daughter bacteria in the
absence of the mitotic spindle found in higher organisms.

### Higher Levels of Organization

Jacob et al.[123] tried to apply the replicon model to higher organisms.
Each mammalian chromosome must contain several replicons, since DNA
synthesis appears to begin simultaneously at several points along the chromosome. The generally similar labeling patterns of homologous chromosomes
and asynchronous DNA synthesis of other chromosomes suggested to them
that the control of DNA synthesis in a specific replicon acts simultaneously
on both copies in a diploid cell. In view of the evidence that such a high
degree of homologue synchrony does not occur, this suggestion may have to
be modified, perhaps along the lines of Ockey's suggestion[195] that replication
is delayed in the more-peripheral, and condensed, member of each homologous pair. The markedly asynchronous duplication of the two X chromosomes in the diploid mammalian complement cannot be accounted for by
the replicon model either, unless is it modified in exactly the same way. In
short, this model does not provide for perhaps the most important controlling
factor in the chromosomes of higher organisms: the existence of euchromatin
and heterochromatin. An earlier proposal of episomal control of the
facultative heterochromatization of the mammalian X chromosome[103]
meets this difficulty, but appears to be untestable in a mammalian system;
at least, it has apparently led to no attempts at experimental verification or
disproof.

Further information about the organization of replicating units in the
chromosomes of higher organisms has come from applications of the same
technique used by Cairns in his studies of phage and bacterial DNA.
Relatively short replicating units have been observed in DNA-containing
fibers from human and other mammalian chromosomes. The nature of these
replicating units has been studied using short incubation of cells with
$^3$H-TdR. Cairns[37] found autoradiograms 10–30 $\mu$ long after 45 min labeling
of HeLa cells, and 50–100 $\mu$ long after 180 min (Fig. 15). He concluded that
human DNA is replicated by a process that moves no more than 0.5 $\mu$/min,
which is much slower than the rate of 20–30 $\mu$/min observed in E. coli
DNA.[36]

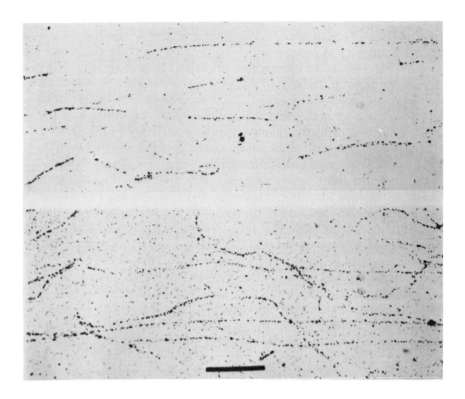

Fig. 15. HeLa cell DNA extracted from cells immediately after labeling with ³H-thymidine for 3 hr (above) and 24 hr (below). Exposed under Kodak AR-10 stripping film for two months. The scale shows 50 μ. (From Cairns.[37])

Replicating sites appear to be joined in series,[37,119] so that each represents a short section of some much longer structure. By using much longer periods of incubation of cells with ³H-TdR, very long autoradiograms representing chromosomal DNA have been obtained. Maximum fiber lengths of 500 μ (0.5 mm) have been observed in material from HeLa cells,[37] 1.8 mm from Chinese hamster cells,[119] and more than 2 cm from human lymphocytes lysed without a detergent.[240] It seems likely that each chromosome contains a single long fiber containing a series of separately replicated regions that are joined end to end, and that this accounts for the observed pattern of segregation of labeled chromatids from one cell generation to the next.[37]

Huberman and Riggs[119] devised a method for lysing single mammalian metaphase cells, and carried out quantitative studies on the autoradiographs prepared from such lysates, using Chinese hamster cells grown in the presence of ³H-TdR for 35–40 hr. They found linear tracks of silver grains up to 1.8 mm in length, although most tracks were less than 0.2 mm. Equally long tracks were found after pronase digestion prior to autoradiography, indicating that the DNA fibers producing the autoradiograms do not contain protein linkers susceptible to pronase under the conditions employed. Despite this evidence, Huberman and Riggs considered that each grain track was produced by a separate DNA molecule, and that each chromosome contained many DNA molecules. Replication could begin at one end of each of these, thus accounting for the common observation that DNA synthesis is initiated and continues at many sites along a chromosome.[89,118a,203,212,242]

Sasaki and Norman[240] obtained much longer tracks of silver grains using a similar but milder technique. Their longest tracks were about 1.8 cm long, which led them to conclude that each mamalian chromosome may consist of a single long DNA molecule, and that the much smaller grain tracks represented technical artifacts, with breakage of the continuous strand during the procedure. Sasaki and Norman also observed apparently circular grain tracks approximately 1 cm long. The significance of these is unclear, unless they represent sister strands with terminal DNA replication not completed. They do not correspond in size to the circular DNA of mitochondria[121] or of boar sperm,[116] nor to the circular DNA postulated by Callan[38] and Whitehouse[283] to exist in all eukaryotic organisms at certain stages of their life cycle. Development of better methods of cell lysis, chromosome degradation, and preparation for autoradiography may resolve this problem.

The most detailed study of the replicating units in higher organisms is that of Huberman and Riggs[120] using Chinese hamster and human cells. In pulse-chase experiments with ³H-TdR they noted decreasing grain counts along chromosomal fibers replicated early in the chase due to reduced incorporation of label as the pool of labeled precursors was diluted by cold thymidine. Since the decrease occurred at both ends of most silver grain tracks, they concluded that DNA synthesis proceeds in both directions in a replicating unit. That is, the long fibers of chromosomal DNA are made up of tandemly joined sections. Even prolonged pronase treatment failed to alter the size of the replicating units, which therefore appear to contain no protein linkers. They also showed that replication proceeds at a fork, as in bacteria, although this is more difficult to visualize by autoradiography in higher organisms because of the necessity for label to be incorporated during successive S periods to see the complete fork, and this is difficult because the amount of label incorporated in the first S period inhibits the cell cycle. Nevertheless, the fork has now been clearly demonstrated in both hamster and man.[120]

Replication proceeds usually, or always, in opposite directions at adjacent growing points. Huberman and Riggs call the smallest unit of replication a replication section, and an adjacent pair of replicator sections,

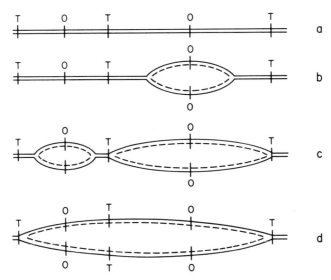

Fig. 16. Model of chromosomal DNA replication. Synthesis proceeds in both directions from each site of initiation of synthesis, and in opposite directions in neighboring replication units. (From Huberman and Riggs.[120])

which share an origin and replicate in divergent directions, a replication unit. By measuring the distance between the center of adjacent replication units, these investigators were able to determine the distribution of lengths of such units. Most were 15–60 $\mu$ long, so that most replication sections are 7–30 $\mu$ long (equivalent to 3–15 genes the size of the hemoglobin chain loci). The rate of replication was found to vary between units, ranging from 0.4 $\mu$ to 2 $\mu$ per minute. Neighboring replication sections sometimes began DNA synthesis at different times, and regions of DNA synthesis were not distributed evenly along chromosomes. A model of DNA replication based on these findings is shown in Fig. 16. A consequence of this model is that closed, somewhat ringlike structures (sister double helices) must occur, and these have been observed.[120]

## Number of Replication Units

Various ways have been devised to calculate the number of replicating units per genome. Cairns[37] determined an average rate of DNA replication along chromosomal fibers of HeLa cells, assumed an S period of 6 hr for such cells and an average length of DNA double helix per chromosome of 3 cm, and concluded that at least 100 sites are required if all replicate throughout the S period; if not all are active at the same time, more would be needed. Huberman and Riggs[120] obtained similar estimates of the rate of DNA replication in Chinese hamster cells, but by directly measuring the length of replicating units, found them most frequently to be only 15–60 $\mu$, long rather than the 720 $\mu$ (about the size of the bacterial "chromosome") required by the hypothesis that each replicating unit continues DNA synthesis throughout an S period of 6 hr. Huberman and Riggs did not estimate the total number of replicating units in either Chinese hamster cells or HeLa cells, perhaps because their observations indicated that neighboring replicating units could begin synthesis at different times. However, their data are clearly incompatible with less than about 1000 replicating units per average mammalian chromosome, a figure that agrees fairly well with other estimates.

Comings[52] estimated the number of replicating units in man as nearly $4 \times 10^4$ from the proportion of cells with unlabeled sex-chromatin bodies after a 3-min incubation of cultured fibroblasts with ³H-TdR, assuming the same rate of DNA synthesis in diploid cells as observed by Cairns[37] in HeLa cells. Painter et al.,[205] using a double-labeling technique involving density-gradient centrifugation and scintillation counting (BUdR as the density label and ³H-TdR as the radioactive label) estimated that HeLa cells have $10^3$–$10^4$ replicating units and that the average size of a replicating unit was $10^9$–$10^{10}$ daltons, which is the same order of magnitude as the "chromosome" of E. coli.

### The Control of DNA Replication

The bidirectional model of Huberman and Riggs[120] has implications for the control of DNA replication, since it postulates that DNA synthesis is initiated in two adjacent replicating sections at the same time and at the same site. While it is unclear what controls the initiation of replication in higher forms, there is some evidence that the cell wall plays such a role in bacteria. In higher organisms the state of chromosome condensation is of primary importance, while the nuclear membrane and cytoplasmic factors also play a role.

Recently Comings and Kakefuda[56] have proposed an exciting modification of the replicon model. They suggested that the nuclear membrane in higher organisms serves the same function as the bacterial surface in the regulation of DNA replication. Each chromosome is thought to contain a number of replicons, with each one attached to the nuclear membrane at a specific site. Analogous to the simple replicon model, DNA replication in each replicon is thought to be initiated at its site of attachment.

If this is correct, DNA replication should be initiated at the nuclear membrane. Comings and Kakefuda[56] tested this hypothesis by synchronizing human cells and labeling DNA synthesized in the first 10 min of the S period with ³H-TdR. Electron-microscope autoradiography of ultra-thin sections showed silver grains restricted to the nuclear membrane or periphery of the nucleolus in 90 % of the cells. A more-homogenous distribution was observed in most of the cells exposed to ³H-thymidine for the first 20 min of the S period and in cells from unsynchronized cultures, as in (Fig. 11), but even under these conditions some of the cells, presumably those just entering the S period, showed the restriction of grains to the nuclear membrane. Moses[181] described similar findings in electron-microscope autoradiographic preparations of HeLa cells pulse-labeled with ³H-thymidine (Fig. 12). He showed this to be true replication by demonstrating the same proportion of nuclei with peripheral grains after following the pulse by a 30-min chase with an excess of unlabeled thymidine before terminating the unsynchronized culture.

Dewey and Thompson[70] used light-microscope autoradiography of thin sections of nuclei (20–25 sections per nucleus) to study the distribution of newly synthesized DNA in logarithmically growing Chinese hamster cells. Using a 10-min labeling with tritiated thymidine, they observed a peripheral distribution of label in 70 % of the nuclei, and widely dispersed label in 30 % of the nuclei. After 4 hr incubation with ³H-TdR 95 % of the cells showed

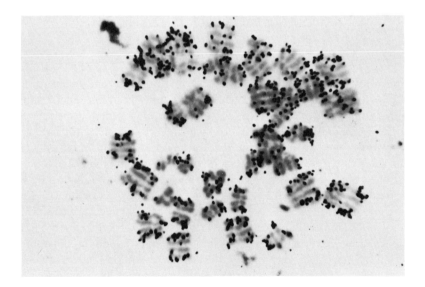

Fig. 17. Endoreduplicated cell exposed to ³H-TdR in the first two rounds of DNA synthesis preceding this mitosis. Note the presence of silver grains over only two of the four chromatids of each diplochromosome, usually the two outer chromatids. Exceptions represent sister strand exchanges. (From Schwarzacher and Schnedl.[251])

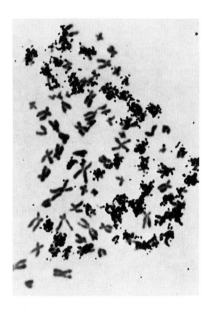

Fig. 18.  Metaphase in a formerly binucleate cell. Note the heavy terminal labeling
of one complete diploid set of chromosomes. (From Sandberg *et al.*[239])

peripheral distribution of label; after 6–7 hr this figure had fallen to 80 %.
After 40 hr incubation with labeled thymidine 84 % of the nuclei showed
peripheral location of label, with only 16 % showing widely dispersed label.

Dewey and Thompson[70] interpreted their findings as indicating the
existence of a limited time during the S period (less than 2 hr) in which the
DNA has a dispersed distribution, probably near the middle of the S period.
Since the resolution possible with light-microscope autoradiography, even
with tissue sections only 0.3 $\mu$ thick, is probably little better than 1 $\mu$, it is
impossible to distinguish between label at the nuclear membrane and label
in a rather thick peripheral zone. Nevertheless, these results clearly indicate
a nonrandom location of chromosomal material throughout most of the
S period of interphase, even though the lack of resolution renders impossible
any statement about sites of synthesis. Similar results of Moses and Coleman
(Fig. 13)[182], using electron-microscope autoradiography and a 30-min
exposure of cells to $^3$H-TdR, have confirmed the frequently peripheral
localization of DNA in fixed interphase nuclei and cast some doubt on
the interpretation of the observations of Comings and Kakefuda,[56] who
claimed that while DNA replication is initiated at the nuclear membrane, it

does not continue there but takes place thoughout the nucleus. This would be an important difference from the situation in bacteria, where the enzyme system necessary for replication is attached to the cell wall, so that DNA synthesis always occurs at this point.[85]

Comings and Kakefuda[56] have tried to account for the late replication of heterochromatin in terms of their model by assuming that DNA replication is initiated at the nuclear membrane even in replicons that start their DNA synthesis after the beginning of S. The two X chromosomes in XX cells are markedly asynchronous in their replication; the late-replicating X chromosome appears to carry out its DNA replication in a shorter period of time than its euchromatic homologue. This is particularly apparent in mammals with easily identifiable X chromosomes,[245] and indicates that the rate of DNA synthesis is not dependent solely on the *number* of replicons, since this is presumably the same in both X chromosomes. This can be accounted for if the replicons duplicate themselves in greater unison in the inactive X chromosome. Comings' model even suggests a possible mechanism for this, i.e., that the sites of attachment may be closely bunched, and that the nuclear membrane regulates DNA synthesis in some way.

This model postulates that each of the many replicons in higher organisms is attached to the nuclear membrane. There is some evidence consistent with this. DuPraw[71] showed by electron microscopy that chromosomal fibers in interphase nuclei of man, like those of the honeybee, are attached to the nuclear envelope. In some preparations the sites of attachment are clearly seen to be adjacent to the circular holes, or annuli, in the nuclear membrane. Whether these are specific sites along the chromosome remains to be seen. Woollam et al.[290] found attachments of the synaptinemal complex of mouse spermatocytes to the nuclear membrane in electron micrographs. However, these attachments, which are of two types, probably represent chromosome ends. One was surrounded by clumped chromatin, thought to represent the centromeric end of a telocentric chromosome with its adjacent heterochromatin. The attachments of the centromeric ends were clustered around the part of the nucleus where the sex vesicle is attached, while attachments of the second type, presumably representing the opposite ends of the chromosomes, were clustered in the opposite portion of the nucleus. This placement finds its expression later as the classical "pachytene bouquet." It is possible that the nuclear membrane may play a role in regulating such events.

There is, of course, abundant evidence that heterochromatin, including sex chromatin, usually lies adjacent to the nuclear membrane, and this gross microscopic feature is in some way correlated with events at the molecular level. Several investigators have noted that the late-replicating X chromosome tends to lie at or near the periphery of the metaphase spread,[4,7,8,9,180,187] and this has been regarded as confirmatory evidence that the late-replicating X chromosome forms the sex chromatin. Not all observers have observed a peripheral location of the late-replicating X, e.g., German;[90] the reason for this apparent discrepancy is not clear, but probably reflects technical differences in preparation of material, differences in scoring, and the relatively slight difference between location of this X and other chromosomes.

Miller *et al.*[173] found that the Y chromosome also tends to occupy a peripheral position, and that certain other chromosomes have a nonrandom location in relation to each other. They reported, for example, that chromosome 13 was further from the center than 14 and 15, and suggested that heteropycnotic chromosomes, or those with the greatest amounts of heterochromatin, tend to be peripheral.[169] This claim did not receive general acceptance because of the possible inaccuracy in identification of individual chromosomes within the B, D, or G groups. Autoradiography should permit an extension of these studies because of the greatly increased number of recognizable chromosome pairs, but few such studies have yet been made. German[90] observed that chromosome 15 and 21 (and, to a lesser extent, 13) are less often at the periphery of the metaphase spread than expected by chance, whereas chromosome 22, the late-replicating, shorter G-group chromosome, is not. He also observed that chromosome 13, determined autoradiographically (with the identification confirmed by its generally greater length than the other D-group chromosomes) is more frequently involved in satellite association than chromosome 15. This is somewhat surprising, since such associations are thought to predispose to translocations between satellited chromosomes and a 13/G translocation has not yet been found. It will be of great interest to know whether chromosome 14, which is most often involved in D/G translocation,[26,63,168] is most often associated with G-group chromosomes.

Ockey[195] reported that chromosomes 4, 13, and 16 are more often at the periphery of flattened metaphase spreads than the morphologically similar but earlier-replicating chromosomes 5, 14, 15, and 17. He also noted that when homologues of chromosomes 4, 13, 16, 18, 22, and the X had different grain densities, the more heavily labeled homologue tended to be more peripheral. He suggested this could be explained if the beginning of DNA synthesis is localized to the center of the nucleus, which now appears to be an untenable hypothesis. Another explanation, that there may be greater thickness of the overlying cytoplasm near the center of the metaphase spread, with greater self-absorption of radiation and consequent lower grain densities near the center, is ruled out by the observation[195] that in cells labeled relatively early in the S period the more centrally placed chromosome 1 is more heavily labeled than its homologue. Ockey[195] suggested that homologous chromosomes probably differ slightly in their time of DNA synthesis and that the homologue showing a delay in DNA synthesis is more peripherally located in metaphase spreads and is also more condensed, suggesting that the delay in replication is related to the degree of condensation. This idea was supported by his observations on length and grain count of the two presumably genetically identical arms of an isochromosome X. When one arm was more peripheral than the other it was usually also shorter and more heavily labeled. No such relation to location was found for the two arms of chromosome 3, although the shorter arm was again more heavily labeled.

### Chromosome Duplication and Segregation

Taylor et al.,[276] Taylor,[273,274] and Prescott and Bender[220] have shown that the DNA of both plant and animal (including human) chromosomes is replicated semiconservatively, with a conserved unit serving as a template for the synthesis of a new unit. At the first division after incorporation of tritiated thymidine both chromatids of each chromosome in the complement are labeled. At the second division each chromosome is still labeled, but usually in only one chromatid at any level along the chromosome. Rarely, both chromatids show labeling at the same level, so-called isolabeling.[208,278] This may indicate that each chromatid is not single-stranded, i.e., made up of a single Watson–Crick double helix, but is double or multistranded. This point will be discussed after consideration of exchanges of labeled material between the two chromatids.

Sister chromatid exchanges occur frequently and lead to interchange of labeled and unlabeled segments of chromatid. Taylor[273] found that sister chromatid exchanges always involve breakage of whole chromatids and exchange of segments of the double chromatid structure rather than breakage and rejoining involving single strands. Marin and Prescott[163] noted in a Chinese hamster cell line that sister chromatid exchanges occur at a rate somewhat higher than one per three chromosomes per cell cycle. The exchanges were detected at the second and third metaphases after labeling with ³H-TdR. The amount of ³H-TdR (over a 100-fold range) had no effect on the exchange frequency, and only a slight increase over the value with ³H-thymidine alone occurred with 50 R of acute X-irradiation, with no further increase to 200 R. Marin and Prescott[163] concluded that most sister chromatid exchanges are probably spontaneous, but Olivieri and Brewen[201] have challenged this interpretation on the basis of observations on endore-duplicated cells, and Wolff[289] has offered further reasons for considering sister chromatid exchanges as radiation-induced. This is an important point which influences our concepts of the etiology of chromosomal abnormalities. For example, Cuevas-Sosa[60] showed in both C-metaphase and C-anaphase preparations that sister chromatid exchanges in human cells frequently occur at the centromere, and suggested such breakage and reunion at the centromere as a possible source of isochromosome formation.

Taylor[273] obtained further information about chromosome structure by studying tetraploid cells that had incorporated tritium into their DNA in the first of the two rounds of DNA synthesis, preceding the observed metaphase. He noted twin exchanges, involving sister chromatid exchanges at the same site on two homologous chromosomes (a sister chromatid exchange involves only the chromatids of one chromosome). Single exchanges can arise from breakage and reunion of subunits at any time before examination of the tetraploid metaphase, but a twin exchange must have occurred when the two homologous chromosomes involved were still joined as chromatids of the same chromosome, i.e., before the second round of DNA synthesis. Taylor noted that the relative frequencies of single and twin exchanges should be 10:1 if rejoining of broken subunits can occur at random, but only 2:1 if reunion were restricted because the two subunits have opposite polarity, comparable to that of the two strands of DNA. The observed relative frequencies in the plant Bellevallia were 1:2.7 (30 single to 81 twin exchanges), pretty well ruling out random rejoining, but offering rather weak support for Taylor's hypothesis of subunits of opposite polarity. A better fit is obtained if one assumes that sister chromatid exchanges are radiation-induced,[289] because the reduction in tritium to half after a round of DNA replication in the absence of tritiated thymidine would therefore reduce the frequency of single exchanges occurring after this second round of synthesis. Wolff[289] calculated an expected ratio of 1:2 in this way, which is much closer to the observed 1:2.7.

Walen[278] discovered in endoreduplicated cells of the marsupial *Potorus tridactylis* that when ³H-TdR was incorporated into DNA in the first but not the second of the two successive DNA replications that occur prior to the observed endoreduplicated metaphase, the label is always found in the two outer chromatids, except for the occasions when sister chromatid exchange leads to inner chromatid labeling of the diplochromosomes. Schwarzacher and Schnedl[251] and Schnedl[248] confirmed this in cells of human origin, using mercaptoethanol to induce endoreduplication (Fig. 17).

These findings have implications for chromosome structure and the nature of chromosome duplication. The observations on the diplochromosomes of endoreduplicated cells provide an excellent demonstration of the semiconservative replication and distribution of the subunits comprising each chromatid. Label was present in all four chromatids of the diplochromosomes of cells that took up ³H-TdR during the second of the two successive chromosome duplications, but only in one of the two chromatids making up each of the two chromosomes in diplochromosomes when ³H-TdR was incorporated during the first cycle of duplication.

This appearance of diplochromosomes offers some support to the notion that the centromere has a front-to-back organization and that at chromosome duplication the centromeric portion of each new half-chromatid is laid down at the opposite face of the chromosome from that occupied by the other new subunit rather than side-by-side. Both occupy a place that is also defined by the persistent connection between the two preexisting half-centromeres. The result is that the centromeres of the four chromatids of a diplochromosome lie in one plane; this has the practical consequence that analysis of chromosome structure and function can be investigated more easily. The analysis of centromere structure and function is still in its early descriptive phase. Comings[53] used autoradiography to show that the delayed separation at the centromere, relative to the arms, is probably not due to delayed completion of DNA replication in the centromere into mitosis.

## Chromatid Segregation and Assortment

Autoradiography can be used to study the segregation of tritium-labeled chromosomes in both mitosis and meiosis. Data from meiotic experiments can be used in the analysis of chiasmata, i.e., by observing the distribution of the label in bivalents at diplotene with one labeled and one unlabeled homologue.[176] In order to have observable segregation of label during the meiotic divisions, the label must be incorporated during earlier mitotic interphases in the germ line. Taylor[275] has shown, using $^3$H-TdR autoradiography, that the distribution is regularly semiconservative in spermatocytes of a species of grasshopper, as had been previously shown by mitosis. He found all chromatids labeled when $^3$H-TdR were incorporated into DNA during the last premeiotic interphase. When incorporation occurred at the interphase preceding this one the meiotic chromosomes had the equivalent of one chromatid of each homologue labeled. Chromatid exchanges were recognizable in such preparations, and a quantitative analysis of the frequency and pattern of exchanges was interpreted by Taylor as indicating that most of the exchanges were the result of breakage and reciprocal exchange between homologous chromosomes (crossing over), with sister chromatid exchanges much less common, and possibly even limited to premeiotic stages.

Taylor et al.[276] and Prescott and Bender[220] found evidence of random segregation of chromatids to daughter nuclei. They observed, at the third division after tritiated thymidine incorporation, one chromatid labeled in about half the chromosomes, and at the fourth division one chromatid labeled in only about a quarter of the chromosomes. The number of unlabeled chromosomes observed was somewhat less than expected because of the frequent occurrence of sister chromatid exchanges.

Lark et al.[149] have challenged the above interpretation and presented evidence for a nonrandom segregation of sister chromatids in cultured embryonic mouse cells, and to a lesser extent in Chinese hamster cells. They found unequal distribution of labeled chromatids to daughter nuclei at the second and third mitosis after labeling with [3]H-TdR and explained this in terms of an extrachromosomal controlling mechanism. They postulated that the first time a conserved unit of a chromosome is used as a template for DNA replication it is attached permanently to a structure distinct from that to which its parent chromosomal conserved unit was attached. This structure could be the nuclear membrane.[56,267] The new segregation structure and its attached chromatids would separate at division from the old, thus giving each daughter cell an exact diploid complement of chromosomes.

Lark[148,149] has extended this hypothesis of the nonrandom segregation of chromatids to *Vicia faba* (broad bean) and *Tritium boeticum* (wheat) on the basis of rather indirect observations, and the implication is clear that this phenomenon may be general in mitotic divisions. However, Heddle et al.[111] have been unable to confirm these results in *Vicia faba*, and have presented strong evidence that labeled chromatids are distributed randomly at the second mitosis after labeling with tritiated thymidine in both *Vicia faba* and the rat kangaroo, *Potorus tridactylis*. The experiments of Heddle et al.[111] differed from those of Lark and his associates in that they examined the labeling of metaphase centromeres and tips of chromatids at the third mitosis after pulse labeling with tritiated thymidine for 2 hr in the broad bean and for only 20 min in the rat kangaroo. In none of the approximately 100 cells of each type scored were all the centromeres or tips labeled or all unlabeled. A binomial distribution of labeled and unlabeled centromeres and tips was observed, as expected if segregation was occurring at random.[59] One criticism of this approach is that sister chromatid exchanges, because of their high frequency,[220] would tend to produce the same, or at least a very similar, distribution of cells with various numbers of labeled centromeres or tips whether segregation occurred randomly or nonrandomly. A direct analysis of segregation through the study of cells in anaphase or telophase would seem to be a better approach than the indirect method of examining the chromosomes at the next metaphase. Shikes and Priest,[252] using the direct comparison of grain counts over second division anaphases, confirmed the significantly unequal distribution of label, using human cells. Nevertheless, the question of whether chromatid segregation is a random process cannot be regarded as settled.

### Chromosome Structure

Is the chromosome a unineme (single-stranded) structure, bineme, or polyneme? Taylor, et al.[276] showed by means of autoradiography that, functionally, the chromatid replicates semiconservatively, and this is compatible with unineme structure, or a single Watson–Crick double helix.

Peacock[208] has raised objections to the unineme structure on the basis of further analysis of the distribution of grains along sister chromatids. Taylor pointed out that at the second metaphase following incorporation of label only one of the two sister chromatids was labeled at any level along the chromosome. Peacock observed apparant exceptions to this generalization, i.e., isolabeling (both chromatids labeled at the same level, or even along their entire length), and concluded from the existence of such isolabeling that the chromosome was at least bineme. If so, such isolabeled chromatids should have only half the grain density of chromatids without isolabeling. Although others have observed this so-called isolabeling (see, e.g., Walen[278]), quantitative data sufficient to resolve this point have not, to my knowledge, been published. Wolff[289] has pointed out that interchromosomal exchanges, which could only occur if there is somatic pairing, could lead to isolabeling and isounlabeling without requiring a multistranded chromosome.

Heddle and Trosko[110] have questioned the unineme structure on other grounds. They used a combined autoradiographic–fluorescent tagging technique to show that single-stranded DNA is not the unit of chromosome breakage by radiation and similar agents. Earlier workers had shown that a rapid changeover from chromosome to chromatid-type aberrations occurs at some point in the cell cycle, since only a very small percentage of cells show both types of aberrations. This change of response to radiation, thought to reflect a functional splitting of each chromosome, is known to occur in a period of very short duration at the beginning of S or the end of the $G_1$ phase. Evans and Savage[75] suggested that this was the result of the separation of the two halves of the DNA double helix, in preparation for replication. If this were so, a proportion of the cells in an asynchronously growing culture should have most or all of their DNA in the single-stranded state. Single-stranded nucleic acids fluoresce red with acridine orange, while double-stranded nucleic acids fluoresce yellow-green. Heddle and Trosko[110] detected no cells with mostly red fluorescence in asynchronous quasidiploid Chinese hamster cell cultures, and concluded that single-stranded DNA is not the unit of breakage of the chromosomes. If this interpretation is correct, and if the unit of breakage is DNA rather than protein or some other chromosomal element, then the chromosome must be multistranded at interphase. Certainly, confirmation by some other technique would seem necessary before such an important conclusion can be accepted.

## Time of Crossing Over

Callan[38] has summarized the evidence that the genome of chromosomal organisms contains serially repeated units of genetic information, of which only the terminal unit serves as the master sequence within which genetic recombination can occur. Only the remaining copies of the gene, which are made congruent to the master copy once per lifecycle in the lampbrush loops of meiotic prophase, serve as templates for RNA synthesis. This hypothesis accounts for the autoradiographic findings in the study of lampbrush chromosomes, which are found in most, if not all, eukaryotic organisms.

Whitehouse[283] has extended Callan's hypothesis, proposing a cycloid model of the chromosome. He has postulated that each replicon consists of a master gene and all of its copies, and has proposed a mechanism by which genetic recombination is restricted to the sequence of master genes. The process involves intrachromatid crossing over between the first and last genes of serially repeated series so as to excise all but one gene per series This will give rise to a greatly shortened linear chain of master genes and series of rings of DNA, each containing all the slave sequences of one gene. After recombination between the paired master gene chains the slave rings are reincorporated by the same process of breakage and reunion, i.e., intrachromatid crossing over of the DNA chain. Such a process might account for the small amount of DNA synthesis which occurs in meiotic prophase or late premeiotic prophase or late premeiotic interphase.[284]

## OTHER APPLICATIONS OF AUTORADIOGRAPHY

### The Genic Content of Specific Chromosomes

The primary contribution of autoradiography to the mapping of human chromosomes has been to increase the accuracy of chromosome identification. Only one gene locus has been localized to any autosome by linkage studies with a chromosomal marker (*Duffy* to chromosome 1 using *uncoiler*[298]) but this approach or others, such as deletion mapping, should be quite productive. There is some evidence that the haptoglobin locus, or perhaps the locus of a controlling gene, is on a D-group chromosome which has been identified by autoradiography as a number 13.[27] This locus is not near the tip of the short or long arm, since one individual with a ring 13 chromosome is a heterozygote,[115] and a larger segment of the long arm has been similarly excluded by studies in a patient with an unbalanced B/D translocation.[237]

Somatic cell genetic approaches are increasingly utilizing autoradiographic techniques, e.g., in the development of methods for identifying[160] or selecting[156] cell lines with specific genetic enzyme variants.

Mendelsohn and his colleagues[166] used autoradiography to check the effectiveness of a method for separating isolated Chinese hamster metaphase chromosomes into three size groups. They found the late-replicating chromosomal material concentrated almost exclusively in the fraction containing the very smallest chromosomes or chromosome fragments. Because of the general finding that late replication is restricted to the relatively long Y chromosome and the long arm of the even longer X chromosome,[274] this finding indicates that their method of isolating and separating chromosomes disrupts both X and Y chromosomes, and is therefore not yet suitable for isolation of intact chromosomes. The importance of the physical separation of chromosomes for human cytogenetics can hardly be overestimated, since this approach offers perhaps the best hope of mapping the chromosomes of any organism that does not have a short life span, large numbers of progeny, or controlled matings.

## Etiology of Chromosome Breaks

### Chemical Agents, Radiation, and Viruses

The effects of chemical agents and radiation upon the genetic material and their mechanism of action in producing chromosome breaks have been studied extensively by means of autoradiography (see, e.g., Brewen,[29] Kihlman,[133] and Monesi et al.[178]). Virus-chromosome interactions have also been studied in this way. Many viruses produce chromosome breaks, but it is unclear whether this is a direct or an indirect effect, the latter perhaps mediated by lysosomes.[2] Studies with tritium-labeled polyoma virus indicate that the viral DNA localizes in mammalian-cell nuclei.[132] Polyoma virus DNA is also known to bind preferentially to single-stranded host DNA, thereby stimulating host DNA synthesis,[137] and perhaps providing a mechanism for a direct breaking effect.

Zur Hausen [297] observed disturbed DNA replication patterns in seven established cell lines derived from the peripheral blood of patients with leukemia. The cells contained incompletely condensed or pulverized chromosome segments which were very late-replicating, continuing their DNA synthesis into what was normally $G_2$. Kato and Sandberg[130] observed similar changes in a herpeslike-virus-containing cell line derived from a male with Burkitt's lymphoma, and suggested that these pulverized chromosomes might arise from micronuclei, which were abundant in this cell line and have been shown to undergo asynchronous DNA synthesis in relation to the main nucleus of the cell.[263] This is analogous to the occurrence of whole diploid sets of pulverized chromosomes in multinucleate cells in which asynchronous DNA synthesis has occurred (Fig. 18).[239] In these cells, too, the pulverized chromosomes are late-replicating, and it has been suggested[239] that the premature, synchronized occurence of mitosis in these multinucleate cells is responsible for the pulverization phenomenon. However, Nichols *et al.*[194] have shown that the stage of the cell cycle susceptible to virus-induced chromosome pulverization is the S period.

## Defective Repair Replication

Under certain conditions DNA synthesis can take place in cells not in their S period. Usually, this appears to be repair replication, in which small numbers of bases are inserted into DNA molecules as replacement for damaged bases that have been excised.[225,226] Radiation stimulates DNA synthesis (reviewed by Shooter[253]), e.g., after exposure to u.v. light virtually 100 % of cultured cells from normal individuals show DNA synthesis, as indicated by the incorporation of ³H-thymidine.[48,68] The same is true of cells from an individual with ataxia telangiectasia, an autosomal recessive condition associated with increased frequencies of chromosome breaks and leukemia. In cells from individuals with xeroderma pigmentosum, on the other hand, such repair replication does not take place, and exposure to u.v. light does not increase the percentage of cells undergoing DNA synthesis.[48] The lack of repair of DNA defects in such individuals may be responsible for the marked increase in malignant disease which is present.

### Control of Gene Action in Development

It has been known for many years that thyroxine speeds up amphibian larval metamorphosis, but the mechanism of action of thyroxine is unclear. Does it act directly or indirectly to activate some genes and turn others off? Moss and Ingram[183] have recently shown that the action is probably indirect, at least as regards thyroxine's effect on hemoglobin synthesis. They found that the hemoglobin synthesized *in vitro* by red blood cells from thyroxine-treated *Rana catesbiana* tadpoles is identical with adult frog hemoglobin and different from normal tadpole hemoglobin. The cells responsible for the synthesis of adult hemoglobin were identified by auto-radiography after incubation with ⁵⁹Fe, and were different from the red blood cells of nonmetamorphosizing tadpoles, being rounder, with larger nuclei and lower amounts of hemoglobin. Moss and Ingram suggested that the cells which synthesize adult hemoglobin were derived, not from the preexisting differentiated red blood cells, but from stem cells that are clonally distinct from tadpole erythropoietic cells. If their interpretation is correct, then metamorphosis involves clonal selection of erythropoietic cells under the influence of thyroxine, with the hormone having no direct action on the hemoglobin structural genes, but causing inhibition of proliferation of the larval red cell line, and, simultaneously, or subsequently, stimulation of the proliferation of a new cell line in which different genes are active, and synthesis of frog hemoglobin occurs. It remains to be seen whether other hormones act in the same manner. Perhaps they do, and perhaps the reason for this is that differentiation is an essentially irreversible process. This is supported by the unchanging replication patterns of the X chromosome in somatic tissues and the different pattern seen in the germ line. However, autoradiographic replication patterns have been uninformative in relation to tissue differentiation, perhaps because they are too crude, with a resolution no better than about 1 $\mu$ by light microscope. In any case, there is overwhelming evidence for the existence of many different types of stem cells, e.g., spermatogonia and the basal layer of cells in all kinds of epithelia. The stem cell concept makes cell division a necessary step in achieving the end result; therefore, factors influencing differentiation are those that control cell division, whether by way of inhibiting or stimulating protein synthesis, RNA synthesis, or DNA synthesis.

Further evidence in favor of this concept has been provided by a study of the development of antibody-forming cells. Szenberg and Cunningham[268] have shown that during the early development of the immune response, cells produce antibody only after first synthesizing DNA, and concluded that most antibody-forming cells arise by mitotic division after exposure to antigen.

## Chromosomes and Evolution

### Replication Patterns

No comparison of the replication patterns of human chromosomes with those of another primate have been reported. Graves[101] compared two marsupial species and found a common replication pattern in the two, with the exception of chromosome 1, which has undergone a rearrangement between the species.

Hayman and Martin[109] found similar replication patterns in two marsupial species that have $XX/XY_1Y_2$ sex determining mechanisms. In each the X chromosome has one very short and one very long arm, with the $Y_1$ chromosome almost equalling the long arm, and the small $Y_2$ the short arm, of the X. In females of both species only the short arm of one X is late-replicating, supporting the hypothesis that the short arm of the X was derived from the original X chromosome and that the long arm was derived, by an evolutionarily recent translocation, from an autosome.

### The Mammalian X Chromosome

Comparisons of the replication pattern of the X chromosomes of many mammals[243,274,286] have led to the realization that the heteropycnotic, late-replicating portions of the X show great changes in mammalian evolution, while the amount of euchromatic or active X chromosome is nearly the same in all placental mammals, comprising about 5% of the haploid complement.[199] Ohno has postulated that this euchromatic segment has been remarkably stable in mammalian evolution, so that it contains virtually the same gene loci in every mammal.

## ACKNOWLEDGMENTS

I should like to acknowledge the critical and generous assistance of D. Warburton, D. A. Miller, M. V. R. Freeman, and P. Kisloff in the preparation of this review.

## BIBLIOGRAPHY

1. Allderdice, P. W., J. Davis, O. J. Miller, H. P. Klinger, C. Abrams, E. McGilvray, D. A. Miller, and D. Warburton, Partial long-arm deletion of chromosome D₁(13) as a cause of absent thumbs and associated anomalies, *Am. J. Human Genet.*, in press.
2. Allison, A. C., and G. R. Paton, Chromosome damage in human diploid cells following activation of lysosomal enzymes, *Nature* **207**:1170 (1965).
3. Amano, M., and C. P. Leblond, Comparison of the specific activity time curves of ribonucleic acid in chromatin, nucleolus and cytoplasm, *Exp. Cell Res.* **20**:250 (1960).
4. Atkins, L., J. A. Book, K. H. Gustavson, O. Hansson, and M. Hjelm, A case of XXXXY chromosome anomaly with autoradiographic studies, *Cytogenetics* **2**:208 (1963).
5. Atkins, L., J. A. Book, and B. Santesson, Chromosome DNA synthesis in the cells of a human triploid/diploid mosaic, *Hereditas* **55**:55 (1966).
6. Atkins, L., S. S. Pant, G. W. Hazard, and E. M. Ouellette, Two cases with a C-group ring autosome, *Ann. Hum. Genet. Lond.* **30**:1 (1966).
7. Atkins, L., and B. Santesson, The pattern of DNA synthesis in the chromosomes of human cells containing an isochromosome for the long arm of an X chromosome, *Hereditas* **51**:67 (1964).
8. Atkins, L., and B. Santesson, Chromosome DNA synthesis in cultured normal human female skin cells, *Hereditas* **55**:39 (1966).
9. Atkins, L., B. Santesson, and H. Voss, Partial deletion of an X chromosome, *Ann. Hum. Genet. (London)* **29**:89 (1965).
10. Atkins, L., P. D. Taft, and K. P. Dalal, Asynchronous DNA synthesis of sex chromatin in human interphase nuclei, *J. Cell Biol.* **15**:390 (1962).
11. Bachmann, L., and M. M. Salpeter, Autoradiography with the electron microscope. A quantitative evaluation, *Lab. Invest.* **14**:1041 (1965).
12. Back, F., and P. Dormer, X-chromosome activity in lymphocytes, *Lancet* **1**:385 (1967).
13. Back, F., P. Dormer, P. Baumann, and E. Olbrich, Zur problematik der chromosomen-autoradiographie. Autoradiographische untersuchungen an den G-chromosomen bei Mongolismus, *Humangenetik* **4**:305 (1967).

14. Bader, S., O. J Miller, and B. B. Mukherjee, Observations on chromosome duplication in cultured human leucocytes, *Exp. Cell Res.* **31**:100 (1963).
15. Balodinos, M. C., H. Lisco, I. Irwin, W. Merrill, and J. F. Dingman, XYY karyotype in a case of familial hypogonadism, *J. Clin. Endocr.* **26**:443 (1966).
16. Baserga, R., R. D. Estensen, and R. O. Petersen, Delayed inhibition of DNA synthesis in mouse jejunum by low doses of actinomycin D, *J. Cell Physiol.* **68**:177 (1966).
17. Bender, M. A., P. C. Gooch, and D. M. Prescott, Aberrations induced in human leukocyte chromosomes by $^3$H-labeled nucleosides, *Cytogenetics* **1**:65 (1962).
18. Bettecken, F., H. Reinwein, W. Kunzer, U. Wolf, and H. Baitsch, Klinische und genetische Untersuchungen an einem Patienten mit Cri-du-chat-Syndrom, *Deutsch. med. Wschr.* **90**:2008 (1965).
19. Bianchi, N. O., and M. S. A. de Bianchi, DNA replication sequence of human chromosomes in blood cultures, *Chromosoma* **17**:273 (1965).
20. Bianchi, N., A. Lima-de-Faria, and H. Jaworska, A technique for removing silver grains and gelatin from tritium autoradiographs of human chromosomes, *Hereditas* **51**:207 (1964).
21. Bias, W. B., and B. R. Migeon, Haptoglobin: a locus on the $D_1$ chromosome? *Am. J. Hum. Genet.* **19**:393 (1967).
22. Bishop, A., and O. N. Bishop, Analysis of tritium-labeled human chromosomes and sex chromatin, *Nature* **199**:930 (1963).
23. Bishop, A. M., C. E. Blank, K. Simpson, and C. J. Dewhurst, An XO/Xring X-chromosome mosaicism in an individual with normal secondary sexual development, *J. Med. Genet.* **3**:129 (1966).
24. Bishop, A., M. Leese, and C. E. Blank, The relative length and arm ratio of the human late-replicating X chromosome, *J. Med. Genet.* **2**:107 (1965).
25. Bloch, D. P., R. A. MacQuigy, S. D. Brack, and J. R. Wu, The synthesis of deoxyribonucleic acid and histone in the onion root meristem, *J. Cell Biol.* **33**:451 (1967).
26. Bloom, G. E., and P. S. Gerald, Autoradiographic studies of D chromosomes, Abstr. Meeting Am. Soc. Hum. Genet., Dec. 1–3, 1967, Toronto.
27. Bloom, G. E., P. S. Gerald, and L. E. Reisman, Ring D chromosome: a second case associated with anomalous haptoglobin inheritance, *Science* **156**:1746 (1967).
28. Boczkowski, K., and M. D. Casey, Pattern of DNA replication of the sex chromosomes in three males, two with XYY and one with XXYY karyotype, *Nature* **213**:928 (1967).
29. Brewen, J. G., The induction of chromatid lesions by cytosine arabinoside in post-DNA-synthetic human leukocytes, *Cytogenetics* **4**:28 (1965).
30. Bryant, B. J., The incorporation of tritium from thymidine into proteins of the mouse, *J. Cell. Biol.* **29**:29 (1966).
31. Buchner, T., and R. A. Pfeiffer, Reduplikationsverhalten der chromosomen der Gruppe D (13-15) und Identifikation des Extrakromosoms bei Trisomie D, *Klin. Wschr.* **43**:1062 (1965).
32. Buchner, T., A. Wilkens, and R. A. Pfeiffer, Asynchrone Reduplikation bei Langenunterschied zwischen den homologen Chromosomen Nr. 1 beim Menschen, *Exp. Cell Res.* **46**:58 (1967).
33. Buchner, T., A. Wilkens, and R. A. Pfeiffer, Autoradiographisches Markierungsmuster der Chromosomen Nr. 1, 2, 3, 4, 5, 13–15, 16 und Grad der Ubereinstimmung der Homologen noch Einbau von H3-Thymidine wahrend der spaten S-Phase. Quantitative Untersuchungen an Zellen der Blutkulture, *Klin. Wschr.* **46**:187 (1968).

34. Buhler, U. K., E. M. Buhler, J. Sartorius, and G. R. Stalder, Multiple Missbildungen bei partieller Trisomie C(12) als Manifestation einer erblichen E/C (18/12) Translokation, *Helv. Paediat. Acta* **22**:41 (1967).

35. Cairns, J., Proof that the replication of DNA involves separation of the strands, *Nature* **194**:1274 (1962).

36. Cairns, J., The bacterial chromosome and its manner of replication as seen by autoradiography, *J. Mol. Biol.* **6**:208 (1963).

37. Cairns, J., Autoradiography of HeLa cell DNA, *J. Mol. Biol.* **15**:372 (1966).

38. Callan, H. G., The organization of genetic units in chromosomes, *J. Cell. Sci.* **2**:1 (1967).

39. Carneiro Leao, J., G. J. Bargman, R. L. Neu, T. Kajii, and L. I. Gardner, New syndrome associated with partial deletion of short arms of chromosome 4, *J. AMA* **202**:434 (1967).

40. Caro, L. G., High-resolution autoradiography, *in* "Methods in Cell Physiology" (D. M. Prescott, ed.), Vol. 1, p. 327, Academic Press, New York (1964).

41. Caro, L. G., and M. Schnos, Tritium and phosphorus-32 in high-resolution autoradiography, *Science* **149**:60 (1965).

42. Castilla, E. E., W. R. Breg, and O. J. Miller, unpublished observations.

43. Cave, M. D., Incorporation of tritium-labeled thymidine and lysine into chromosomes of cultured human leukocytes, *J. Cell Biol.* **29**:209 (1966).

44. Cave, M. D., Reverse patterns of thymidine-$H^3$ incorporation in human chromosomes, *Hereditas* **54**:338 (1966).

45. Cave, M. D., and J. M. Levitsky, Tritiated thymidine uptake by group G chromosomes of female individuals with Down's syndrome, *Exp. Cell Res.* **43**:210 (1966).

45a. Chandra, H. S., and D. A. Hungerford, Identification of the human X chromosome: a reconciliation between results obtained from morphological and from radioautographic studies, *Ann. Genet. (Paris)* **10**:13 (1967).

46. Chicago Conference: Standardization in Human Cytogenetics, Birth Defects Original Article Series, Vol. 2, No. 2, 1966.

47. Cleaver, J. E., "Thymidine Metabolism and Cell Kinetics." North Holland Research Monographs: Frontiers of Biology, Vol. 6, North Holland Publishing Company, Amsterdam (1967).

48. Cleaver, J. E., Defective repair replication of DNA in Xeroderma pigmentosum, *Nature* **218**:652 (1968).

49. Cohen, M. M., and T. S. Bumbalo, Double aneuploidy, trisomy-18 and Klinefelter's syndrome, *Am. J. Dis. Child.* **113**:483 (1967).

50. Cohen, M. M., V. Capraro, and N. Takagi, Pericentric inversion in a group D chromosome (13–15) associated with amenorrhea and gonadal dysgenesis, *Ann. Hum. Genet.* **30**:313 (1967).

50a. Cohen, M. M., A. A. Sandberg, N. Takagi, and M. H. MacGillivray, Autoradiographic investigations of centric fragments and rings in patients with stigmata of gonadal dysgenesis, *Cytogenetics* **6**:254 (1967).

51. Comings, D. E., $H^3$-uridine autoradiography of human chromosomes, *Cytogenetics* **5**:247 (1966).

52. Comings, D. E., Uridine-5-$H^3$ radioautography of the human sex chromatin body, *J. Cell Biol.* **28**:437 (1966).

53. Comings, D. E., Centromere absence of DNA replication during chromatid separation in human fibroblasts, *Science* **154**:1463 (1966).

54. Comings, D. E., Sex chromatin, nuclear size and the cell cycle, *Cytogenetics* **6**:120 (1967).

55. Comings, D. E., The duration of replication of the inactive X chromosome in humans based on the persistance of the heterochromatic sex chromatin body during DNA synthesis, *Cytogenetics* **6**:20 (1967).

56. Comings, D. E., and T. Takefuda, Initiation of deoxyribonucleic acid replication at the nuclear membrane in human cells, *J. Mol. Biol.* **33**:225 (1968).

57. Crippa, L., and J. German, Autoradiographic estimation of DNA content in a variant No. 16 chromosome, Abstr., Meeting Am. Soc. Hum. Genet., Dec. 1–3, 1967, Toronto.

58. Crippa, M., The rate of ribonucleic acid synthesis during the cell cycle, *Exp. Cell Res.* **42**:371 (1966).

59. Cronkite, E. P., T. M. Fliedner, S. A. Killman, and J. R. Rubini, *in* "Tritium in the Physical and Biological Sciences," Vol. 11, p. 189, International Atomic Energy Agency, Vienna (1962).

60. Cuevas-Sosa, A., Crossing-over and the centromere, *Cytogenetics* **6**:331 (1967).

61. Davies, D. R., and D. E. Wimber, Studies of radiation-induced changes in cellular proliferation, using a double-labelling autoradiographic technique, *Nature* **200**:229 (1963).

61a. de Capoa, A., F. H. Allen, Jr., A. Gold, R. Koenigsberger, and O. J. Miller, Presumptive C/15 translocation and familial large Y identified by autoradiography, *J. Med. Genet.* **6**:89 (1968).

62. de Capoa, A., D. A. Miller, O. J. Miller, and W. R. Breg, Asynchronous DNA replication and discordant length of homologous autosomes demonstrated by the use of markers, *Nature* **220**:264 (1968).

63. de Capoa, A., W. R. Breg, T. Kushnick, and O. J. Miller, Autoradiographic identification of chromosomes involved in the centric fusion type of D/G translocation, *Ann. Hum. Genet.* **32**:191 (1968).

64. de Capoa, A., O. J. Miller, B. B. Mukherjee, and D. Warburton, Autoradiographic studies on a mother and aborted fetus from a family with four mongoloid children and a presumptive 21/21 translocation, *Ann. Hum. Genet.* **31**:243 (1968).

65. de Capoa, A., D. Warburton, W. R. Breg, D. A. Miller, and O. J. Miller, Translocation heterozygosis: a cause of five cases of the cri du chat syndrome and two cases with a duplication of chromosome number five in three families, *Am. J. Hum. Genet.* **19**:586 (1967).

66. Dekaban, A., Transmission of a D/D reciprocal translocation in a family with high incidence of mental retardation, *Am. J. Hum. Genet.* **18**:288 (1966).

67. de la Chapelle, A., J. Wennstrom, H. Hortling, and C. H. Ockey, Isochromosome-X in Man, *Hereditas* **54**:277 (1966).

68. Dendy, P. P., and J. E. Cleaver, An investigation of (a) variation in rate of DNA-synthesis during S-phase in mouse L-cells. (b) Effect of ultraviolet radiation on rate of DNA synthesis, *Int. J. Rad. Biol.* **8**:301 (1964).

69. Dewey, W. C., R. M. Humphrey, and B. A. Jones, Comparisons of tritiated thymidine, tritiated water, and cobalt-60 gamma rays in inducing chromosomal aberrations, *Radiation Res.* **24**:214 (1965).

70. Dewey, W. C., and R. P. Thompson, Distribution of DNA in Chinese hamster cells, *Exp. Cell Res.* **48**:605 (1967).

71. DuPraw, E. J., Evidence for a folded-fibre organization in human chromosomes, *Nature* **209**:577 (1966).

72. Ebstein, B. S., Tritiated actinomycin D as a cytochemical label for small amounts of DNA, *J. Cell Biol.* **35**:709 (1967).

73. El-Alfi, O. S., J. J. Biesele, and P. M. Smith, Trisomy 18 in a hydrocephalic fetus, *J. Pediat.* **65**:65 (1964).

74. El-Alfi, O. S., H. C. Powell, and J. J. Biesele, Possible trisomy in chromosome group 6–12 in a mentally retarded patient, *Lancet* **1**:700 (1963).
75. Evans, H. J., and J. R. K. Savage, The relation between DNA synthesis and chromosome structure as resolved by x-ray damage, *J. Cell Biol.* **18**:525 (1963).
76. Falk, G. K., and R. C. King, Radioautographic efficiency for tritium as a function of section thickness, *Radiation Res.* **20**:466 (1963).
77. Feinendegen, L. E., "Tritium-Labeled Molecules in Biology and Medicine," Academic Press, New York (1967).
78. Field, E. O., K. B. Dawson, and J. E. Gibbs, Autoradiographic differentiation of tritium and another β-emitter by a combined colour-coupling and double stripping film technique, *Stain Tech.* **40**:295 (1965).
79. Fraccaro, M., L. Tiepolo, J. Lindsten, M. Hulten, T. Linne, and D. Andrews, DNA replication patterns of chromosomes numbers 21–22 in female mosaic mongols, *in* "Mongolism" (G. E. W. Wolstenholme and R. Porter, eds.), p. 62, Ciba Foundation Study Group No. 25, London (1967).
80. Franks, R. C., K. W. Bunting, and E. Engel, Male pseudohermaphroditism with XYY sex chromosomes, *J. Clin. Endocr.* **27**:1623 (1967).
81. Frenster, J. H., Correlation of the binding to DNA loops or to DNA helices with the effect on RNA synthesis, *Nature* **208**:1093 (1965).
82. Froland, A., Internal asynchrony in late replicating X chromosomes, *Nature* **213**:512 (1967).
83. Fujita, S., O. Takeoka, M. Kaku, and Y. Nakajima, Synthesis of ribonucleic acid by human chromosomes and a possible mechanism of its repression, *Nature* **210**:446 (1966).
84. Gall, J. G., and H. G. Callan, H³-uridine incorporation in lampbrush chromosomes, *Proc. Natl. Acad. Sci. U.S.* **48**:562 (1962).
85. Ganesan, A. T., and J. Lederberg, A cell-membrane bound fraction of bacterial DNA, *Biochem. Biophys. Res. Commun.* **18**:824 (1965).
86. Gavosto, F., L. Pegoraro, G. Rovera, and P. Masera, Time sequence of DNA replication in heteropycnotic X, *Nature* **215**:535 (1967).
87. Gendel, E., P. W. Allerdice, C. Zelson, and O. J. Miller, Clinical and autoradiographic studies in a 14-trisomic mosaic, in preparation.
88. German, J. L., III, DNA synthesis in human chromosomes, *Trans. N.Y. Acad. Sci.* **24**:395 (1962).
89. German, J. L., III, The pattern of DNA synthesis in the chromosomes of human blood cells, *J. Cell Biol.* **20**:37 (1964).
90. German, J., Identification and characterization of human chromosomes by DNA replication sequence, *Symp. Int. Soc. Cell Biol.* **3**:191 (1964).
91. German, J. L., J. Lejeune, N. M. Macintyre, and J. de Grouchy, Chromosomal autoradiography in the cri du chat syndrome, *Cytogenetics* **3**:347 (1964).
92. Gey, W., Untersuchungen über die DNS—Replikationsmuster der Chromosomengruppen 4–5, 13–15 und 21–22 an *in vitro* gezuchteten menschlichen Lymphocyten, *Humangenetik* **2**:246 (1966).
93. Giannelli, F., The pattern of X-chromosome deoxyribonucleic acid synthesis in two women with abnormal sex chromosome complements, *Lancet* **1**:863 (1963).
94. Giannelli, F., Autoradiographic identification of the D(13–15) chromosome responsible for D₁-trisomic Patau's syndrome, *Nature* **208**:669 (1965).
95. Giannelli, F., and R. M. Howlett, The identification of the chromosomes of the D-group (13–15) Denver: an autoradiographic and measurement study, *Cytogenetics* **5**:186 (1966).

96. Giannelli, F., and R. M. Howlett, The identification of the chromosomes of the E-group (16–18 Denver): an autoradiographic and measurement study, *Cytogenetics* **6**:420 (1967).

97. Gilbert, C. W., L. G. Lajtha, S. Muldal, and C. H. Ockey, Synchrony of chromosome duplication, *Nature* **209**:537 (1966).

98. Gilbert, C. W., S. Muldal, and L. G. Lajtha, Rate of chromosome duplication at the end of the deoxyribonucleic acid synthetic period in human blood cells, *Nature* **208**:159 (1965).

99. Gilbert, C. W., S. Muldal, L. G. Lajtha, and J. Rowley, Time-sequence of human chromosome duplication, *Nature* **195**:869 (1962).

100. Graham, C. F., The regulation of DNA synthesis and mitosis in multinucleate frog eggs, *J. Cell Sci.* **1**:363 (1966).

101. Graves, J. A. M., DNA synthesis in chromosomes of cultured leucocytes from two marsupial species, *Exp. Cell Res.* **46**:37 (1967).

102. Grumbach, M. M., and A. Morishima, X-chromosome abnormalities in gonadal dysgenesis, DNA replication of structurally abnormal X chromosomes; relation to thyroid diseases, *J. Pediat.* **65**:187 (1964).

103. Grumbach, M. M., A. Morishima, and J. H. Taylor, Human sex chromosome abnormalities in relation to DNA replication and heterochromatinization, *Proc. Natl. Acad. Sci. U.S.* **49**:581 (1963).

104. Haines, M., Autoradiographic studies of the chromosomes in chronic granulocytic leukemia, *Nature* **207**:552 (1967).

105. Harris, H., Breakdown of nuclear ribonucleic acid in the presence of Actinomycin D, *Nature* **202**:1301 (1964).

106. Harris, H., and J. F. Watkins, Hybrid cells derived from mouse and man: artificial heterokaryons of mammalian cells from different species, *Nature* **205**:640 (1965).

107. Harris, H., J. F. Watkins, C. E. Ford, and G. I. Schoefl, Artificial heterokaryons of animal cells from different species. *J. Cell Sci.* **1**:1 (1966).

108. Hay, E. D., and J. P. Revel, The fine structure of the DNP component of the nucleus. An electron-microscopic study utilizing autoradiography to localize DNA synthesis, *J. Cell Biol.* **16**:29 (1963).

109. Hayman, D. L., and P. G. Martin, An autoradiographic study of DNA synthesis in the sex chromosomes of two marsupials with an $XX/XY_1Y_2$ sex chromosome mechanism, *Cytogenetics* **4**:209 (1965).

110. Heddle, J. A., and J. E. Trosko, Is the transition from chromosome to chromatid aberrations the result of the formation of single-stranded DNA? *Exp. Cell Res.* **42**:171 (1966).

111. Heddle, J. A., S. Wolff, D. Whissell, and J. E. Cleaver, Distribution of chromatids at mitosis, *Science* **158**:929 (1967).

112. Higurashi, M., Y. Nakagome, T. Nagao, M. Naganuma, and I. Matsui, Identification of translocated chromosomes by means of autoradiography, *Paediatria Universitatis Tokyo* **14**:14 (1967).

113. Hill, D. K., Resolving power with tritium autoradiographs, *Nature* **194**:831 (1962).

114. Hill, R. N., and J. J. Yunis, Mammalian X-chromosomes: change in patterns of DNA replication during embryogenesis, *Science* **155**:1120 (1967).

115. Hollowell, J. G., L. G. Littlefield, and G. E. Bloom, personal communication.

116. Hotta, Y., and A. Bassel, Molecular size and circularity of DNA in cells of mammals and higher plants, *Proc. Natl. Acad. Sci. U.S.* **53**:356 (1965).

117. Hsu, L. Y. F., J. Geller, and I. Nemhauser, Triple chromosomal mosaicism XY/XXY/XXxY in Klinefelter's syndrome, *J. Clin. Endocrinol.* **26**:104 (1966).

118. Hsu, T. C., Differential RNA synthesis between euchromatin and heterochromatin, *Exp. Cell Res.* **27**:332 (1962).

118a. Hsu, T. C., and L. H. Lockhart, The beginning and the terminal stages of DNA synthesis of human cells with an XXXXY constitution, *Hereditas* **52**:320 (1965).

119. Huberman, J. A., and A. D. Riggs, Autoradiography of chromosomal DNA fibers from Chinese hamster cells, *Proc. Natl. Acad. Sci. U.S.* **55**:599 (1966).

120. Huberman, J. A., and A. D. Riggs, On the mechanism of DNA replication in mammalian chromosomes, *J. Mol. Biol.* **32**:327 (1968).

121. Hudson, B., and J. Vinograd, Catenated circular DNA molecules in HeLa cell mitochondria, *Nature* **216**:647 (1967).

122. Hugh-Jones, K., J. Wallace, J. M. Thornber, and N. B. Atkin, Gonadal dysgenesis with unusual abnormalities, *Arch Dis. Child.* **40**:274 (1965).

123. Jacob, F., S. Brenner, and F. Cuzin, On the regulation of DNA replication in bacteria, *Cold Spring Harbor Symp. Quant. Biol.* **28**:329 (1963).

124. Jacob, F., and J. Monod, Genetic regulatory mechanisms in the synthesis of proteins, *J. Mol. Biol.* **3**:318 (1961).

125. Jacobs, P. A., G. Cruikshank, M. J. W. Faed, A. Frackiewicz, E. B. Robson, H. Harris, and I. Sutherland, Pericentric inversion of a group C autosome: a study of three families, *Ann. Hum. Genet.* **31**:219 (1968).

126. Jacobsen, P., and M. Mikkelsen, Chromosome 18 abnormalities in a family with a translocation $t(18p-, 21p+)$, *J. Ment. Def. Res.* **12**:144 (1968).

127. Jacobsen, P., M. Mikkelsen, A. Froland, and A. Dupont, Familial transmission of a translocation between two non-homologous large acrocentric chromosomes. Clinical, cytogenetic and autoradiographic studies, *Ann. Hum. Genet.* **29**:391 (1966).

128. Kajiwara, K., and G. C. Mueller, Molecular events in the reproduction of animal cells. III. Fractional synthesis of DNA with 5-bromodeoxyuridine and its effect on cloning efficiency, *Biochem. Biophys. Acta* **91**:486 (1964).

129. Kasten, F. H., and F. F. Strasser, Nucleic acid synthetic patterns in synchronized mammalian cells, *Nature* **211**:135 (1966).

130. Kato, H., and A. A. Sandberg, Chromosome pulverization in human cells with micronuclei, *J. Natl. Cancer Inst.* **40**:165 (1968).

131. Kelly, S., R. Almy, and M. Barnard, Another XYY phenotype, *Nature* **215**:405 (1967).

132. Khare, G. P., and R. A. Consigli, Multiplication of polyoma virus. I. Use of selectively labeled ($H^3$) virus to follow the course of infection. *J. Bact.* **90**:819 (1965).

133. Kihlman, B. A., "The Actions of Chemicals on Dividing Cells," Prentice-Hall, Englewood Cliffs, N. J. (1966).

134. Kikuchi, Y., and A. A. Sandberg, Chronology and pattern of human chromosome replication. I. Blood leukocytes of normal subjects, *J. Natl. Cancer Inst.* **32**:1109 (1964).

135. Kikuchi, Y., and A. A. Sandberg, Chronology and pattern of human chromosome replication. II. Autoradiographic behavior of various Y and X chromosomes. *J. Natl. Cancer Inst.* **34**:795 (1965).

136. Kinsey, J. D., X-chromosome replication in early rabbit embryos, *Genetics* **55**:337 (1967).

137. Kit, S., R. de Torres, D. Dubbs, and M. Salvi, Induction of cellular DNA synthesis by simian virus 40 (SV 40), *J. Virol.* **1**:738 (1967).

138. Klinger, H. P., H. G. Schwarzacher, and J. Weiss, DNA content and size of sex chromatin positive female nuclei during the cell cycle, *Cytogenetics* **6**:1 (1967).

139. Kopriwa, B. M., and C. P. Leblond, Improvements in the coating techniques of radioautography, *J. Histochem. Cytochem.* **10**:269 (1962).

140. Kornberg, A., "Enzymatic Synthesis of DNA," John Wiley and Sons, New York (1962).

141. Kosenow, W., and R. A. Pfeiffer, YY syndrome with multiple malformations, *Lancet* **1**:1375 (1966).

142. Krause, M. O., Tritiated thymidine effects on DNA, RNA, and protein-synthetic rates in synchronized L-cells, *J. Cell Physiol.* **70**:141 (1967).

143. Lajtha, L. G., and C. W. Gilbert, Kinetics of cell proliferation, *Adv. Biol. Med. Physics* **11**:1 (1967).

144. Lajtha, L. G., and R. Oliver, The application of autoradiography in a study of nucleic acid metabolism, *Lab. Invest.* **8**:215 (1959).

145. Lajtha, L. G., R. Oliver, R. J. Berry, and E. Hell, Analysis of metabolic rates at the cellular level, *Nature* **187**:919 (1960).

146. Lamerton, L. F., and R. J. M. Fry, (eds.), "Cell Proliferation," Blackwell Scientific Publications, London (1963).

147. Lang, W., D. Muller, and W. Maurer, Determination of thymidine metabolism in HeLa cell cultures by a combined electrophoretic and paper-chromatographic method, *Exp. Cell Res.* **44**:645 (1966).

148. Lark, K. G., Nonrandom segregation of sister chromatids in *Vicia faba* and *Tritium boeticum*, *Proc. Natl. Acad. Sci. U.S.* **58**:352 (1967).

149. Lark, K. G., R. A. Consigli, and H. C. Minocha, Segregation of sister chromatids in mammalian cells, *Science* **154**:1202 (1966).

150. Leblond, C. P., and K. B. Warren, (eds.), "The Use of Radioautography in Investigating Protein Synthesis," Academic Press, New York (1965).

151. Lieber, E., K. Hirschhorn, W. Seegers, P. Allderdice, A. de Capoa, and O. J. Miller, An anomaly of chromosome 13 in four generations, Abstr., Meeting Am. Soc. Hum. Genet., Dec. 1–3, 1967, Toronto.

152. Lima-de-Faria, A., Differential uptake of tritiated thymidine into hetero- and euchromatin in Melanoplus and Secale, *J. Biophys. Biochem. Cytol.* **6**:457 (1959).

153. Lima-de-Faria, A., N. O. Bianchi, and P. C. Nowell, Patterns of chromosome replication in a patient with chronic granulocytic leukemia, *Hereditas* **58**:31 (1967).

154. Lima-de-Faria, A., and H. Jaworska, Late DNA synthesis in heterochromatin, *Nature* **217**:138 (1968).

155. Littau, V. C., V. G. Allfrey, J. H. Frenster, and A. E. Mirsky, Active and inactive regions of nuclear chromatin as revealed by electron microscope autoradiography, *Proc. Natl. Acad. Sci. U.S.* **52**:93 (1964).

156. Littlefield, J. W., Hybridization of quasidiploid hamster fibroblasts, Abstr., Meeting Am. Soc. Hum. Genet., Dec. 1–3, 1967, Toronto.

157. Lubs, H. A., personal communication.

158. Lyon, M. F., Sex chromatin and gene action in the mammalian X-chromosome, *Am. J. Hum. Genet.* **14**:135 (1962).

159. Lyon, M. F., A. G. Searle, C. E. Ford, and S. Ohno, A mouse translocation suppressing sex-linked variegation, *Cytogenetics* **3**:306 (1964).

160. Magrini, U., M. Fraccaro, L. Tiepolo, S. Scappaticci, L. Lenzi, and G. P. Perona, Mucopolysaccharidoses: autoradiographic study of sulphate-$^{35}$S uptake by cultured fibroblasts, *Ann. Hum. Genet.* **31**:231 (1967).

161. Mann, J. D., A. Valdmanis, S. C. Capps, and R. H. Puite, A case of primary

amenorrhea with a translocation involving chromosomes of groups B and C, *Am. J. Hum. Genet.* **17**:377 (1965).

162. Marden, P. M., and J. J. Yunis, Trisomy $D_1$ in a 10-year-old girl. Normal neutrophils and fetal hemoglobin, *Am. J. Dis. Child.* **114**:662 (1967).

163. Marin, G., and D. M. Prescott, The frequency of sister chromatid exchanges following exposure to varying doses of $H^3$-thymidine or x-rays, *J. Cell Biol.* **21**:159 (1964).

164. Martin, P. G., The pattern of autosomal DNA replication in four tissues of the Chinese hamster, *Exp. Cell Res.* **45**:85 (1966).

165. Maurer, W., and E. Primbsch, Grosse den β-Selbstabsorption bei der $^3$H-Autoradiographie, *Exp. Cell Res.* **33**:8 (1964).

166. Mendelsohn, J., D. E. Moore, and N. P. Salzman, Separation of isolated Chinese hamster metaphase chromosomes into three size-groups, *J. Mol. Biol.* **32**:101 (1968).

167. Migeon, B. R., Short-arm deletions in group E and chromosomal "deletion" syndromes, *J. Pediat.* **69**:432 (1966).

168. Mikkelsen, M., DNA replication analysis of six 13–15/21 translocation families, *Ann. Hum. Genet.* **30**:325 (1967).

169. Miller, O. J., W. R. Breg, B. B. Mukherjee, A. van N. Gamble, and A. C. Christakos, Nonrandom distribution of chromosomes in metaphase figures from cultured human leucocytes, II. The peripheral location of chromosomes 13, 17–18, and 21, *Cytogenetics* **2**:152 (1963).

170. Miller, O. J., W. R. Breg, D. Warburton, D. A. Miller, A. de Capoa, P. W. Allderdice, J. Davis, E. McGilvray, and C. W. Stimson, Partial deletion of the short arm of chromosome 4 (4p−): Clinical, measurement, autoradiographic, dermatoglyphic, and genetic studies in six unrelated cases, in preparation.

171. Miller, O. J., W. R. Breg, D. Warburton, D. A. Miller, I. L. Firschein, and K. Hirschhorn, Alternative DNA replication patterns associated with long arm length of chromosome 4 and 5 in the *cri du chat* syndrome, *Cytogenetics* **5**:137 (1966).

172. Miller, O. J., B. B. Mukherjee, S. Bader, and A. C. Christakos, Autoradiographic studies of X-chromosome duplication in an XO/X-isochromosome X mosaic human female, *Nature* **200**:918 (1963).

173. Miller, O. J., B. B. Mukherjee, W. R. Breg, and A. van N. Gamble, Nonrandom distribution of chromosomes in metaphase figures from cultured human leucocytes. 1. The peripheral location of the Y chromosome, *Cytogenetics* **2**:1 (1963).

174. Miller, O. J., D. Warburton, D. A. Miller, A. de Capoa, P. W. Allderdice, and W. R. Breg, Two functional states for autosomes?, *J. Cell. Biol.* **39**:91A (1968).

175. Mittwoch, U., N. B. Atkin, and J. R. Ellis, Barr bodies in triploid cells, *Cytogenetics* **2**:323 (1963).

176. Moens, P., Segregation of tritium-labeled DNA at meiosis in *Chorthippus*, *Chromosoma* **19**:277 (1966).

177. Monesi, V., Differential rate of ribonucleic acid synthesis in the autosomes and sex chromosomes during male meiosis in the mouse, *Chromosoma* **17**:11 (1965).

178. Monesi, V., M. Crippa, and R. Zito-Bignami, The stage of chromosome duplication in the cell cycle as revealed by x-ray breakage and $^3$H-thymidine labeling, *Chromosoma* **21**:369 (1967).

179. Moorhead, P. S., and V. Defendi, Asynchrony of DNA synthesis in chromosomes of human diploid cells, *J. Cell Biol.* **16**:202 (1963).

180. Morishima, A., M. M. Grumbach, and J. H. Taylor, Asynchronous duplication of human chromosomes and the origin of sex chromatin, *Proc. Natl. Acad. Sci. U.S.* **48**:756 (1962).

181. Moses, M. J., Application of autoradiography to electron microscopy, *J. Histochem. Cytochem.* **12**:115 (1964).

182. Moses, M. J., and J. R. Coleman, Structural patterns and the functional organization of chromosomes, *in* "The Role of Chromosomes in Development" (M. Locke, ed.), pp. 11–49, Academic Press, New York (1964).

183. Moss, B., and V. M. Ingram, Hemoglobin synthesis during amphibian metamorphosis. II. Synthesis of adult hemoglobin following thyroxine administration, *J. Mol. Biol.* **32**:493 (1968).

184. Mueller, G. C., and K. Kajiwara, Early- and late-replicating deoxyribonucleic acid complexes in HeLa nuclei, *Biochem. Biophys. Acta* **114**:108 (1966).

185. Mukherjee, B. B., G. D. Burkholder, A. K. Sinha, and S. K. Ghosal, Sequence of DNA replication in the iso-X chromosomes from the X/iso-X human females during the initial stages of the synthetic period, *Canad. J. Genet. Cytol.* **8**:631 (1966).

186. Mukherjee, B. B., and S. K. Ghosal, Replicative differentiation of mammalian sex-chromosomes during spermatogenesis, *Exp. Cell. Res.* **54**:101 (1969).

187. Mukherjee, B. B., O. J. Miller, W. R. Breg, and S. Bader, An autoradiographic study of chromosome duplication in cultured leucocytes from XXX and XXXXY human subjects, *Exp. Cell Res.* **34**:333 (1964).

188. Mukherjee, B. B., and A. K. Sinha, Single-active X hypothesis: cytological evidence for random inactivation of X-chromosomes in a female mule complement, *Proc. Natl. Acad. Sci. U.S.* **51**:252 (1964).

189. Mukherjee, B. B., and A. K. Sinha, Patterns of initiation of DNA replication in cultured cells from human females, *J. Med. Genet.* **2**:157 (1965).

190. Mukherjee, B. B., W. C. Wright, S. K. Ghosal, G. D. Burkholder, and K. E. Mann, Further evidence for the simultaneous initiation of DNA replication in both X-chromosomes of bovine female, *Nature* **220**:714 (1968).

191. Mukherjee, D., and W. J. Burdette, Multiple congenital anomalies associated with a ring 3 chromosome and translocated 3/X chromosome, *Nature* **212**:153 (1966).

192. Muldal, S., C. W. Gilbert, L. G. Lajtha, J. Lindsten, J. Rowley, and M. Fraccaro, Tritiated thymidine incorporation in an isochromosome for the long arm of the X-chromosome in man, *Lancet* **1**:861 (1963).

193. Neuhäuser, G., and F. Back, X-Autosom-Translokation bei einem Kind mit multiplen Missbildungen, *Humangenetik* **3**:300 (1967).

194. Nichols, W. W., P. Aula, A. Levan, W. Heneen, and E. Norrby, Radioautography with tritiated thymidine in measles and Sendai virus-induced chromosome pulverization, *J. Cell Biol.* **35**:257 (1967).

195. Ockey, C. H., The behavior of sex chromatin (heterochromatin) from DNA-labelling experiments, *in* "Symposium on the Early Conceptus, Normal and Abnormal," (W. W. Park, ed.), p. 98, D. C. Thomson and Co., Dundee (1965).

196. Ockey, C. H., and A. de la Chapelle, Autoradiographic reappraisal of an XXXxY male as a probable XXXXY with 4/11 translocation, *Cytogenetics* **6**:178 (1967).

197. Ockey, C. H., G. V. Feldman, M. E. Macauley, and M. J. Delaney, A large deletion of the long arm of chromosome No. 4 in a child with limb abnormalities, *Arch. Dis. Child.* **42**:428 (1967).

198. Ockey, C. H., J. Wennstrom, and A. de la Chapelle, Isochromosome-X in man. Part II, *Hereditas* **54**:277 (1966).

199. Ohno, S., W. Becak, and M. L. Becak, X-autosome ratio and the behavior pattern of individual X-chromosomes in placental mammals, *Chromosoma* **15**:14 (1964).

200. Okazaki, R., T. Okazaki, K. Sakabe, K. Sugimoto, and A. Sugino, Mechanism of

DNA chain growth. I. Possible discontinuity and unusual secondary structure of newly synthesized chains, *Proc. Natl. Acad. Sci. U.S.* **59**:598 (1968).

201. Olivieri, G., and J. G. Brewen, Evidence for nonrandom rejoining of chromatid breaks and its relation to the origin of sister-chromatid exchanges, *Mutation Res.* **3**:237 (1966).
202. Overman, R. T., and H. M. Clark, "Radioisotope Techniques," McGraw-Hill, New York (1960).
203. Painter, R. B., and R. M. Drew, Studies on deoxyribonucleic acid metabolism in human cancer cells (HeLa). I. The temporal relationship of deoxyribonucleic acid synthesis to mitosis and turnover time, *Lab. Invest.* **8**:278 (1959).
204. Painter, R. B., R. M. Drew, and B. G. Giaque, Further studies on deoxyribonucleic acid metabolism in mammalian cell cultures, *Exp. Cell Res.* **21**:98 (1960).
205. Painter, R. B., D. A. Jermany, and R. E. Rasmussen, A method to determine the number of DNA replicating units in cultured mammalian cells, *J. Mol. Biol.* **17**:47 (1966).
206. Palmer, C. G., N. Fareed, and A. D. Merritt, Ring chromosome 18 in a patient with multiple anomalies, *J. Med. Genet.* **4**:117 (1967).
207. Patau, K., Identification of chromosomes, *in* "Human Chromosome Methodology" (J. J. Yunis, ed.), pp. 155–186, Academic Press, New York (1965).
208. Peacock, W. J., Chromosome duplication and structure as determined by autoradiography, *Proc. Natl. Acad. Sci. U.S.* **49**:793 (1963).
209. Pegoraro, L., A. Pileri, R. Bernardelli, G. Rovera, and F. Gavosto, Sintesi dell'ARN nei chromosomi umani in periodo premitotico, *Bull. Soc. Ital. Biol. sper.* **41**:751 (1965).
210. Pelc, S. R., T. C. Appleton, and M. E. Welton, State of light autoradiography, *Symp. Int. Soc. Cell Biol.* **4**:9 (1965).
211. Perry, R. P., Quantitative autoradiography, *in* "Methods in Cell Physiology" Vol. 1, p. 305, (D. M. Prescott, ed.), Academic Press, New York (1964).
212. Petersen, A. J., DNA synthesis and chromosomal asynchrony, *J. Cell Biol.* **23**:651 (1964).
213. Pfeiffer, R. A., Neue Dokumentation zur Abgrenzung eines Syndroms der Deletion des kurzen Arms eines Chromosoms Nr. 4, *Z. Kinderheilk.* **102**:49 (1968).
214. Pfeiffer, R. A., K. D. Bachmann, and K. Bartel, Missbildungsyndrom bei autosomaler Defizienz ($D_2/G_1$), *Z. Kinderheilk.* **100**:279 (1967).
215. Pfeiffer, R. A., T. Buchner, W. Scharfenberg, and I. Schluter, Morphologie und DNS-synthese eines ringformigen Geschlecht-Chromosoms bei einem Kind mit Turner-Syndrom, *Klin. Wchsch.* **43**:521 (1965).
216. Pfeiffer, R. A., W. Scharfenberg, T. Buchner, and H. Stolecke, Ringchromosomen und zentrische Fragmente bei Turner-Syndrom, *Geburtshilf u. Frauenheilk.* **28**:12 (1968).
217. Pitt, D. B., G. C. Webb, J. Wong, M. K. Robson, and J. Ferguson, A case of translocation (C/14) with mental retardation in two offspring. *J. Med. Genet.* **4**:177 (1967).
218. Pogo, A. O., V. C. Littau, V. G. Allfrey, and A. E. Mirsky, Modification of ribonucleic acid synthesis in nuclei isolated from normal and regenerating liver: some effects of salt and specific divalent cations, *Proc. Natl. Acad. Sci. U.S.* **57**:743 (1967).
219. Prescott, D. M., and M. A. Bender, Synthesis of RNA and protein during mitosis in mammalian tissue culture cells, *Exp. Cell Res.* **26**:260 (1962).
220. Prescott, D. M., and M. A. Bender, Autoradiographic study of chromatid distribution of labeled DNA in two types of mammalian cells *in vitro*, *Exp. Cell Res.* **29**:430 (1963).
221. Prescott, D. M., and L. Goldstein, Nuclear-cytoplasmic interaction in DNA synthesis, *Science* **155**:469 (1967).

222. Priest, J. H., J. E. Heady, and R. E. Priest, Synchronization of human diploid cells by fluorodeoxyuridine. The first ten minutes of synthesis in female cells, *J. Natl. Cancer Inst.* **38**:61 (1967).

223. Priest, J. H., J. E. Heady, and R. E. Priest, Delayed onset of replication of human X chromosomes, *J. Cell Biol.* **35**:483 (1967).

224. Puck, T. T., and J. Steffen, Life cycle analysis of mammalian cells. I. A method for localizing metabolic events within the life cycle, and its application to the action of colcemide and sublethal doses of x-irradiation, *Biophys. J.* **3**:379 (1963).

225. Rasmussen, R. E., and R. B. Painter, Evidence for repair of ultraviolet-damaged deoxyribonucleic acid in cultured mammalian cells, *Nature* **203**:1360 (1964).

226. Rasmussen, R. E., and R. B. Painter, Radiation-stimulated DNA synthesis in cultured mammalian cells, *J. Cell Biol.* **29**:11 (1966).

227. Reinwein, H., L. Z. Gorman, and U. Wolf, Defizienz am langen Arm eines Chromosoms Nr. 18 (46,XX,18q−), *Z. Kinderheilk.* **101**:152 (1967).

228. Reinwein, H., H. Ritter, and U. Wolf, Deletion of short arm of a chromosome 18 (46,XX,18p−), *Humangenetik* **5**:72 (1967).

229. Reinwein, H., R. Schroter, G. Wegner, and U. Wolf, Chromosomenmosaik mit zwei aneuploiden Stammlinien in der Gewebekultur bei einem Patienten mit multiplen Missbildungen, *Helv. Pediat. Acta* **21**:72 (1966).

230. Reitalu, J., The occurrence of 48-chromosome cells in a patient with Klinefelter's syndrome over a six-year period. Identification by autoradiography of the 48th chromosome, *Hereditas* **58**:63 (1967).

231. Revel, J. P., and E. D. Hay, Autoradiographic localization of DNA synthesis in a specific ultrastructural component of the interphase nucleus, *Exp. Cell Res.* **25**:474 (1961).

232. Robbins, E., and T. W. Borun, The cytoplasmic synthesis of histones in HeLa cells and its temporal relationship to DNA replication, *Proc. Natl. Acad. Sci. U.S.* **57**:409 (1967).

233. Robins, A. B., Relative susceptibilities of isotopically labelled and unlabelled nuclei to deoxyribonuclease I, *Nature* **215**:1291 (1967).

234. Rogers, A. W., "Techniques of Autoradiography," Elsevier Publishing Co., Amsterdam (1967).

235. Rowley, J., S. Muldal, C. W. Gilbert, L. G. Lajtha, J. Lindsten, M. Fraccaro, and K. Kaijser, Synthesis of deoxyribonucleic acid on X-chromosomes of an XXXXY male, *Nature* **197**:251 (1963).

236. Rowley, J., S. Muldal, J. Lindsten, and C. W. Gilbert, H³-thymidine uptake by a ring X chromosome in a human female, *Proc. Natl. Acad. Sci. U.S.* **51**:779 (1964).

237. Rowley, J., E. Pergament, W. Yarema, and Sister M. Elizabeth, Autoradiographic analysis of a B/D translocation chromosome present in a child whose mother and grandfather carry a D/D translocation chromosome, Abstr., Meeting Am. Soc. Hum. Genet., Dec. 1–3, 1967, Toronto.

238. Salpeter, M. M., General area of autoradiography at the electron microscope level, *in* "Methods in Cell Physiology" (D. M. Prescott, ed.), Vol. 2, p. 229, Academic Press, New York (1966).

239. Sandberg, A. A., T. Sofuni, N. Takagi, and G. E. Moore, Chronology and pattern of human chromosome replication. IV. Autoradiographic studies of binucleate cells, *Proc. Natl. Acad. Sci. U.S.* **56**:105 (1966).

240. Sasaki, M. S., and A. Norman, DNA fibres from human lymphocyte nuclei, *Exp. Cell Res.* **44**:642 (1966).

241. Schlegel, R. J., R. L. Neu, J. Carneiro Leao, J. A. Reiss, T. B. Nolan, and L. I.

Gardner, *Cri du chat* syndrome in a 10-year-old girl with deletion of the short arms of chromosome No. 5, *Helv. Paediat. Acta* **22**:2 (1967).

242. Schmid, W., DNA replication patterns of human chromosomes, *Cytogenetics* **2**:175 (1963).

243. Schmid, W., Heterochromatin in mammals, *Arch. Jul. Klaus-Stift Vererb. Sozialanthrop u. Rassenh.* **42**:1 (1967).

244. Schmid, W., and J. Carnes, Techniques of Autoradiography of human chromosomes, *in* "Human Chromosome Methodology" (J. J. Yunis, ed.), p. 91, Academic Press, New York (1965).

245. Schmid, W., M. Leppert, and J. J. Yunis, Rates of DNA synthesis in heterochromatin and euchromatic segments of the chromosome complements of two rodents, Abstr., Meeting Am. Soc. Hum. Genet., Dec. 1–3, 1967, Toronto.

246. Schmid, W., and D. Vischer, A malformed boy with double aneuploidy and diploid-triploid mosaicism 48,XXYY/71,XXXYY, *Cytogenetics* **6**:145 (1967).

247. Schmid, W., and D. Vischer, *Cri-du-chat* syndrome, *Helv. Paediat. Acta* **22**:22 (1967).

248. Schnedl, W., Geregelte Anornung der Chromatid untereinheiten in den Diplochromosomen bei der Endoreduplikation, *Humangenetik* **4**:140 (1967).

249. Schultze, B., P. Citoler, K. Hempel, K. Citoler, and W. Maurer, Cytoplasmic protein synthesis in cells of various types and its relation to nuclear protein synthesis, *Symp. Int. Soc. Cell Biol.* **4**:107 (1965).

250. Schwarzacher, H. G., Sex chromatin in living human cells *in vitro*, *Cytogenetics* **2**:117 (1963).

251. Schwarzacher, H. G., and W. Schnedl, Position of labelled chromatids in diplochromosomes of endoreduplicated cells after uptake of tritiated thymidine, *Nature* **209**:107 (1966).

252. Shikes, R. H., and J. H. Priest, Nonrandom mitotic chromosome segregation in synchronized diploid rat and human cell lines, *Fed. Proc.* **27**:720 (1968).

253. Shooter, K. V., The effects of radiation on DNA synthesis and related processes, *Progr. Biophys. Mol. Biol.* **17**:291 (1967).

254. Sigman, B., and S. M. Gartler, Utilization of tritium-labeled cytidine and thymidine in a radioautographic study of human chromosomes, Abstr., Meeting Am. Soc. Hum. Genet., Dec. 1–3, 1967, Toronto.

255. Sisken, J. E., and L. Marasca, Intrapopulation kinetics of the mitotic cycle, *J. Cell Biol.* **25**:179 (1965).

256. Slezinger, S. I., and A. A. Prokofieva-Belgovskaya, Sequence of DNA replication along human chromosomes 1, 2, and 3, *Cytology* (Russian) **8**:187 (1966).

257. Slezinger, S. I., and A. A. Prokofieva-Belgovskaya, Reproduction of human chromosomes in the primary culture of embryonic fibroblasts. I. Interchromosomal asynchrony of DNA replication, *Cytogenetics*, **7**:337 (1968).

258. Sofuni, T., and A. A. Sandberg, Chronology and pattern of human chromosome replication. VI. Further studies, including autoradiographic behavior of normal and abnormal No. 1 chromosomes, *Cytogenetics* **6**:357 (1967).

259. Sparkes, R. S., R. E. Carrel, and S. W. Wright, Absent thumbs with a ring $D_2$ chromosome: a new deletion syndrome, *Am. J. Hum. Genet.* **19**:644 (1967).

260. Steinberger, E., A. Steinberger, K. D. Smith, and W. H. Perloff, Apparent deletion of X chromosome in a prepuberal girl, *J. Med. Genet.* **3**:226 (1966).

261. Stevens, A. R., High-resolution autoradiography, *in* "Methods in Cell Physiology" (D. M. Prescott, ed.), Vol. 2, p. 255, Academic Press, New York (1966).

262. Stratton, L. P., and E. Frieden, Autoradiographic detection of reactive protein-SH and its application to Anuran haemoglobin chains, *Nature* **216**:932 (1967).

263. Stubblefield, E., DNA synthesis and chromosomal morphology of Chinese hamster cells cultured in media containing N-deacetyl-N-methyl-colchicine (Colcemid), *Symp. Int. Soc. Cell Biol.* **3**:223 (1964).
264. Stubblefield, E., Quantitative tritium autoradiography of mammalian chromosomes. I. The basic method, *J. Cell Biol.* **25**:137 (1965).
265. Stubblefield, E., R. Klevecz, and L. Deaven, Synchronized mammalian cell cultures. I. Cell replication cycle and macromolecular synthesis following brief colcemid arrest of mitosis, *J. Cell Physiol.* **69**:345 (1967).
266. Stubblefield, E. S., and G. C. Mueller, Molecular events in the reproduction of animal cells. II. The focalized synthesis of DNA in the chromosomes of HeLa cells, *Cancer Res.* **22**:1091 (1962).
267. Sved, J. A., Telomere attachment of chromosomes. Some genetical and cytological consequences, *Genetics* **53**:747 (1966).
268. Szenberg, A., and A. J. Cunningham, DNA synthesis in the development of antibody-forming cells during the early stages of the immune response, *Nature* **217**:747 (1968).
269. Taft, P., and S. E. H. Brooks, Late labelling of Iso-X chromosome, *Lancet* **2**:1069 (1963).
270. Takagi, N., and A. A. Sandberg, Chronology and pattern of human chromosome replication. VII. Cellular and chromosomal DNA behavior, *Cytogenetics* **7**:118 (1968).
271. Takagi, N., and A. A. Sandberg, Chronology and pattern of human chromosome replication. VIII. Behavior of the X and Y in the early S-phase, *Cytogenetics* **7**:135 (1968).
272. Tauro, P., H. O. Halvorsen, and R. L. Epstein, Time of gene expression in relation to centromere distance during the cell cycle of *Saccharomyces cereviseae*, *Proc. Natl. Acad. Sci. U.S.* **59**:277 (1968).
273. Taylor, J. H., Sister chromatid exchanges in tritium-labeled chromosomes, *Genetics* **43**:515 (1958).
274. Taylor, J. H., Asynchronous duplication of chromosomes in cultured cells of Chinese hamster, *J. Biophys. Biochem. Cytol.* **7**:455 (1960).
275. Taylor, J. H., Distribution of tritium-labeled DNA among chromosomes during meiosis. I. Spermatogenesis in the grasshopper, *J. Cell Biol.* **25**:57 (1965).
276. Taylor, J. H., P. S. Woods, and W. L. Hughes, The organization and duplication of chromosomes as revealed by autoradiographic studies using tritium-labeled thymidine, *Proc. Natl. Acad. Sci. U.S.* **43**:122 (1957).
276a. Tiepolo, L., M. Fraccaro, M. Hulten, J. Lindsten, A. Manninni, and P. M. L. Ming, Timing of sex chromosome replication in somatic and germ-line cells of the mouse and the rat, *Cytogenetics* **6**:51 (1967).
277. Utakoji, T., and T. C. Hsu, DNA replication patterns in somatic and germ-line cells of the male Chinese hamster, *Cytogenetics* **4**:295 (1965).
278. Walen, K. H., Spatial relationships in the replication of chromosomal DNA, *Genetics* **51**:915 (1965).
279. Warburton, D., D. A. Miller, O. J. Miller, W. R. Breg, A. de Capoa, and M. W. Shaw, Distinction between chromosome 4 and chromosome 5 by replication pattern and length of long and short arms, *Am. J. Hum. Genet.* **19**:399 (1967).
280. Waterman, D. F., J. London, A. Valdmanis, and J. D. Mann, The XXYY chromosome constitution, *Am. J. Dis. Child.* **111**:421 (1966).
281. Watson, J. D., "Molecular Biology of the Gene," W. A. Benjamin, Inc., New York (1965).
282. Wennstrom, J., and A. de la Chapelle, Elongation as the possible mechanism of origin of large human Y chromosomes, *Hereditas* **50**:345 (1963).

282a. Wennstrom, J., and A. de la Chapelle, Autoradiographic studies of chromosomal DNA synthesis in two males with female karyotypes, *Hereditas* **57**:411 (1967).
283. Whitehouse, H. L. K., A cycloid model for the chromosome, *J. Cell. Sci.* **2**:9 (1967).
284. Wimber, D. E., and W. Prensky, Autoradiography with meiotic chromosomes of the male newt (Triturus viridiscens) using $H^3$-thymidine, *Genetics* **48**:1731 (1963).
285. Winter, G. C. B., and J. M. Yoffey, Incorporation of $^3H$-5-uridine by human peripheral mononuclear leucocytes changing from the nonmultiplying to the multiplying state, *Exp. Cell Res.* **43**:84 (1966).
286. Wolf, U., G. Flinspach, R. Bohm, and S. Ohno, DNS-Reduplikationsmuster bei den Riesen-Geschlechtschromosomen von Microtus agrestis, *Chromosoma* **16**:609 (1965).
287. Wolf, U., H. Reinwein, W. Gey, and J. Close, Cri-du-chat syndrome mit Translokation $5/D_2$, *Humangenetik* **2**:63 (1966).
288. Wolf, U., H. Reinwein, R. Porsch, R. Schroter, and H. Baitsch, Defizienz an den kurzen Armen eines Chromosoms Nr. 4, *Humangenetik* **1**:397 (1965).
289. Wolff, S., Are sister chromatid exchanges sister strand crossovers or radiation-induced exchanges? *Mutation Res.* **1**:337 (1964).
290. Woollam, D. H. M., J. W. Millen, and E. H. R. Ford, Points of attachment of pachytene chromosomes to the nuclear membrane in mouse spermatocytes, *Nature* **213**:298 (1967).
291. Yunis, J. J., M. Alter, E. B. Hook, and M. Mayer, Familial D-D translocation. Report of a pedigree and DNA replication analysis, *New Engl. J. Med.* **271**:1133 (1965).
292. Yunis, J. J., and E. B. Hook, Deoxyribonucleic acid replication and mapping of the $D_1$ chromosome, *Am. J. Dis. Child.* **111**:83 (1966).
293. Yunis, J. J., E. B. Hook, and M. Mayer, Deoxyribose-nucleic acid replication pattern of trisomy-18, *Lancet* **2**:286 (1964).
294. Yunis, J. J., E. B. Hook, and M. Mayer, Deoxyribonucleic acid replication pattern of trisomy $D_1$, *Lancet* **2**:935 (1964).
295. Yunis, J. J., E. B. Hook, and M. Mayer, Identification of the mongolism chromosome by DNA replication analysis, *Am. J. Hum. Genet.* **17**:191 (1965).
296. Zaleski, W. A., C. S. Houston, J. Pozsonui, and K. L. Ying, The XXXXY chromosome anomaly. Report of three new cases and review of 30 cases from the literature, *Canad. Med. Assoc. J.* **94**:1143 (1966).
297. Zur Hausen, H., Chromosomal changes of similar nature in seven established cell lines derived from the peripheral blood of patients with leukemia, *J. Nat. Cancer Inst.* **38**:683 (1967).
298. Renwick, J. H., Progress in mapping human autosomes, *Brit. Med. Bull.* **25**:65 (1969).

*Chapter 3*

# Genetics of Immunoglobulins*

## H. Hugh Fudenberg
*Department of Medicine*
*University of California, San Francisco*
*and Department of Bacteriology and Immunology*
*University of California, Berkeley*

## and Noel L. Warner
*Cancer Research Unit*
*The Walter and Eliza Hall Institute of Medical Research*
*Victoria, Australia*

## INTRODUCTION

The introduction of a foreign protein or antigenic material into any vertebrate organism rapidly results in the development of an immune response which is specifically directed toward that particular antigen. It is the remarkable specificity of this response to each different antigen which presents one of the most intriguing current problems in immunogenetics.

The immune response can be divided into cellular and humoral immunity, which are characterized, respectively, by a lymphocytic infiltration and the production of specific antibody molecules. Since both forms of the immune response can show a similar wide range of specificity, it is probable that the same or a similar genetic mechanism for determining specificity is involved. However, in the virtual absence of any data regarding the nature of the recognition site on lymphocytes, the present discussion on the genetic control of the immune response will be restricted to the circulating antibody molecules found in serum and many body fluids.

*The original work reported in this review was supported by research grants HE–05677 and HE–05997 from the United States Public Health Service, Contract Nonr 3656 (12) from the Office of Naval Research, and the Northern California Chapter of the Arthritis and Rheumatism Foundation. This is publication number 1245 from the Walter and Eliza Hall Institute.

131

All protein molecules having antibody activity, as well as structurally related molecules such as myeloma proteins, Waldenström macroglobulins and Bence–Jones proteins found in various pathological conditions, are collectively referred to as immunoglobulins. One of the most characteristic features of this group of proteins is the extreme heterogeneity of antibody molecules. This heterogeneity is of two basic types: (1) the specificity to react with a given antigenic determinant can be carried on molecules which, although of basically similar polypeptide chain structure, differ markedly in size, shape, charge, composition, and biological function; and (2) molecules of virtually identical amino acid sequence and structure can have differing antibody specificities.

This review is basically concerned with the genetic control of the synthesis of immunoglobulin molecules and the different genes concerned in the synthesis and expression of the different types of immunoglobulin molecules. Several other recent reviews have dealt more fully with structural and chemical aspects of the immunoglobulins.[46,47,95,97,111,198]

## I. SEROLOGY AND PHENOGROUPS OF IMMUNOGLOBULINS*

All immunoglobulins have the basic structure of a four-polypeptide-chain molecule composed of two of each of two types of chains termed the light (L) and heavy (H) chains. Widespread interest in the structure of the molecule was initiated by Porter,[284] who showed that treatment of the IgG molecule with papain in the presence of cysteine led to its breakdown into three fragments, two Fab and one Fc. The Fab fragments retain all antibody-combining specificity for the antigen, and are each composed of one L chain and the N-terminal half of the H chain (Fd fragment). The Fc fragment is the C-terminal half of the H chain and carries most of the regions involved in different biological properties of the differing immunoglobulins.[274]

Treatment of the intact molecule with pepsin, in the absence of a reducing agent, cleaves the H chain at a point slightly nearer the C terminus than the point attacked by papain.[251] This results in a fragment F(ab)2 which, as well as retaining all antibody-combining activity, is still divalent. Separation of the light (L) and heavy (H) polypeptide chains has been achieved by reduction of interchain disulphide bonds and disruption of the noncovalent interchain bonds by either urea,[71] acid,[96] or detergent,[68] followed by passage through gel-filtration columns. The light chain has a molecular weight of about 25,000

---

*The terminology used for the immunoglobulins and their fragments is that proposed by the committee on nomenclature of human immunoglobulins, World Health Organization [377]

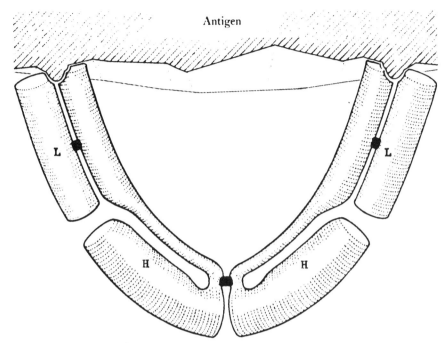

Fig. 1a. Diagrammatic model of the IgG antibody molecule, in combination with antigen. The two heavy (H) and two light (L) chains are held together by disulfide bonds indicated by ■. [From A. Nisonoff, "Hospital Practice" (1967), with permission of the author.]

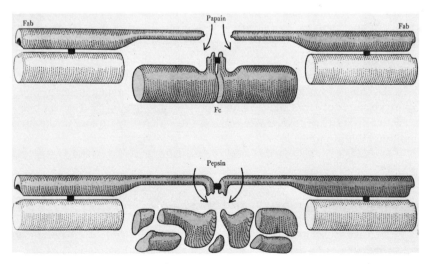

Fig. 1b. Diagrammatic model of the effect of papain and pepsin on the IgG molecule. [From A. Nisonoff, "Hospital Practice" (1967), with permission of the author.]

and the heavy chains about 50,000.[277,321] The unit structure of the IgG molecule is summarized in Fig. 1.

Despite all molecules having this basic structure two types of chains, the immunoglobulins of most vertebrate species exist in several distinct groups. These groups, termed immunoglobulin classes, differ from each other in molecular weight, amino acid composition, carbohydrate content, biological function, and antigenic composition.

Of greatest practical use in detecting and defining the different classes is the serological analysis of antigenic determinants. This section will examine the different classes of mouse, rabbit, and human immunoglobulins as determined by antigenic analysis of their light and heavy chains. Immunoglobulin classes represent different H-chain genes all present within the same individual: superimposed upon this class heterogeneity is a heterogeneity within a class, in that different individuals of the same species may have a different gene at the particular L- or H-chain locus. This genetic polymorphism—termed allotypy for serum proteins—has also been studied principally by serological methods.

Before reviewing the present state of immunoglobulin classes and allotypes in mice, rabbits, and man it is pertinent to examine the various types of antigenic determinants carried on immunoglobulin molecules. Antigenic determinants which have been detected at present include: (1) the L-chain antigen (either $\kappa$ or $\lambda$) present in all immunoglobulin classes of a species, (2) H-chain antigens present in more than one, but not all, H-chain classes of a species, (3) the H-chain antigen-defining specificity, which is present in only one H-chain class, (4) allotypic antigens, which are associated with a given allele at the particular locus, and (5) idiotypic antigenic determinants, which are unique to each molecule with a given antibody specificity. Within each of these categories three types of antigenic determinant are possible, although all 15 theoretical types have not been detected: (a) dependent upon combination with the other polypeptide chain, e.g., conformational antigens on light chains expressed only when combined with a particular heavy chain; (b) expressed only on the isolated polypeptide chain (buried antigenic determinants), and (c) expressed both on the isolated chain and in the intact immunoglobulin molecule.

## Mouse

### Immunoglobulin Classes—Light Chains

Extensive physicochemical and antigenic studies on both human and mouse light chains have been made possible through the availability of plasma cell tumors in these species.

Although spontaneous plasma cell tumors are relatively rare in mice ($\sim 1\%$ incidence in C3H mice for plasmacytomas arising at the ileocecal junction,[69,282] and occasional plasma cell leukemias in some strains[308]), they can be successfully induced in BALB/c mice by various treatments. Plasmacytomas were first induced in BALB/c mice by the intraperitoneal placement of diffusion chambers containing various tumor tissues.[236] If was subsequently found that even empty diffusion chambers would lead to plasmacytoma development in this strain, but rarely in any other mouse strain.[237] At about the same time Potter and co-workers found that the injection of paraffin oil, adjuvant, heat-killed staphylococcus mixtures,[297] or even mineral oil,[287,296] would also lead to a high incidence of plasmacytoma development. The incidence of plasma-cell-tumor development is much higher in males than in females, and is very sensitive to endocrine factors.[342-344]

It was recognized by all workers in this field that these transplantable plasma cell neoplasms in mice resembled the malignant plasmacytomas in man, in that they were virtually all associated with either homogenous serum myeloma proteins,[291,304] or with a Bence-Jones proteinuria.[86] Analysis of the proteins produced by plasmacytomas revealed a very high incidence of IgA[292] and of Bence-Jones protein[216] producing tumors, with a lower incidence of IgG myeloma producing tumors. Recent studies on plasma cell tumor induction in (NZB $\times$ BALB/c)$F_1$ hybrid (Goldstein et al.,[129] and N. L. Warner, unpublished observations), and in NZB (N. L. Warner, unpublished observations) mice has revealed a basically similar pattern of myeloma incidence. Since Bence-Jones proteins[22] have been shown to be identical to the serum immunoglobulin light polypeptide chain,[71,259,301] they provide a suitable source for chemical and antigenic analysis of the light chain.

Thirty different Bence-Jones protein producing tumors were studied by McIntyre and Potter.[216] The Bence-Jones proteins fell into three different groups; 22 of them consisted of variations of the L chain, five consisted of an L-chain variant plus the peptides of the H chain of IgA globulin (probably a monomer of one light plus one IgA heavy chain), and the remaining three were similar to each other but markedly different from the other two groups. This latter group, termed the RPC-20 group after the protein first detected to show these particular features,[19] does not cross-react antigenically with the other mouse Bence-Jones proteins.[216] Further studies revealed that RPC-20 has a molecular weight of about 24,000,[192] which placed it in the size range for light chains. It thus appeared that two types of mouse light chains existed.

From the peptide maps of about 20 mouse Bence-Jones proteins it was shown that each protein contained 11 peptides which were common to all (except RPC-20), as well as several spots which were unique to each protein.[288,289] The individuality of each protein has been shown to remain constant through repeated transplantation, although sublines may occasionally arise, differing in the expression of the light and heavy chains.[293] It was concluded from these studies that each protein consisted of a large sequence which was common to all as well as a part unique to itself.[284] Further studies of peptide maps and amino acid composition[25] presented convincing evidence for the presence of a common sequence localized in a particular region, which was subsequently shown to be the carboxyl-terminal 107 residues of the protein, supplemented by a unique stretch of polypeptide chain in the N-terminal region.[165]

These data, together with similar extensive studies on human $\kappa$ and $\lambda$ Bence-Jones proteins, have led to the conclusion that light chains are composed of about 214 amino acid residues divided at or near the midpoint of each protein into a variable region which is different for each light chain, and a common region which is essentially invariant for all light chains of a given species and type ($\kappa$ or $\lambda$).[132,162,164,241,352] The specificity for a given antigenic determinant hence probably resides in the variable halves of the light chains of antibody molecules (as well as in a region of the heavy chain).

Analysis of the peptide maps of RPC-20 confirmed the antigenic studies by showing that this Bence-Jones protein was unrelated to virtually all other mouse Bence-Jones proteins.[216,289] Proteins of the first Bence-Jones light-chain type, which were antigenically related to the light chain most commonly found in IgA and IgG myeloma proteins, were designated as $\lambda$-type light-chain globulins, and the RPC-20 group were termed $\kappa$-type light-chain globulins.[215] (The nomenclature of $\kappa$ and $\lambda$ derived from the original Korngold–Lipari K–L antigenic groups of human light chains, see below.) One of the three RPC-20 group of tumors, MOPC-104, was subsequently found to also produce an anomalous serum protein which proved antigenically to be IgM.[215] This is the only intact myeloma protein at present known to be of the RPC-20 light-chain type.

Amino acid sequence studies of mouse Bence-Jones proteins were compared to the sequences of human Bence-Jones proteins. Striking similarities were evident at both the N-terminal[165] and C-terminal ends[281] of human $\kappa$-type light chains and of the mouse light chains of type "$\lambda$" in the terminology of McIntyre et al.[215] In contrast, there was only a very slight resemblance between the mouse "$\lambda$" type and the human $\lambda$ type.[240] It was therefore suggested that it would be appropriate to reverse the proposed nomenclature of mouse L chains.[165] Hence, mouse light chains are of two types, $\kappa$ and $\lambda$. The $\kappa$ type is far more predominant in both mouse Bence-Jones proteins and in intact myelomas. The $\lambda$ type is represented by RPC-20 and is quite rare, being found associated only with a myeloma H chain in the IgM protein MOPC-104. The two groups $\kappa$ and $\lambda$ are antigenically unrelated. Present preliminary sequence analysis[8] of the $\lambda$ light chains of RPC-20 and

MOPC-104 have shown that they have identical peptide maps and C-terminal sequence. Complete sequence analysis will be necessary to determine if they are in fact fully identical. Unlike $\kappa$ chains, there is so far little direct homology between mouse and human $\lambda$ chains. The distribution of mouse $\lambda$ and $\kappa$ light-chain types in normal immunoglobulin classes or in specific antibody responses is not presently known, but, on the incidence in myeloma proteins, would not be expected to show the proportion of approximately two-thirds of molecules of $\kappa$ type seen in both human[221] and guinea pig immunoglobulins.[256]

## Immunoglobulin Classes—Heavy Chains

The immunoglobulins of all higher vertebrate species can be subdivided into immunoglobulin classes on the basis of many properties. The division into classes is based on differing heavy-chain genes coding for the heavy polypeptide chains of the respective classes. Thus, molecules of different immunoglobulin classes all have the same light chain, but different heavy chains. Differences in heavy chains can be recognized by physicochemical criteria, such as net electrophoretic charge, molecular size, amino acid composition; by biological properties, such as placental transfer, skin fixation to heterologous or homologous tissues, complement binding, and rate of catabolism; and by genetically determined antigens characteristic of the given heavy chain. In view of these many different properties, it is most important for many biological studies involving functional, genetic, and structural aspects of the immune response to have a clear definition of the various heavy-chain classes.

**Antigenic Analysis of Mouse H-Chain Classes.** Clear delineation of the major immunoglobulin classes in mice was greatly aided by the availability of many inbred strains, considerable data on the immune response of mice, and the existence of plasma cell tumors producing relatively (but not absolute[76]) homogenous proteins.

The initial studies on electrophoretic analysis of mouse myeloma proteins revealed that, like human myeloma proteins, mouse myelomas were usually of either $\beta$ or $\gamma$ mobility,[41,290,304] and immunoelectrophoretic studies[131,150] of normal mouse serum showed many precipitation lines including $\beta$ and $\gamma$ arcs. Immunochemical studies with rabbit antisera prepared against either normal mouse $\gamma$-globulin, mouse myeloma protein, or microsomes from plasma cell tumors were carried out with two series of, respectively, thirteen[292] and twenty[75] mouse myeloma proteins. Together with other studies on the molecular size of antibodies in immune responses in mice,[83] and by analogy with human immunoglobulins, these results indicated that mouse immunoglobulins existed in three classes, namely, $7S$ ($6.6S$) $\gamma$-globulins, $\beta_{2A}$-globulins, and $18S$, $\beta_{2M}$-globulins equivalent to human IgG, IgA, and IgM globulins (in the current terminology).

Several observations on the electrophoretic behavior of mouse antibodies indicated that mouse $7S$ $\gamma$-globulin might include more than one immunoglobulin type.[84,235] Further immunoelectrophoretic studies with purified anti-hapten antibodies and rabbit antisera to normal mouse serum[257] showed that two precipitation lines in the gamma region were present, indicating the presence of two antibody types. Since neither of these proteins reacted with specific anti-$\beta_{2A}$, they were termed, by analogy to guinea pig globulins, [23,29,275,348] mouse $\gamma_1$- and $\gamma_2$-globulins. Immunochemical studies with a series of antisera prepared against different mouse myeloma proteins and appropriately absorbed with other myelomas to remove antibodies to common, i.e., light chain, antigens has clearly demonstrated the existence of four distinct immunoglobulin classes in normal mouse serum,[90] and in myeloma proteins. These were accordingly termed $\gamma_{1M}$, $\gamma_{1A}$, $7S$ $\gamma_1$, and $7S$ $\gamma_2$. Previous studies[79] with antisera prepared against two $7S$ $\gamma_2$ myeloma proteins had shown that $7S$ $\gamma_2$ myelomas from BALB/c mice had distinctive as well as common antigenic determinants. This suggested the possibility of further subgroups of $7S$ $\gamma_2$, which was demonstrated by a later study[91] with absorbed rabbit antisera to other $7S$ $\gamma_2$ mouse myeloma proteins. These two subclasses were termed $7S$ $\gamma_{2a}$ and $7S$ $\gamma_{2b}$.

Since rabbit antisera directed to mouse $7S$ $\gamma_2$ will react with both $7S$ $\gamma_{2a}$ and $7S$ $\gamma_{2b}$ molecules, but not with the other immunoglobulin classes, it appears that there are common regions on the H chains of $7S$ $\gamma_{2a}$ and $7S$ $\gamma_{2b}$ in addition to their distinctive regions. Studies with $7S$ $\gamma_{2a}$ myelomas from (NZB $\times$ BALB/c)$F_1$ hybrid mice[153,370] have shown that there is more than one $7S$ $\gamma_{2a}$ class-defining specificity. A myeloma protein (GPC-5) was found which appears to have been derived by recombination between the $7S$ $\gamma_{2a}$ and $7S$ $\gamma_{2b}$ loci. Although nonreactive in the $7S$ $\gamma_{2a}$ class-specific assay employing antiserum made to normal mouse $7S$ $\gamma_2$ globulin, a $7S$ $\gamma_{2a}$ specific assay was still developed with this myeloma and an antiserum to GPC-7 (NZB-type $7S$ $\gamma_{2a}$ myeloma) in which RPC-5 (BALB/c $7S$ $\gamma_{2a}$) and 5563 (C3H $7S$ $\gamma_{2a}$ myeloma) myeloma proteins reacted. Myelomas of the other four classes did not react at all. Hence GPC-5 carries only one of two $7S$ $\gamma_{2a}$ class specific antigens.

In a study on the immunoglobulins of thymectomized mice Arnason et al.[9] have reported that $\gamma$A levels are subnormal. They have designated the protein described by Clausen and Heremans[39] (called $\beta_{3-II}$) as $\gamma$A, and state it is distinct from the protein $\beta_{2A}$ described by Fahey et al.[90] However, in three other studies normal or elevated levels of the protein designated $\gamma_{1A}$ by Fahey et al.[89] were found in thymectomized mice (Fahey and Solomon,[88]

**TABLE I.   Mouse Immunoglobulin Nomenclature, Properties, and Myeloma Proteins**

| Nomenclature | | | | | | |
|---|---|---|---|---|---|---|
| 1. | | $\gamma_M$ | $\gamma_A$ | $\gamma_{G_1}$ | $\gamma_{G_{2a}}$ | $\gamma_{G_{2b}}$ |
| 2. | | IgM | IgA | IgG$_1$ | IgG$_{2a}$ | IgG$_{2b}$ |
| | | | | $\gamma_F$ | $\gamma_G$ | $\gamma_H$ |
| 3. | | $18S\,\gamma_{1M}$ | $\gamma_{1A}$ | $7S\,\gamma_1$ | $7S\,\gamma_{2a}$ | $7S\,\gamma_{2b}$ |
| 4. | | $\beta_{2M}$ | $\beta_{2A}$ | — | — | — |
| 5. | | — | — | — | $\gamma$G-Be1 | $\gamma$G-Be2 |
| Sedimentation coefficient ($S_{20,w}$) | | 18$S$ | 7, 9, 11, 13$S$ | 7$S$ | 7$S$ | 7$S$ |
| Electrophoretic mobility | | mid $\gamma$ | $\beta$ | fast $\gamma$ | slow $\gamma$ | slow $\gamma$ |
| Representative myeloma proteins | BALB/c | MOPC-104 | MPC-1 | MPC-25 | RPC-5 | MPC-11 |
| | | | RPC-6A | MOPC-21 | MOPC-173 | MOPC-141 |
| | C3H | — | X-5647 | — | X-5563 | — |
| | NZB | — | GPC-3 | — | GPC-7 | — |
| | | | HPC-1 | — | HPC-3 | — |

Humphrey et al.,[170] and N. L. Warner, unpublished observations). Fahey et al.[89] did, however, find a variable reduction in $\gamma_1$- and $\gamma_2$-globulins. Possibly, then, the protein termed $\gamma$A by Arnason et al. is actually $7S\,\gamma_1$. [Nomenclature (1) in Table I will now be used in the remainder of this review.]

**Physicochemical Analysis of Mouse H-Chain Classes.** As mentioned previously, electrophoretic and size differences in mouse immunoglobulin classes have been clearly established for many years (Table I). The IgA globulins are the most rapidly migrating immunoglobulins, the bulk being in the mid-$\beta$ region on zone electrophoresis, with components extending into the $\gamma$ and $\alpha$ regions. Many of the IgA globulin molecules are intermediate in size between 7$S$ and 18$S$; on ultracentrifugation peaks were found at 7, 9, 11, and 13$S$. The IgM macroglobulins are the most rapidly sedimenting with a sedimentation coefficient ($S_{20,w}$) of 18$S$. Most of the IgM molecules migrate in the faster half of the $\gamma$ region. The IgG$_2$ globulins move in the middle and slow $\gamma$ regions on zone electrophoresis, and sediment at 6.7$S$. The electrophoretic mobility of IgG$_1$ globulins overlaps that of the IgG$_2$ globulins, but the bulk of this protein migrates in the middle of the fast $\gamma$ region. A sedimentation coefficient of 6.9$S$ was found for IgG$_1$.

The IgG$_{2a}$ and IgG$_{2b}$ globulins of normal mouse sera show identical electrophoretic heterogeneity and sedimentation coefficients. To date these globulins have not been separated from normal serum.

In order to categorically state that the different immunoglobulin classes are products of different genetic loci, it should be shown that the individual members of a given class have an identical (or near-identical, in view of antibody specificity variability) sequence which is different from that of another immunoglobulin class. Heavy chains were isolated from several myeloma proteins of each of the classes $IgG_1$, $IgG_{2a}$, and $IgG_{2b}$ and were subjected to tryptic peptide map analysis.[286] Despite variations between the myelomas of the same class, many common peptides were present. Marked differences were present between the groups, except that there were several common peptides between the $IgG_{2a}$ and $IgG_{2b}$ groups. The individual variations in each protein are probably due to the antibody specificity region. Mapping of the tryptic peptides of the Fc fragments[295] has shown that all $IgG_{2a}$ myelomas tested gave identical maps to one another, and all $IgG_{2b}$ Fc maps were identical. However, the $IgG_{2a}$ and $IgG_{2b}$ patterns were distinctly different in the position of some 18 peptides, but were identical for about 12. This offers considerable support for the immunochemical findings of cross-reactions between $IgG_{2a}$ and $IgG_{2b}$ Fc fragments.

Several recent observations have shown a difference between $7S$ antibodies in their susceptibility to 2-mercaptoethanol treatment, both in early phases of the $7S$ antibody response to sheep red blood cells[1,2] and very late in the same type of immune response.[73] Eighty days after primary immunization with dinitrophenolhemocyanin a 2-mercaptoethanol-sensitive antibody was still present in DBA and C57 mice, but not in A, AKR, or C3H mice.[372] Further studies are needed to determine whether these effects are related to a different immunoglobulin class, or to changes in some other activity of molecules within the same class, e.g., binding affinity.

**Biological Activities of Mouse Immunoglobulin Classes.** Both IgM and $IgG_2$ antibodies,[257] but not $IgG_1$ or IgA globulins, possess the ability to fix complement and thus cause passive lysis, IgM being far more efficient than IgG. Both $IgG_{2a}$ and $IgG_{2b}$ molecules have the complement-fixing site (H. J. Mueller–Eberhard and H. Grey, personal communication). Although the catabolic rates of the three IgG immunoglobulins are different (13 % per day for $IgG_{2a}$, 25 % for $IgG_{2b}$, and 17 % for $IgG_1$), all three seem to share a common catabolic control mechanism.[87] This mechanism is influenced by the serum level of each of these IgG components, but is independent of the serum level of IgA and probably of IgM. Catabolism of IgA and IgM globulins is much more rapid than that of the IgG globulins.

Preliminary studies on sera from mice immunized to transplantation antigens indicate that the antibodies responsible for enhancement of tumor growth are restricted to the fast $\gamma$ region on zone electrophoresis, whereas cytotoxic activity measured against the same tumor cell population is located in the slow $\gamma$ region.[363] The results would suggest that the enhancing antibodies are possibly of $IgG_1$ type (although the term IgY) is used in the report cited). However, this does not necessarily imply that the ability to give immunological enhancement is to be considered a biological property of the $\gamma G_1$ class in the sense that a specific region on the molecule is involved; instead, it may imply that antibodies incapable of fixing complement would give protection rather than a cytotoxic action. Recent studies have not confirmed a localization of enhancement activity to the $IgG_1$ globulins, but have implicated $IgG_2$ globulins.[173]

Newborn mice have low but detectable levels of $IgG_1$ and $IgG_2$ globulins in their serum, but no detectable IgA or IgM globulins.[80] This would indicate that as in guinea pigs,[30] rabbits,[32] and man,[125] IgG globulins have been selectively transmitted from the maternal circulation across the placenta or yolk sac into the embryo. Transfer of immunoglobulins *via* the colostum also appears selective, since there is a rapid rise in serum levels only of $IgG_1$ and $IgG_2$ after the onset of nursing. Furthermore, both IgG globulins and IgA globulins are found in colostum, but since no rapid rise in IgA serum levels occurs in newborn mice after nursing, there must either be a selective transfer across the gatrointestinal tract, or a very rapid catabolism of IgA. Two to three weeks after birth there is also a decrease in permeability to the IgG globulins, probably contributing to the transient low immunoglobulin level around the 3–4-week age.

One of the best-studied biological properties of the immunoglobulin is the ability of the globulin molecule to bind to homologous or heterologous tissues, thus sensitising them for anaphylactic reactions. Use of the technique of passive cutaneous anaphylaxis (PCA)[270,271] has clearly shown that mouse $IgG_1$ antibody is the only immunoglobulin class capable of giving PCA in the mouse, and $IgG_2$ antibody is the only class capable of giving PCA in the guinea pig.[18,257,372] Further studies[275] with reverse PCA (RPCA)[273] using myeloma proteins have shown that only the $IgG_{2a}$ class (and not $IgG_{2b}$) carries the Fc receptor site[272] for attachment to heterologous tissues. *In vitro* fixation of mouse antibody to mouse mast cells has also been found to be a property exclusively of $IgG_1$ globulins.[371a]

Recent studies[214,245,246] (also N. H. Vaz and Z. Ovary, personal communication) on PCA with mouse antibodies have indicated that existence of a sixth mouse immunoglobulin class. To date no purification of this class or demonstration of unique antigenic determinants has been made. However, the functional evidence is quite convincing that a mouse reaginic antibody, analogous to rat reaginic[27,244] and human IgE,[174] does exist. Mouse $IgG_1$ globulins have the characteristics of being heat stable, of short persistence in skin-binding activity, and are continuously formed throughout most of an immune response. Recently a mouse antibody was described which is

TABLE II.   Biological Properties of Mouse Immunoglobulins

| Class | Complement fixation | Placental transfer | Catabolism T 1/2 days | Guinea pig PCA or RPCA | Mouse PCA (4 hr) | Mouse PCA (72 hr) |
|---|---|---|---|---|---|---|
| IgM | + | − | 0.5 | − | − | − |
| IgA | − | − | 1.3 | − | − | − |
| IgG$_1$ | − | + | 4.0 | − | + | − |
| IgG$_{2a}$ | + | + | 5.4 | + | − | − |
| IgG$_{2b}$ | + | + | 2.5 | − | − | − |
| "Early antibody" | ? | ? | ? | ? | + | + |

detected by homologous PCA reactions even after 72 hr of sensitization,[245,246] this antibody is heat labile,[213,245] and the PCA reaction is not abolished by mepyramine[254] (whereas IgG$_1$ PCA reactions are prevented). This antibody seems to be formed only during the early stages of an immune response,[245,246] and hence has been referred to as mouse "early" antibody.

Mast cells taken from mice producing "early antibody" and challenged *in vitro* with specific antigen will release histamine. Prior extensive washing of these mast cells will not prevent this reaction, whereas histamine release on antigenic challenge with *in vitro* sensitization of normal mast cells by IgG$_1$ antibodies will not occur if the cells are washed (N. M. Vaz and Z. Ovary, personal communication). It thus appears that the binding properties of IgG$_1$ and "early antibodies" to mast cells differ. A summary of the biological properties of mouse immunoglobulins is given in Table II.

## Allotypes of Mouse Immunoglobulins

Superimposed upon genetic variations of immunoglobulins into distinct classes is the existence of genetic polymorphisms of some (if not all) of these classes. A gene locus is defined as the length of DNA which codes for a species of polypeptide chain. Thus, in the mouse there are at least five heavy-chain genes and two light-chain genes. Multiple alleles at some of these loci have been demonstrated, principally through the detection of genetically controlled isoantigens (allotypes). We will use the terms alloantigen or allotypic specificities in referring to these antigenic determinants which are characteristic of a given allele at a particular locus, and to the antisera produced against them in mice as alloantisera (rather than isoantisera).

### Production of Antisera to Mouse Immunoglobulin Alloantigens:

*Immunization with Normal Immunoglobulin.* Immunization of mice of one strain with a normal serum from another rarely leads to the production of good high-titer alloantibodies.[154] Several workers have previously found that antigen–antibody complexes are far more effective as antigens than the antigen alone.[346,357] This is also the case in allotype immunization, one of the most effective means for the production of alloantibodies is to use bacteria coated with donor-type antibacterial antibodies. Agglutinins to *Proteus mirabilis*, as well as to *Bordetella pertussis*, have been reported to be highly efficient in this regard.[153,294] Alternatively, an antigen which is itself an antibody directed to some protein or tissue component in the host was found to be far more immunogenic than γ-globulins from normal sera in all cases when direct comparison has been made.[154] The antibodies most commonly used in this manner are antibodies directed to either H2 or non-H2 histocompatibility antigens. Effective immunization has also been obtaiden using antibody directed to the HC' complement component. Regardless of the type of the immunizing globulin, the primary injection is given with complete Freund's adjuvant followed 3–4 weeks later by one or more booster injections. When whole normal serum or serum containing anti-H2 antibodies is used for immunization a dose of 10–20 $\mu$l has generally been found far more successful than amounts of 100 $\mu$l.[151] Myeloma proteins have also been used to prepare alloantisera and have the added advantage that the immunization is made with an immunoglobulin population of only one H-chain class.[295]

*Immunization of Rabbits with Mouse Proteins.* The production of class-specific sera involves the immunization of another species (usually rabbits) with either purified mouse myeloma proteins or normal mouse globulins. Although the majority of the antibodies produced react with the appropriate immunoglobulin class derived from all mouse strains, a small proportion of alloantibodies may be present. In many cases these are not detected by such techniques as immunoelectrophoresis or Ouchterlouny testing, as they form such a small proportion of the total antibody population. However, with appropriately sensitive techniques and absorption to remove antibodies specific for immunoglobulin class antigens, specific antiallotype antisera can be produced using heterologous immunization.[44,368]

*Alloantibodies to Maternally Derived Incompatible Gammaglobulin.* Several studies have shown that antibodies to the genetic factors of human IgG globulins are found in normal human sera. Since the IgG globulins which carry the Gm antigens have been shown in man to cross the maternal fetal barrier in both directions,[230] Gm incompatibility between the mother and fetus could lead to anti-Gm production by the mother in a manner analogous to the production of anti-Rh antibodies in an Rh-negative mother of an Rh-positive child. Conversely, the production of antibody in the child directed against maternal Gm factors is possible. Evidence for each of these possibilities has recently been advanced. Direct experimental support for this concept has also been shown in inbred mice.[367a] Female mice heterozygous at the immunoglobulin H-chain locus Ig-1 were mated to homozygous male mice carrying a third allelic type at this locus. During fetal and neonatal life the mice were exposed to γ-globulin of the maternal type which they did not genetically inherit. The results showed that a large proportion of these mice made antibody at some stage of their life to the maternally derived incompatible γ-globulin. In all cases the antibody produced was extremely weak and could only be detected by sensitive precipitation assays. In view of the relatively weak immune response in these mice (approximately 1 % of the immune response made by mice specifically immunized with the usual adjuvant scheme), it could be speculated that the true incidence may have been 100 %. Further studies are needed to determine whether these mice would be extremely good responders to a subsequent immunization with the allotypic gammaglobulin of incompatible type.[367a]

**Detection of Alloantibodies.** Since mice are known to generally produce good precipitating antibodies, most assays for the detection of alloantibodies are based on some form of precipitation technique. It is important to realize that since most immunizations have been performed with globulins or whole serum from normal or immunized mice, the antiserum produced might contain antibodies directed to more than one immunoglobulin class. These antisera may also identify more than one determinant on a single immunoglobulin class. Both these factors must be considered in attempting to characterize the specificity of the antibody or antibodies present in the serum.

Routine testing is usually performed by Ouchterlouny analysis.[263] Sera which give precipitin lines against the whole serum from the immunizing strain are then tested against the sera of mice of other strains to determine the strain distribution of the antigen or antigens being detected. The sera must also be tested against purified preparations of each immunoglobulin class or myeloma proteins, in order to determine which immunoglobulin class carries the determinant or determinants being detected. A more-sensitive method for detecting alloantibodies has been described by Herzenberg et al.,[154] complete details of which are published elsewhere.[153] Tests sera are reacted with small amounts, usually about 0.01 $\mu$g, of purified myeloma proteins of the different immunoglobulin classes, which have been previously labeled with $^{125}$I at high specific activity. This method is capable of detecting antibodies, presumably of low binding affinity, which fail to give detectable precipitin lines in Ouchterlouny analysis. It is often necessary to determine whether all molecules of the labeled immunoglobulin preparation are precipitated by a given antigen. At least three successive precipitations must be employed using carrier globulin, in order to bring down any soluble complexes which may be formed. An alternative method employs the application of mixtures of antiserum and labeled globulins to either gel-filtration columns or acrylamide-gel electrophoresis, which will detect even bimolecular complexes of antigen and antibody. The inclusion of a final concentration of 5 % normal rabbit serum in the direct precipation technique using [125]I labeled globulin greatly aids precipitation. It has been suggested that this effect has been caused by the presence of a natural antiantibody in normal rabbit serum which binds to the soluble complexes formed in the higher dilutions of antibody. This greatly aids sedimentation of the complexes which otherwise would have remained in the supernatant.[370a] Alloantibodies have also been detected by their ability to cause the hemagglutination of mouse red blood cells previously coated with anti-H2 globulin.[379] Alloantisera can also cause strong hemagglutination of red cells from old mice of the NZB strain which have an autoimmune hemolytic anemia. These reactions are of great value in examining the expression of the two parental chromosomes in the autoimmune response in heterozygous NZB mice.[371]

**Mouse Allotypic Antigens** The first allotype of mouse immunoglobulins was described by Kelus and Moor - Jankowski,[184] who showed that immunization of C57B1 mice with antibody of BALB/c mice coated on *Proteus vulgaris* gave rise to an isoprecipitin which reacted with a determinant in the sera of all BALB/c and C3H mice, but not with the sera of C57B1 mice. Since that time a large number of mouse allotypic antigens have been described. Potter and Lieberman have identified 14 immunoglobulin heavy-chain determinants in inbred strains and studied their distribution in 39 different mouse strains. In an independent study and using a different method for analyzing allotypic antigens Herzenberg and Warner have described the existence of 19 separate allotypic antigens. In the absence of direct experimental comparisons, it is very difficult at the present time to determine which antigenic determinants in these two sets of data are actually identical. We will therefore treat these two sets of data separately in the initial analysis.

At the present time a genetic polymorphism has been described for the three mouse IgG heavy chains and for mouse IgA heavy chain, but not for the macroglobulin heavy chain nor for either of the two mouse light-chain types. The three gene loci identified by genetically determined allotypic antigens have been termed, respectively, the Ig-1 locus, coding for mouse $IgG_{2a}$ H chain,[154] the Ig-2 gene locus, coding for IgA heavy chain,[148] and the Ig-3 locus, coding for mouse $IgG_{2b}$ heavy chain.[385]

*Ig-1 Locus.* The first results from four separate laboratories reported the existence of two $\gamma$-globulin isoantigens which were controlled by alleles of a single gene locus.[59,66,184,379] Subsequent studies showed that this locus is actually highly polymorphic with eight recognized alleles, and the allotypes serologically cross-react with each other, thus showing multiple antigenic specificities. These are inherited as a single unit, and therefore constitute a phenogroup.[341] The nomenclature used by the various groups for mouse allotypic antigens is shown in Table III. In order to further investigate the genetic control of these allotypic antigens, a highly sensitive method was developed to test the degrees of cross-reactivity of allotypic antigens of the different strains. This assay was based on the inhibition of precipitation of $^{125}$I-labeled $\gamma$-globulins, using allotypic antisera to precipitate the labeled globulins. These assays test for the ability of whole sera from different inbred mouse strains to inhibit the precipitation of the labeled globulin prepared from a single mouse strain and precipitated by an alloantiserum. Several basic rules have been followed in analyzing the antigenic specificities. Strains producing an alloantiserum have none of the specificities recognized by the antiserum; the immunizing strain has all the specificities recognized by the antiserum, regardless of the labeled antigen used to detect the antibody; the specificities detected in the immunizing strain by an antiserum made against it are not necessarily all of the antigenic specificities present in that immunizing strain; the specificities detected by an antiserum when used with a labeled antigen from a strain other than the immunizing strain represent the specificities detected by the antiserum minus those specificities which are present in the immunizing strain and absent in the labeled antigen. A test

TABLE III.   Mouse Immunoglobulin H-Chain Gene Loci and Alleles

| Ref. | | Immunoglobulin class | | | |
|------|------|------|------|------|------|
| | | IgG$_{2a}$ | IgA | IgG$_{2b}$ | IgG$_1$ |
| 75, 109 | Locus | Ig-1 | Ig-2 | Ig-3 | Ig-4 |
| 113, 131, 137 | Alleles | a-h | a-c | a-h* | Phenotypes Em-1, 2 |
| 127 | | $\beta a$ | — | — | — |
| 128 | | MuA2 | — | — | — |
| 125 | | Gg-1, 2 | — | — | — |
| 140 | | Ig-a$^{1,2}$ | — | — | — |
| 141 | | Asa$^{1-5}$ | — | — | — |
| 142 | | MuAsa$^{1,2}$ | MuAsb$^1$ | — | — |
| 112 | | G$^{(5)}$ † | A$^{(4)}$ † | H$^{(3)}$ † | — |

* Listed as a-h by analogy with Ig-1 locus, in view of close linkage.[369] Only four distinct alleles have, however, been identified serologically.

† Number in brackets indicates the number of distinct alleles recognized on basis of patterns of antigenic determinants.

**TABLE IV.** Allotypic Determinants of $IgG_{2a}$ Immunoglobulins

| Type strain | Ig-1 allele | Antigenic determinants[153,154,369] | Asa allele* | G determinants † | | |
|---|---|---|---|---|---|---|
| | | | | Assigned | Not definitely assigned to G | Probably equivalent determinants |
| BALB/c | a | 1 2 – – – 6 7 8 10 – | 1 | 1, 6, 7, 8 | — | — |
| C57B1/10 | b | – – – 4 – – 7 – – – | 2 | — | 2 | G1 Ig-1.10 |
| DBA/2 | c | – 2 3 – – – 7 – – – | 3 | 8 | 3 | G6 — |
| AKR | d | 1 2 – – 5 – 7 – – – | 4 | 6, 7, 8 | 4, 10 | G7 Ig-1.1 |
| A/J | e | 1 2 – – 5 6 7 8 – – | 4 | — | — | G8 Ig-1.2 |
| CE | f | 1 2 – – – – – – – – 11 | 5 | 7, 8 | 5 | G2 Ig-1.4 |
| R III | g | – 2 3 – – – – – – – | 3 | — | — | 3 Ig-1.3 |
| SEA | h | 1 2 – – – 6 7 – 10 – | 1 | — | — | 5 Ig-1.11 |
| | | | | | | 10 — |
| | | | | | | 4 Ig-1.5 or Ig-3.3 |

* Asa-1 allele includes mice of Ig-1$^a$ and Ig-1$^h$, Asa 3 includes Ig-1$^c$ and Ig-1$^g$, Asa 4 includes Ig-1$^d$ and Ig-1$^e$.[204]

† Assigned determinants are those which were definitely found to be on $IgG_{2a}$ myelomas. Not assigned to G are determinants in strains for which no myelomas are available.[207,294,295]

serum which completely inhibits precipitation has all the specificities detected by the antiserum in that assay, while a test serum which does not inhibit at all has none of the specificities; a test serum which partially inhibits the reaction has some, but not all of the specificities detected in that assay, and, accordingly, indicates that the particular assay detects more than one antigenic determinant: as a corollary to this, two strains which each partially inhibit a given reaction need not share any specificities with each other, but each must share at least one specificity with the labeled antigen strain and the immunizing strain. The number of antigenic specificities described is always a minimum estimation of the number compatible with the result. Accordingly, numerical designations were given to the various antigenic determinants. For example, Ig-1.1 indicates the presence of an antigenic determinant in all strains listed as having antigenic determinant 1. The reasons used for allocating given antigenic specificities to the Ig-1 locus rather than to the other loci are given in Section II. The allotypic specificities presently allocated to the Ig-1 locus are listed in Table IV. Ten distinct allotypic specificities have been identified by Herzenberg and Warner.[154,369,370] In independent studies using Ouchterlouny analysis with homologous sera prepared against either mixtures of normal immunoglobulins or against myeloma immunoglobulins four distinct $IgG_{2a}$ heavy-chain determinants have been identified. These are also listed in Table IV.

*Ig-2 Locus.* Several isoantisera which form two lines of precipitation on Ouchterlouny tests with DBA/2 mouse serum were found by Herzenberg;[151] one line corresponded to $IgG_{2a}$ globulin and the other to IgA globulin. Subsequently another alloantiserum was found which recognized an IgA alloantigen in the C3H strain. Genetic tests showed that these two IgA alloantigens were controlled by genes at a single locus, which was designated Ig-2. In separate studies six inbred strains of mice were immunized with BALB/c IgA myeloma globulin. The results[207] showed that three of these strains produced antisera that precipitated both normal sera and myeloma IgA proteins of BALB/c mice. These were therefore designated as allotype isoantisera. Three distinct allotypic specificities of IgA were identified using these antisera.

*Ig-3 Locus.* Several alloantisera have been obtained which were found to react solely with $IgG_{2b}$ myeloma proteins and not with $IgG_{2a}$ myeloma proteins. Six distinct $IgG_{2b}$ alloantigenic determinants were identified by Warner et al.[370] and two distinct determinants were identified by Lieberman et al.[61,206,294] Table V shows the present status of the $IgG_{2b}$ allotypic antigens.

*Ig-4 Locus.* Analysis of the electrophoretic mobility of antibodies from different inbred strains of mice has shown that there are characteristic electrophoretic mobility differences. This was shown for both precipitating and skin-sensitizing antibodies. It was therefore suggested that genetic

**TABLE V. Allotypic Determinants of $IgG_{2b}$ Immunoglobulins**

| Type strain | Ig-3 allele | Antigenic determinants* | | | | | | H determinants[294,295] | Probable equivalent determinants |
|---|---|---|---|---|---|---|---|---|---|
| BALB/c | a | 1 | 2 | – | 4 | 7 | 8 | 9, 11 | H 9–Ig-3.4 |
| C57B1/10 | b | – | – | – | 4 | 7 | 8 | 9, | H 11–Ig-3.2 |
| DBA/2 | c | 1 | 2 | – | 4 | 7 | 8 | 9, 11 | — |
| AKR | d | 1 | – | 3 | – | 7 or 8 | | — | — |
| A/J | e | 1 | – | 3 | – | 7 | – | — | — |
| CE | f | 1 | 2 | – | 4 | – | – | 9, 11 | — |
| R III | g | 1 | 2 | – | 4 | ? | – | 9, 11 | — |
| SEA | h | 1 | 2 | – | 4 | 7 | 8 | 9, 11 | — |

* Alleles are listed similar to Ig-1, although only four distinct alleles have been identified, (1) a, c, h; (2) b; (3) d, e; (4) f, g.[153,369]

factors influence the electrophoretic mobility of antibodies in mice.[82] In a subsequent study strain differences in the electrophoretic mobility of both whole $IgG_1$ and $IgG_1$ Fc fragments were described.[42] The study was in turn confirmed by Minna et al.,[242] who used the mobility differences as genetic markers in order to study the segration of this $IgG_1$ heavy-chain locus through an intercross. The results from tests with 201 animals showed that the $IgG_1$ heavy-chain locus designated Ig-$4_1$ was tightly linked to the other heavy chain loci Ig-1, -2, -3. A concordance of $IgG_{2a}$ allotypic antigens and the $IgG_1$ allelic type was also found in analyzing 34 different inbred strains. This is consistent with the linkage data. Serological analysis has not yet revealed polymorphism of the $IgG_1$ immunoglobulin. A few antisera have been prepared against $IgG_1$ myeloma proteins. All of these antisera were found to precipitate both $IgG_2$ globulin and one $IgG_1$ Fc fragment. Accordingly, they do not detect a unique $IgG_1$ allotypic antigen. Results of experiments using these antisera are discussed in Section II.

**Linkage of Immunoglobulin Heavy Chain Genes.**   Using alloantisera specific for Ig-1 and Ig-2 determinants, linkage of the Ig1 and Ig2 locus was demonstrated by Herzenberg.[151] No recombinations of alleles of these two loci were seen in 149 animals tested, an indication of quite close linkage. Recent data of a similar nature in tests of many hundreds of mice still disclose no evidence of recombination. Similarly, genetic linkage between allotypic specificities of the $IgG_{2a}$ and $IgG_{2b}$ globulins have been demonstrated by Lieberman et al.[61,206] In a more recent study by Lieberman and Potter[215] alloantisera specific for determinants on the IgA and the $IgG_{2a}$ heavy chain of BALB/c were used in genetic tests to test the sera of 758 backcross progeny for possible recombination. Sera of 366 of the progeny showed neither the IgA nor $IgG_{2a}$ determinants, whereas sera of 392 of the progeny showed both determinants, indicating very close linkage. At present no recombinants have been found. When a large number of inbred mouse strains were typed for the Ig-3 determinants the strains were found to fall into exactly the same groups as had previously been shown for the Ig-1 alleles. These data provide even stronger evidence for the extremely close linkage between the $IgG_{2a}$ and $IgG_{2b}$ heavy-chain genes.

The possible linkage of genes controlling antigenic determinants on immunoglobulin heavy chains to other genes in the mouse has been sought for, but not found. The genes controlling the immunoglobulin heavy-chain determinants are not sex-linked, and no apparent close linkage was found to a wide collection of other mouse genetic loci.[59,154]

**Heavy Chain Genes in Immunoglobulins of Wild Mice.**   The sera of 123 wild mice from six geographic locations in the United States were analyzed for $IgG_{2a}$ and $IgG_{2b}$ allotypic antigens.[208] Fifty four samples behaved like known homozygous inbred strains. Forty six of the mice were judged to be probable heterozygotes of chromosome types identified in inbred mice. One of these determinants, determinant 2 in Lieberman and Potter's nomenclature, was not found in any of the 123 mice. This is somewhat surprising, since the incidence of determinant 2 is quite high in inbred mouse strains. This would suggest that immunoglobulins carrying determinant 2 are the result of extensive mutations from the ancestral wild type. Two of the 123 mice had combinations of determinants that were not found in any inbred strain. It is likely that these mice have a new heavy-chain linkage group which could be the result of a recombination, so that the particular determinants detected are now linked on the same chromosome.

## Rabbit

### Immunoglobulin Classes—Light Chains

Since the first study by Porter on the fractionation of rabbit $\gamma$-globulin a considerable amount of data has become available on the chain structure and fragmentation of this molecule.[46,47] However, considerably less attention has been given to antigenic studies as compared to human and mouse immunoglobulins. This in part is due to the absence of myeloma proteins in rabbits, thus making the isolation of a purified immunoglobulin class considerably more difficult.

Several studies have shown that not all light chains in a single rabbit carry the allotypic markers characteristic of that rabbit,[124,337] thus suggesting the possible existence of two light-chain types, one lacking these allotypic markers. Studies of amino acid sequence on human $\kappa$ and $\lambda$ light chains has shown a unique amino acid sequence for the C-terminal half of the chain.[162,353] Comparative studies of the amino acid sequence from mouse and human L chains have shown that there are many sequence identities in the C-terminal half, which clearly allows assigment of the bulk of mouse Bence-Jones proteins to the $\kappa$ class.[132,165] Sequence analysis of rabbit light chains has not as yet been as extensive; however, preliminary studies have shown that of the seven C-terminal amino acid residues of rabbit L chains (from normal rabbit $\gamma$-globulin) six were in common with human $\kappa$ and five with mouse $\kappa$. The human $\lambda$ was distinctly different. It was suggested that the bulk of rabbit L chains are of the $\kappa$ variety.[55]

One recent study has reported the existence of two antigenic types of rabbit L chain.[212] A goat antiserum to the Fab fragment of rabbit $\gamma$-globulin was prepared, and on Ouchterlouny analysis was shown to give two distinct precipitin bands against normal rabbit IgG, Fab fragments, and isolated rabbit L chains. When monomer and dimer preparations of rabbit L chains were tested against this serum two bands were found with the dimer preparation, but only one band was present with a monomer preparation—indicating that only one of these light-chain types forms a stable antigenic monomer. Treatment of rabbit L chains with cyanogen bromide resulted in the disappearance of the precipitin line corresponding to the stable monomer, whereas the other precipitin line was not affected by this treatment. This suggests a difference in the methionine content or localization in the two light-chain types. It was suggested that the rabbit has two light chain types, $\lambda$ and $\kappa$, and, by analogy with human $\kappa$ chain, the $\kappa$ is the one susceptible to cyanogen bromide treatment, and is also the one which forms stable monomers when light chains are isolated without alkylation. Purified antibodies to DNP and arsenilic acid haptens were tested against this goat antiserum. Both preparations showed the presence of only one precipitin band, the $\lambda$ light-chain type. This result is quite analogous to studies on guinea pig L chain types,[256] which have shown that quantitative variations in L-chain types occur in specific antibody preparations as compared to the normal $\gamma$-globulin content of $\kappa$ and $\lambda$ types. In guinea pigs, however, antibodies with $\kappa$-type light chains were found to predominate in purified anti-DNP antibody.[253,255]

Further studies are clearly indicated to confirm the existence of these rabbit L-chain types and to study the distribution of allotypic markers.

## Immunoglobulin Classes—Heavy Chain

As in other species, the immunoglobulins of rabbits exist in several distinct classes, all present in all normal rabbits. Detection, purification, and, hence, detailed characterization of these classes have suffered from the unavailability of myeloma protein. Delineation of these classes has accordingly been made by studies employing antisera to several specific antigens followed by attempts to fractionate out the antibody activity into different groups on the basis of either physicochemical properties such as molecular weight or electrophoretic charge, or by techniques employing specific biological properties of the various antibody molecules. Rabbit immunoglobulins were initially found to fall into three major groups: IgM, IgG, and a class presumed to be analogous to human IgA. Rabbit IgG globulin has a molecular weight of 140,000,[197,277,321] and IgM 850,000–900,000.[197] The IgM molecule is split by reducing agents and reducing enzyme systems into monomer units having molecular weights of 180,000.[197] IgM is therefore probably made of five 7S units linked together by interchain disulphide bonds which appear to be located between the C-terminal cysteine residues.[56]

When a highly specific goat antiserum to chromatographically purified γ-globulin was tested in immunoelectrophoresis against rabbit colostum, as well as the γ-globulin arc, a second arc with a mobility of a fast β-globulin was detected. Absorption with several γ-globulin fractions showed that the β-globulin possessed light chains antigenically identical with those of γ-globulin, but lacked other structural components of γ-globulin. It was distinguishable from IgM by its faster mobility and was thought to correspond to the third immune globulin IgA globulin identified in human serum.[92] Independent studies on rabbit anti-P-azobenzene arsenate showed by the technique of radioimmunoelectrophoresis that the antibodies were to be found in 3 different protein components. These components were identified as the 6S γ-type, a 16S $β_2$ type, and a $β_1$ type, possibly of 9S and 6S size. It was also suggested that this $β_1$ type was the counterpart of human IgA.[261] In two other independent studies[36,316] IgA immunoglobulin was isolated from rabbit colostrum. It was shown to have a molecular weight of about 370,000, corresponding to a sedimentation coefficient of about 10.8S. Human salivary IgA has been shown to be associated with an antigenically distinct fragment termed the transport or T piece which is not present in 7S colostral IgA nor in the polymeric IgA of myeloma and normal serum.[356] This T piece dissociates from the IgA of rabbits in the presence of 5M guanidine.[37] The dissociated material has a molecular weight of about 50,000 and contains light-chain determinants which are presumably present either on the T piece[167] or on dissociated light chains.[37] As in other species, IgA immunoglobulin differs from IgG in its β-mobility, in possessing a unique IgA antigenic site, and also a higher carbohydrate content. IgA globulin is present in a higher concentration in colostrum than in serum.

Onoue et al.[62] isolated two IgA antibody fractions, one 7S and one 9S, from rabbit antibodies to P-azobenzene arsonate. When these fractions, as well as fractions containing IgM and IgG antibodies, were tested in homologous rabbit skin for PK and PCA reactivity only the 7S IgA fraction was found to give activity. In contrast, when the same fractions were tested for PCA activity in guinea pigs only the IgG fraction was shown to be active. Ohter studies by Onoue et al.[261] had previously demonstrated two chormatographically distinct fractions of γ type, one of a $γ_1$ and the other of $γ_2$ mobility. These two γ-globulins were, however, not distinguished antigenically at that time. In a further detailed study rabbit anaphylactic antibodies were shown to have the following characteristics: appearance early in immunization with a peak activity about day 9 often disappearing about the third week; heat lability; and a long latent period in PCA tests, often activity persisting in the skin for 17 days. This antibody was also shown to have a faster electrophoretic mobility than IgG.[381] The term rabbit anaphylactic antibody was suggested for this homologous skin-fixing class,[381] and it was found in

TABLE VI.   Rabbit Immunoglobulins

| Immunoglobulin class | Molecular weight | Carbohydrate content | PCA in guinea pig | PCA in rabbit | Allotype locus | |
|---|---|---|---|---|---|---|
| | | | | | $a_1$ | $a_2$ |
| IgM | 850–900,000 | High | − | − | + | − |
| IgG$_1$ | 140,000 | 2.4 %* | +* | − | + | − |
| IgG$_2$ | ? | ? | ? | − | − | + |
| IgA | 370,000 | 6.4 % | − | − | + | − |
| "Anaphylactic" | ? (7S) | ? | − | + | ? | ? |

* These values refer to experiments using rabbit IgG which probably contained mainly IgG$_1$.

approximately one half of a group of rabbits after primary immunization with a hapten antigen.[382] These properties of heat lability, appearance early in immunization, and long skin fixation correspond exactly to the properties of rat and human anaphylactic antibodies and differ from the homologous anaphylactic antibodies of mice and guinea pigs.[23,28] To recapitulate, rabbit immunoglobulins include IgG, IgM, IgA, and a homologous anaphylactic antibody equivalent to the reaginic antibody of rats and rabbits. The possibility that rabbits possess $\gamma_1$-globulin analogous to $\gamma_1$ in guinea pigs and mice cannot be dismissed, particularly since two different IgG classes have been reported to exist in rabbits on the basis of presence or absence of the presently known allotypic specificities.[142] Several properties of rabbit immunoglobulins are listed in Table VI. Radioimmunoelectrophoretic analysis of the sera of rabbits immunized with bovine fibrinogen has demonstrated an antibody globulin located in the medium-mobility area, but clearly distinct from IgA or IgM. A provisional name of Ig(DK) has been given to this new type of antibody.[232] Further studies are clearly necessary to determine whether this antibody is in fact the $\gamma$G described by Hamers et al.[142] or the rabbit anaphylactic antibody.[381]

## Allotypes of Rabbit Immunoglobulins

Allotypes of rabbit immunoglobulins were first described in 1956 when Oudin[264,265] immunized rabbits with immune globulins purified as antibodies from other rabbits, and showed the presence of immunogenic determinants. These were called allotypes and the phenomenon was termed allotypy. Since that time many rabbit allotypic specificities have been described, and the genetic control and molecular localization of these allotypic specificities have recently been reviewed.[182,269] A summary of rabbit allotypic specificities is given in Table VII.

TABLE VII.   Allotypic Specificities of Rabbit Immunoglobulins

| Allotypic specificity | Gene locus | Immunoglobulin class localization | Submolecular localization |
|---|---|---|---|
| As1, As2, As3 | $a_1$ | IgM, IgA, IgG$_1$ | Fd |
| As8 | $a_2$ | IgG$_2$ | Fc |
| As4, As5, As6, As9 | $b$ | All classes | L |
| Ms1, Ms2, Ms3 | — | IgM | ? |

**Detection of Rabbit Allotypes.**   Rabbit alloantisera are usually strong precipitating sera. Accordingly, most of the work on rabbit allotypes has been performed with precipitation techniques. These involve either the liquid precipitation system of Oudin,[266] or precipitation in agar by Ouchterlouny or immunoelectrophoretic techniques. Ouchterlouny tests of new alloantisera are performed against a panel of known sera. Examination is carefully made for spurs, indicative of cross-reactions, and for double bands, possibly indicative of multiple antibodies to antigens in different immuno-globulin classes. Hemagglutination and hemagglutination inhibition have been reported to provide a convenient assay for work with allotype sera. Agglutination titers with alloantisera to such coated red cells are usually in the thousands, and high sensitivity can be achieved with this technique.

For the production of monospecific sera the recipient rabbit should have all the allotypes of the donor except the particular one concerned. As previously mentioned for mouse alloantisera production, immunization with normal whole serum rarely leads to the production of strong precipitating alloantisera. Antibody production is best achieved by the use of antibodies to either protein antigens or to bacterial antigens when complexed with their respective antigen. A detailed description of the production of rabbit alloantisera has recently been published.[182]

It has also been shown that heterologous antisera, such as goat or chicken anti-rabbit IgG, may contain antibodies to allotypic determinants. Careful absorption to remove antibodies to the class-specific antigens is necessary in order to reveal the antiallotype antibodies.[31,201]

**Rabbit Allotypic Antigens.**   In the several years immediately following the first description by Oudin of rabbit allotypes six allotypic specificities were clearly identified.[61,69,180,267] The specificities As1, As2, and As3 were shown to be controlled by three allelic genes at one locus, termed $a$, and the allotypic specificities As4, As5, and As6 by three allelic genes at a second locus, termed the $b$ locus. The two loci are not closely linked. A large amount of material has been published to support this pattern of inheritance;

in all, well over 1000 offspring have been tested by the several groups involved. The detailed molecular localization of these different specificities is discussed more fully in the following section; basically, specificities of the *a* locus are located on the heavy chain, whereas specificities of the *b* locus are located only on light chains. Another specificity termed As9 has recently been described to constitute a fourth allele at the *b* locus.[68] Allotypic specificity As8 has been shown to be present on IgG molecules which do not carry As1, 2, or 3. Molecular localization of this allotypic specificity seems to indicate the existence of distinct IgG subclasses in rabbits. This is also discussed further in the following section. Two other allotype specificities termed P and T were identified by Dray *et al.*;[64] allotype P appears to be determined at a locus distinct from the *a* and *b* loci, whereas genetic control of specificity T is not established.

Double lines have been found by several authors in precipitating systems employing antiallotype antisera.[64,266] A detailed analysis of this situation led Hamers *et al.*[140–142] to describe the existence of a specificity which they termed As8. It was shown that the double-line phenomenon cannot be due to the presence of a new allele of a single *a*- or *b*-chain gene, since it is also present in animals supposedly heterozygous for both loci, and must therefore be attributed to a new locus which is situated in the same linkage group as the *a*-chain gene. Hamers designated the class $IgG_1$ as the class characterized by the allotypic markers As1, 2, and 3, whereas $IgG_2$ would be the class defined by the new allotype termed As8. Anti-DNP antibodies were shown to be present in both $IgG_1$ and $IgG_2$ classes.

During the course of cross immunization of animals with apparently identical allotypes a new alloantiserum was produced. The determinant recognized by this antiserum was shown to be present on the macroglobulin $\gamma_M$ molecule. The allotypic specificity was designated Ms1.[191] In further studies [179a,315] two other distinct macroglobulin allotypes termed Ms2 and Ms3 were identified. Several other macroglobulin specificities are under investigation[179a] in order to determine whether they are carried by the immunoglobulin IgM molecule. At the present time the genetic relationship between Ms1, Ms2, and Ms3 and between the specificities controlled by the *a* and *b* loci have not been clearly determined.

Individual molecules in heterozygous rabbits have been shown to be symmetrical in terms of the genetic markers carried on their $\gamma$-globulin molecules. Individual molecules may carry specificities determined by different loci, the *a* and *b* loci coding for the light and heavy chains, but different alleles at these loci are never found on the same molecule.[60,64,124,268,337] Several quantitative estimations on the proportion of molecules carrying allelic specificities have shown that between 10 and 20 % of molecules do not carry either *a*- or *b*-locus alleles.[60,64,337] In view of the recent description of several new alleles for both light and heavy chains, further studies will be necessary to determine whether molecules lacking all presently known alleles are present in rabbit serum, which would indicate the existence of further subclasses as yet undefined.

### Human

### The Immunoglobulins and Related Proteins

Considerable progress has been made in recent years in elucidating the structure of the immunoglobulins in man and in defining some aspects of their genetic control. Advances in these two areas have proceeded in parallel, and, not infrequently, progress in one area has influenced observations and conclusions in the other. Since an appreciation and understanding of the genetic $\gamma$-globulin factors requires a thorough knowledge of immunoglobulin structure, this section will survey the major immunoglobulin classes now recognized in man and the fundamental structural units of which they are composed. With this as a basis we will then attempt to summarize some of the concepts dealing with the genetic control of the polypeptide chains which constitute some of the immunoglobulins, and, in Section II, to discuss the structural basis of some of the currently recognized genetic factors.

Antibodies in man are associated with at least five major classes of proteins collectively known as the immunoglobulins.[377] These are: (1) $\gamma_G$-globulins (IgG); (2) $\gamma_A$-globulins (IgA); (3) $\gamma_M$-globulins (IgM); (4) $\gamma_D$-globulins (IgD);[313] and (5) the most recently defined fraction, known as the $\gamma_E$-globulin (IgE), which appears to contain the reaginic antibodies.[183] All five of these immunoglobulins have certain structural and functional features in common; yet they differ from each other sufficiently to warrant their separation into five major classes. Some of the more important properties of each class are summarized in Table VIII.

**IgG Globulins.** This is the major immunoglobulin class, making up about 85% of the total. Normally, its concentration in adult Caucasian serum is 1200 mg %.[85,340] The IgG globulins have a molecular weight of about 145,000, a relatively slow electrophoretic mobility, a sedimentation coefficient of 6.7–7$S$, and are relatively poor in carbohydrate (2.5%).[77,101,149] Each IgG globulin molecule has a valence of 2, i.e., it has two combining sites for antigen. Of great practical importance is the fact that this fraction appears to be the only one that can cross the placenta from the maternal to the fetal circulation.[107] Because it is the only immunoglobulin of nonfetal origin in the circulation of the newborn, it can, under certain circumstances, act as a foreign protein and induce the formation of antibodies by the infant to

TABLE VIII. Properties of Human Immunoglobulins*

| Class | Synonyms | Sed. rate | Mol. wt. | Adult serum conc. (mg %) | Percent of total antibody | Complement fixing ability | Distribution |
|---|---|---|---|---|---|---|---|
| $\gamma_A$ | IgA, $\gamma_1$A, $\beta_2$A | 7S (monomer) also 10 and 13S | 160,000 (monomer) | 50–150 | 10 | Absent | External secretions, extracellular and intravascular |
| $\gamma_G$ | IgG, 7S $\gamma_2$, $\gamma_{ss}$ | 7S | 160,000 | 500–1500 | 80 | Present | Extracellular and intravascular |
| $\gamma_M$ | IgM, 19S macro-globulin | 19S | 900,000 | 50–70 | 5–10 | Present | Intravascular |
| $\gamma_D$ | IgD | 7S | 160,000 | 3 | 1–3 | ? | ? |
| $\gamma_E$ | IgE | 8S | ? | ? | <1 | ? | ? |

* From B. R. Anderson, "The Classification of Human Antibodies," prepared for Immunology, Inc., with permission of the author.

antigenic determinants present on the maternal protein which are absent from the fetal IgG globulin fraction. The possible clinical significance of this will be discussed in greater detail later. It should be noted that although significant IgG globulin synthesis had been thought not to begin until a few months after birth,[119] very sensitive techniques have demonstrated that Gm factors characteristic of the fetus can be synthesised *in utero*.[115]

Recently, largely through studies of myeloma proteins, a number of antigenically distinguishable subclasses of IgG globulins have been discovered.[57,134,347] These appear to be under separate genetic control, and will be described in greater detail later.[228]

**IgM Globulins.** The macroglobulin ($\gamma_M$) fraction makes up approximately 5 % of the normal immunoglobulin, and its concentration in normal Caucasian adults averages approximately $100 \pm 25$ mg %.[85,340] Its electrophoretic mobility is somewhat faster, and its molecular weight (approximately 900,000), sedimentation coefficient of 18–20$S$, and carbohydrate content of 10 % are considerably greater than IgG globulin. Each macroglobulin molecule appears to be composed of five (or six) subunits, each with a molecular weight of about 185,000, held together by disulfide bonds. These bonds can be reversibly dissociated under mild conditions by a variety of sulfhydryl reagents,[54] generally with significant loss of antibody activity by most serologic assay systems.[116,138] However, it seems likely that the subunits of at least the majority of IgM antibodies can still bind antigen.[160,238,260] This serologic inactivation by sulfhydryl reagent is often used to distinguish IgM antibodies from IgG antibodies, as the latter generally resist mild reduction.[54,116,138] However, certain exceptions to this rule have been noted, and it should not be used as a sole criterion of molecular size. Recent studies in several species suggest that the IgM fraction has a valence of 5–6, and that each monomeric 8$S$ unit is univalent (one combining site for antigen).[102,159,260] The IgM fraction cannot cross the placental circulation; however, it has been clearly shown that this fraction is synthesized by the fetus as early as the last trimester of pregnancy.[319]

The abnormal protein corresponding to the IgM fraction is the macroglobulin produced in macroglobulinemia of Waldenstrom. Here, too, at least two antigenically distinguishable subclasses appear to exist,[103,145,217,376] and these proteins have been used extensively as models of the normal IgM fraction. In the IgM fraction paraproteins occasionally have been shown to possess antibody activity, the most common specificity being cold agglutinins, rheumatoid factors, and antiantibodies.[106,116]

**IgA Globulins.** This fraction makes up approximately 10 % of the total and is normally present at a concentration of $200 \pm 60$ mg %.[85,340] Its electrophoretic mobility is roughly equal to that of the IgM fraction. Its molecular weight and sedimentation constant are generally similar to those of the IgG fraction; however, some normal IgA molecules, and especially the IgA myeloma proteins, often exist as dimers, trimers, or larger polymers, with sedimentation coefficients of 9, 11, 13, and 15–17$S$.[50,78,361] The IgA globulins resemble the IgM in carbohydrate content (10%) and in inability to cross the placental barrier. However, unlike the IgM fraction, IgA synthesis does not start until a few days after birth. Two antigenically distinguishable subclasses are now known to exist.[94,195,360] Recent studies strongly suggest that the IgA fraction provides antibody activity in a variety of external secretions, that it is synthesized in plasma cells located in the exocrine organs, and that IgA in these secretions contains a "secretory piece" produced in the glandular cells which is subsequently attached to the IgA globulin prior to its secretion.[37,167,356]

**IgD and IgE Globulins.** Little is known about these two fractions in normal serum, and to date there is no knowledge of their genetic control. Both appear to be present in trace amounts; IgD normally has a concentration of 3 mg%.[313] The physical properties of several IgD myeloma proteins closely resemble those of IgG globulins. Not enough IgE is present in normal serum to allow its isolation and analysis at the present time, but it is present in increased concentration in the serum of allergic individuals. The IgE fraction, which contains the reaginic antibodies, is difficult to separate from the IgA fraction and has been recognized only by virtue of its unique antigenic properties.[175] One IgE myeloma (ND) has been described. This protein blocks passive transfer of reagin activity.[177]

**General Comments.** Differences in size, mobility, solubility, and charge have permitted isolation of the three major immunoglobulins from normal serum in a state of great purity, and may also prove useful in the isolation of the IgD and IgE fractions. A combination of precipitation, preparative electrophoresis, gel filtration, ion-exchange chromatography, and ultracentrifugation has been employed for this purpose. The antigenic determinants of these proteins have proved exceedingly useful in analytical studies of these proteins and in determination of their cellular origin. All of the immunoglobulins have certain common antigenic determinants; the additional presence in each immunoglobulin heavy chain of determinants unique to each permits the ready preparation of antisera specific for each of the immunoglobulins. Such antisera have been used to identify each of these proteins in serum and to demonstrate that all the immune globulins are synthesized in cells of the plasma cell and lymphocyte series.

**Minor Immunoglobulin Classes.** In addition to these major classes of immunoglobulins, several minor ones appear to exist. Thus, certain antibodies have been associated with molecules having the antigenic properties of IgM globulins, buth with sedimentation constants of approximately $7S$.[312] Other antibodies are found in a fraction having a sedimentation rate intermediate netween $7S$ and $19S$.[306] The precise relationship of these antibodies to the five major classes remains to be determined.

## Structural Units of the Immunoglobulins

As previously discussed for mouse and rabbit, in man the heavy chains carry those properties which distinguish the different immunoglobulins from each other. In the nomenclature recommended by the WHO Committee on Immunoglobulins[377] the heavy chains are identified by the Greek letter corresponding to the immunoglobulin class ($\gamma$, $\alpha$, $\mu$, $\delta$, and $\epsilon$ for the IgG, A, M, D, and E, respectively of human immunoglobulins). Figure 1, a schematic diagram of the IgG molecule, can be used as a representative of all the currently recognized classes. Table IX lists the structural units and probable molecular formulas for each human immunoglobulin class.

TABLE IX.   Nomenclature of Immunoglobulins

| Immunoglobulins (Ig) | Subunits | |
|---|---|---|
| | Light chains | Heavy chains |
| $(\kappa\gamma)_2$ = IgG | $\kappa$ $\lambda$ | New term. $\gamma_1$, $\gamma_2$, $\gamma_3$, $\gamma_4$ |
| $(\kappa\alpha)_2$ $(\lambda\alpha)_2$ = IgA, etc. | $\kappa$ $\lambda$ | $\alpha$, $\alpha$ |
| $(\kappa\mu)_{10}$ $(\lambda\mu)_{10}$ = IgM | $\kappa$ $\lambda$ | $\mu$ |
| $(\kappa\delta)_2$ $(\lambda\delta)_2$ = IgD | $\kappa$ $\lambda$ | $\delta$ |
| $(\kappa\epsilon)_2$ $(\lambda\epsilon)_2$ = IgE | $\kappa$ $\lambda$ | $\epsilon$ |

Precise characterization of the various subunits has proceeded most effectively with fragments and chains from myeloma proteins and Bence-Jones proteins (light chains), and with the naturally occurring fragments produced in heavy-chain disease.[108] Fortunately, in all instances so far examined findings obtained with the abnormal proteins have been applicable to the normal immunoglobulins as well, thus making these so-called "paraproteins" exceedingly useful as models of the normal immunoglobulins and antibodies. Through immunologic studies and, subsequently, by precise biochemical technique, it was possible to identify two types of human light chains, known as $\kappa$ and $\lambda$, which differ completely in their primary structure and appear to be under separate genetic control.[88,220,239] More recently studies of the almost complete amino acid sequence of several $\kappa$ Bence-Jones proteins have demonstrated the existence in these chains of two distinct regions.[162,353] One of these consists of about 106–108 amino acids at the amino-terminal end, and seems to differ significantly in amino acid sequence for each protein; the other, which consists of a stretch of about 106-108 amino acids at the carboxy-terminal end, appears to be identical for all the proteins studied with the exception of residue No. 189 (or 191), which appears to be related to the Inv type of the molecule.[15,162] On the basis of less-complete studies of several $\lambda$ Bence-Jones proteins it would appear that they have the same overall structural arrangement and also consist of a common and variable region.[302] A single amino acid substitution at position 190 (oz) may be an allotypic variant.[7] The ratio of $\kappa$ to $\lambda$ molecules in the total $\gamma$G of normal individuals is about 2:1, any one molecule having either two $\kappa$ or two $\lambda$ chains and never both.[88,220] More recently at least four subclasses of the $\gamma$ chains, each of which appears to be under separate genetic control, have been defined by immunologic techniques.[57,134,347] They are now called $\gamma G_1$, $\gamma G_2$, $\gamma G_3$, and $\gamma G_4$, and were previously referred to as $\gamma_{2a,b,c,d}$,[57,347] or Ne, We, Vi, and Ge, respectively, in two terminologies. Structural studies have demonstrated that the determinants responsible for subclass specificity are largely in the Fc fragment[134] and that subtle differences exist in the amino acid composition and peptide maps of proteins of different subclasses.[98] Because of their large size and greater complexity, knowledge of the primary structure of the H chain has not progressed as far as that of the light chains. However, the overall arrangement appears to be similar, since the Fc fragment and a part of the Fd fragment appear to be similar for all proteins belonging to one subgroup,[99,100,351] with the exception of a few amino acid residues related to the Gm type.[98,351] The remainder of the Fd fragment, probably located at the amino-terminal end and probably involved in the antigen-binding site, appears to differ for each myeloma protein studied to date.[100]

## Allotypes of Human Immunoglobulins

**History.** A group of anitglobulins present individually or collectively in certain human sera behave as antibodies directed against the $\gamma$-globulin of various species, including man.[112] In 1939 Waaler[365] reported that the sera of certain patients with rheumatoid arthritis agglutinated sheep cells sensitized by subagglutinating doses of rabbit anti-sheep red-cell antibody. Subsequently Rose et al.[311] demonstrated the diagnostic value of this "sensitized sheep cell test" in rheumatoid arthritis, and the factor causing this agglutination became generally designated as "rheumatoid factor." Subsequently sera containing "rheumatoid factor" were shown to react not only with rabbit IgG globulin, but also with human IgG globulin[148] (recent experiments suggest that rheumatoid factor reacts only with aggregated, but not with native human IgG globulin[163]). Subsequently various modifications of diagnostic test systems for rheumatoid factor have been devised, employing human $\gamma$-globulin coated on inert indicator particles, such as tanned cells, latex or bentonite particles, or human Rh+ red cells coated with certain selected incomplete antibodies. However, tests with such systems employing human $\gamma$-globulin as the antigen are often positive in conditions other than rheumatoid arthritis, e.g., cirrhosis, sarcoidosis, lues, kala-azar, leprosy, etc., whereas such sera are only rarely positive in the standard test system for rheumatoid arthritis, employing rabbit $\gamma_G$-globulin as antigen.[16,17,169,367] Thus, if the term "rheumatoid factor" is to retain any significance, it should be restricted to a test system highly specific for the disease process, rheumatoid arthritis, i.e., restricted to sera producing positive results with rabbit $\gamma$-globulin as antigen. Other agglutinating substances in human sera reactive with human $\gamma$-globulin but not with IgG globulin of other species include factors reactive with antigen–antibody complexes but not with nonantibody $\gamma$-globulin (i.e., "antiantibody") and antibodies to buried determinants within the human IgG molecules ("pepsin-agglutinators"). Such antiglobulins are grouped together with the poorly studied factors in liver disease, sarcoid, etc., under the general heading of "antiglobulins."[112]

Rheumatoid factors in sera of patients with rheumatoid arthritis may be heterospecific, isospecific, or autospecific. Heterospecific rheumatoid factors react with IgG globulin of infrahuman species; isospecific rheumatoid factors react with IgG globulin from human sera of genetic type other than that of the individual from whom the "antiiso-$\gamma$-globulin" is obtained. Whether or not rheumatoid factors possess preferential autospecificity for autologous undenatured IgG globulin is still uncertain.[5]

During investigations on rheumatoid factor Grubb[135] in 1956 noted that some sera from patients with rheumatoid arthritis agglutinated Rh+ red cells coated with certain incomplete anti-Rh sera, but did not agglutinate cells coated with other anti-Rh sera of equivalent or greater titer. Certain of the agglutinating systems were inhibited by some human sera, but not by others. Grubb and Laurell[137] showed that the inhibitory activity present in normal sera resided in the $\gamma$-globulins, and hence termed the factor responsible for the inhibition "Gm($a$)(1)," an abbreviation for $\gamma$-globulin. Gm($a$)(1) inhibitory activity was inherited as a simple Mendelian genetic autosomal trait. Soon

TABLE X.  Allotypic Specificities of Human Immunoglobulins

| Original | New | Ref. |
|---|---|---|
| Notation for the factors at the Gm locus* | | |
| $a$ | 1 | 137 |
| $X$ | 2 | 146 |
| $b^w$ and $b^2$ | 3 | 333 |
| $f$ | 4 | 128 |
| $b$ and $b^1$ | 5 | 143 |
| $c$ | 6 | 330 |
| $r$ | 7 | 33 |
| $e$ | 8 | 309 |
| $p$ | 9 | 366 |
| $b\alpha$ | 10 | 308 |
| $b\beta$ | 11 | 308 |
| $b\gamma$ | 12 | 308 |
| $b^3$ | 13 | 331 |
| $b^4$ | 14 | 331 |
| $S$ | 15 | 231 |
| $t$ | 16 | 231 |
| Z-Rockefeller | 17 | 211 |
| Rouen-2 | 18 | 310 |
| Rouen-3 | 19 | 310 |
| Z-San Francisco | 20 | 186 |
| $g$ | 21 | 248 |
| $y$ | 22 | 209 |
| $c^3$ | — | † |
| $c^5$ | — | † |
| $m$ | — | 126 |
| $n$ | — | 196 |
| Notation for the factors at the Inv locus | | |
| 1 | 1 | 309 |
| $a$ | 2 | 307 |
| $b$ | 3 | 334 |

\* A number has not been assigned to Gm(D) because it has been found to be an artifact and not a Gm factor.

† E. van Loghem, and L. Martensson, personal communication.

afterward two other genetically determined, serologically detectable differences in human $\gamma$-globulin were found through the use of different reagent pairs (i.e., anti-Rh "coat" and rheumatoid serum agglutinator); these were termed Gm($x$)(2) and Gm($b$)(5), respectively.[143,146] In family studies the genes determining Gm($a$)(1) and Gm($b$)(5) appeared to be inherited in a manner compatible with autosomal codominant inheritance (at least in Caucasians). However, recent biochemical data (see below) suggest that this simple interpretation may be incorrect and that these two factors are probably determined by two distinct, but possibly closely linked, genetic loci.

Subsequently it became evident that anti-$\gamma$-globulins in nonrheumatoid sera provided sharper delineation between positive (i.e., inhibitory) and negative (i.e., noninhibitory) sera in one or another Gm system[329] (the origin of these nonrheumatoid antiglobulins is discussed below.) Use of such highly specific nonrheumatoid antiglobulin reagents greatly facilitated subsequent studies, and led to the rapid detection of many additional genetically determined differences in human $\gamma$-globulin. Thus, as of January 1968, 25 Gm factors are known (Table X). These Gm factors are all restricted to the heavy (H, $\gamma$) chain of IgG globulin. Table X also lists three additional factors, Inv (1), ($a$), and ($b$). These Inv factors are inherited independently of the Gm factors and are under control of genes at the Inv locus; the Inv factors are present on the light chains and are therefore found in all three major immunoglobulins, IgG, IgA, and IgM. It appears, however, that they are present only in light chains of the $\kappa$ antigenic subgroup. Another factor, the $O_Z$ factor, has recently been found on $\lambda$-type light chains.[7] The factor is present on some, but not all, $\lambda$-type myeloma light chains. So far no genetic factors have been detected for the $\alpha$ and the $\mu$ heavy chains of IgA and IgM.

**Source of Reagents.** Standard test systems for each Gm factor involve as antigen Rh+ cells coated with incomplete Rh antibody of a given Gm specificity, and human antiglobulins specific for the Gm factor. IgG globulin (whether in the isolated state or in whole serum) positive for the factor inhibits the agglutination system, whereas protein lacking this Gm factor fails to inhibit. In general, antiglobulins specific for one or another of the known Gm factors are detected by screening human sera for agglutinating activity against Rh+ red cells coated with IgG incomplete antibodies of known Gm type.[391] As stated above, nonrheumatoid agglutinators ("SNagg's"—serum normal agglutinant)[317] are now generally used as typing reagents in most laboratories, since, in contradistinction to rheumatoid sera ("Ragg"),[328] they are usually monospecific for only one Gm factor, and also because they provide better differentiation between inhibitory (+) and noninhibitory (−) normal sera. For example, nonrheumatoid agglutinators

("SNagg's") can provide test systems in which normal Gm(−) sera produce no inhibition even when undiluted, but which are inhibited by dilutions of Gm(+) sera as great as 1:2000.[117]

SNagg's presumably arise as a result of exposure of an individual to human γ-globulins containing genetically "foreign" Gm determinants. For example, specific anti-Gm reagents are found in high frequency in children with thalassemia who receive multiple blood transfusions.[4,362] (In our own hands the incidence of anti-Gm factors in children with aplastic anemia receiving similar numbers of transfusions is much lower than in thalassemic children, possibly because the enlarged spleen in thalassemia provides an increased mass of reticuloendothelial tissue, so that the incidence of antibody producers is greater (H. H. Fudenberg and H. Pretty, unpublished observations). The incidence of anti-Gm factors is also high in individuals receiving frequent injections and/or large amounts of γ-globulin for other reasons.[117,349] For example, anti-Gm antibodies were present in 13 of 35 infants studied 1–2 years after exchange or simple transfusion for hemolytic disease of the newborn, and in more than 50% of children without agammaglobulinemia receiving repeated injections of γ-globulin for "allergy." The incidence of anti-γ-globulins was much higher in children exposed to these known antigenic stimuli than in their normal sibling controls. In contrast, agammaglobulinemic subjects who lack the ability to form antibodies to any antigen failed to form anti-Gm factors despite their frequent exposure to large doses of parenterally injected γ-globulin.

Anti-Gm factors also occurred frequently in subjects studied after open heart surgery.[299] Such patients received an average of 12 units of blood during the procedure, and samples were obtained about three months after open heart surgery. Approximately 50% of such patients developed anti-γ-globulins, many specific for one or another known Gm factor. The anti-γ-globulins in the remaining subjects presumably reflect antibodies directed to Gm specificities not yet delineated. In all studies anti-Gm($a$) was the antibody most frequently formed. Since Gm($a$−)($1$−) individuals constitute about 40% of the Caucasian population, and since 90% of Caucasian individuals are positive for Gm($b$)(5) and Gm($f$)(4), on a statistical basis anti-Gm($a$)(1) should be found much more frequently than anti-Gm($b$)(5) or anti-Gm($f$)(4).

Anti-Gm antibodies can also be produced by deliberate repeated immunization of humans negative for a given Gm factor with γ-globulin positive for this factor.[118,202] Both whole plasma of incompatible Gm type[118] and isolated IgG globulin[202] have been used for this purpose. However, because of the occasional adverse effects of Gm–anti-Gm interaction, such deliberate immunization appears unethical and contraindicated, since the volunteer recipients might subsequently be exposed to "Gm-incompatible" plasma.

Anti-Gm agglutinators are also frequently present as a transient phenomenon in normal infants.[326,327,332,375] Indeed, recent studies by Speiser strongly suggest that all infants who lack a Gm factor present in the mother produce anti-Gm antibodies specifically directed toward one or another maternal Gm factor.[326] The antibodies first appear during the latter part of the first year of life and gradually disappear by the age of three or four years. However, it is possible that at least in some individuals these antibodies persist throughout life, since about 1–2% of normal individuals without a known disease and without known exposure to transfusion have detectable anti-Gm antibodies in their serum.[114] Since the fetus is exposed to maternal γ-globulin during intrauterine life, the invariable formation of anti-Gm antibodies shortly after birth is of great relevance in evaluating data on immune tolerance in humans. These findings, together with recent findings in immunized rabbits[120] and mice[368a] suggest that allotypic determinants cannot induce tolerance.

Since IgG globulin of the fetus appears to cross the placenta into the maternal circulation, anti-Gm agglutinators can also arise by immunization of the mother by fetal γ-globulin.[115] This occurs in those instances in which the fetus has inherited from the father Gm genes that are not present in the mother's, for example, if the fetus of a Gm($a-$)($1-$) mother inherits a Gm($a$)(1) gene from the father, Gm($a$ +)(1) globulin may enter the maternal circulation. In such circumstances the mother may be immunized by the Gm($a$)(1) antigen. (This postulated mechanism for anti-Gm formation is analogous to formation of anti-Rh antibodies in Rh-negative mothers of Rh-positive infants.) Indeed, the Gm types of one of the present authors [HF-Gm($a+f+$)($1+4+$)] and of his wife [Gm($a-f+$)($1-4+$)] made it likely that half of their offspring would be positive for the Gm($a$) factor present in the father but absent in the mother. Hence, the first search for anti-Gm production due to fetal–maternal incompatibility involved HF, BRF,and their offspring.Serum samples obtained from BRF during and after each of her four pregnancies over an eight-year period were tested for anti-Gm activity. Anti-Gm activity did not appear in maternal serum during or after the first three pregnancies; however, these three offspring were Gm($a-$)($1-$). During the fourth pregnancy an anti-Gm($a$) agglutinator was detected in the maternal serum at the beginning of the third trimester (this fourth pregnancy was uncomplicated; specifically, the mother received no transfusions or injections during its course). Serial serum samples obtained from BRF at term and in weekly intervals thereafter lacked significant amounts of anti-Gm($a$)(1). The serum of the fourth infant at birth was weakly Gm($a+$)($1+$) inhibitory in the Gm($a$)(1) test system and gradually increased in inhibitory capacity over a two-year period. These data indicate that endogenous synthesis of Gm($a+$)($1+$) γ-globulin by the fetus of this Gm($a-$)($1-$) mother was already occurring by the seventh month of gestation, and that the amounts synthesized are sufficient to immunize the mother. The exact incidence of this phenomenon is unknown, but is currently under study.

In addition to human anti-Gm antisera, reagents produced in other species have been used by several groups. Thus, rhesus monkeys, lacking most, if not all, known Gm factors, when immunized with pooled human FII occasionally produce anti-human globulin reagents which are useful for Gm typing when used in conjunction with a highly specific coat.[3,157] Similarly, rabbit antisera produced to myeloma proteins positive for only one Gm factor and subsequently absorbed with myeloma proteins lacking this factor often provide valuable anti-Gm reagents.[211] Indeed, such reagents led to the discovery of factors Gm(17), Gm(21), and Gm($n$).[196,209,210]

For Gm typing of the factors listed in Table X antiglobulins are used to establish an agglutination system for each factor. Proteins and sera are typed by inhibition of agglutination or dispersal of agglutination.[198] The recent delineation of two subclasses of $IgG_2$ myeloma proteins on the basis of precipitation or nonprecipitation with a rabbit antiserum to one $IgG_2$ myeloma protein and the development of a precipitating system for Gm(5) and Gm(21) raises the possibility that in due course precipitating systems may be developed for all Gm factors.[196]

The applicability of Gm typing to many immunologic problems has been hampered by the scarcity not only of anti-Gm reagents, but also by the difficulties in obtaining high-titer anti-Rh sera specific for each of the various Gm factors. Thus, few if any of the laboratories currently active in this field have anti-Rh sera specific for each of the various Gm factors; work at present is consequently dependent on the (thus far) remarkably harmonious interchange of such sera between various laboratories. However, in recent studies chromatographically isolated IgG globulin of one or another Gm type devoid of anti-Rh activity has been coated on tanned red cells, and this antigen used successfully for Gm typing systems with certain anti-Gm reagents (Natvig and Kunkel,[249] and H. Borel and F. H. Allen, Jr., personal communication). If this method proves applicable for typing systems for all Gm factors, it will eliminate the need for anti-Rh sera and thus greatly facilitate Gm typing. Thus far such antigens work effectively with some anti-Gm reagents, but not with all; in particular, SNagg reagents appear to be markedly superior in the tanned cell system than are rheumatoid arthritis anti-Gm's. Other methods of coating IgG globulin on inert cells appear to hold considerable promise of proving stable antigens;[364] however, attempts to use latex or bentonite particles coated with human IgG of appropriate Gm type has thus far been unrewarding.[364]

**Mode of Inheritance.** As stated earlier, two sets of genetically determined antigens are inherited independently of one another in human immunoglobulins (the Gm and Inv factors). The Gm factors are inherited in phenogroups, which vary in different ethnic groups[13,74,110,196,209,210,313,328,377] (also H. H. Fudenberg and H. Pretty, unpublished observations). For example, in Caucasians the various Gm(*b*) determinants together with Gm(4) are inherited as a phenogroup; hence, a normal individual is either positive for all of these factors or negative for all.[331] Similarly, Gm(*a*) [also termed Gm(1)] and Gm(*g*) [Gm(21)] are inherited concordantly in Caucasians, so that a normal Caucasian is either Gm(*a*+*g*+)(1+21+) or Gm(*a*−*g*−)(1−21−).[248] As shown by family studies, a "heterozygous" individual, i.e., Gm(*a*+*g*+, *f*+*b*+) − (1+21+, 4+5+), has inherited the gene(s) for Gm(*a*, *g*)(1, 21) from one parent and for Gm(*f*, *b*)(4, 5) from the other. Thus, the data obtained in family studies are compatible with one genetic locus which determines the elaboration of all Gm factors[229]; however, studies with isolated myeloma proteins have demonstrated that Gm(*a*)(1) and Gm(*f*)(4) and the recently discovered factors 17 and 22 are restricted to proteins of the $IgG_1$ antigenic subclass, and Gm(*g*)(21) and Gm(*b*)(5) to proteins of the $IgG_3$ subclass. Further, Gm(*a*)(1) and (*f*)(4) are present in a much larger percentage of IgG globulin molecules than are Gm(*g*)(21) and (*b*)(5),[348] and the ratio of Gm(*b*)(5) to Gm(*a*)(1) molecules is considerably higher in the newborn than in the adult, implying genetic control by different loci which are "turned on" at different stages in biologic development.[230] These data, especially when taken in combination, suggest that at least two cistrons determine the elaboration of the Gm factors, the $IgG_1$ cistron being represented by the genes $Gm^1$ and $Gm^4$ (as well as other genes allelic with $Gm^1$ and $Gm^4$, e.g., $Gm^{1,2}$), and those at the $IgG_3$ cistron (at least in Caucasians) by $Gm^{21}$ and $Gm^b$ (in this view one $Gm^b$ gene determines the elaboration of a multiplicity of antigenic factors including, $Gm^5$, $Gm^{10}$, $Gm^{11}$, $Gm^{12}$, and $Gm^{13}$. Presumably, according to the proponents of multiple loci, two other genetic loci exist; these cistrons determine the presence or absence of genetically determined antigens on the H chains of IgG globulin molecules of the $IgG_2$ and $IgG_4$ subclasses.

Thus, considerable controversy exists as to the number of Gm loci. Those who define a genetic locus on the basis of the lack of recombination of the measurable factors in family studies hypothesize one Gm locus; those who define it on the basis of antigenic differences in proteins which presumably reflect significant differences in primary structure of polypeptide chains (i.e., those who define a gene as a nucleotide region coding for one given class of polypeptide chains) postulate multiple loci. Though this controversy has not been completely resolved, recent data on the structural bases for the variations in Gm factors and antigenic subclasses of IgG globulin (see below) are of considerable relevance in evaluation of the two contending theories.

## II. RELATION OF GENETIC FACTORS TO POLYPEPTIDE CHAINS AND DIFFERENCES IN PRIMARY STRUCTURE

### Mouse

At the present time no published reports on chemical structure of mouse allotypes are available. This section will therefore be devoted solely to a description of the submolecular localization of the mouse allotypic specificities. As previously mentioned, four immunoglobulin loci have been described: Ig-1 for $IgG_{2a}$ heavy chains, Ig-2 for IgA heavy chains, Ig-3 for $IgG_{2b}$ heavy chains, and Ig-4 for $IgG_1$ heavy chains.

### Ig-1 Locus

Ten antigenic specificities have been assigned by Herzenberg and Warner to this locus (Table IV). Each of these specificities was defined by the pattern of inhibition of precipitation given by normal mouse sera of the eight allelic types in different antigen–antibody precipitation assays. When a specificity was found to be present in mice of allelic types *a* or *e*, a positive assignment of the specificity to a given immunoglobulin heavy chain could be made through the availability of myeloma proteins in each of these allelic groups. Accordingly, specificities 1, 2, 5–8, and 10 were assigned to the Ig1 locus. This leaves specificities Ig1.3, 4, and 11. Iodine-125-labeled preparations of slow-migrating $\gamma$-$G_2$-globulin from C57B1 mice are precipitated by both rabbit antisera to the $IgG_{2a}$ class-defining specificity and by the alloantisera directed to specificity 1.4. Since both these antisera can precipitate at least 80 % of the labeled preparation, Ig1.4 must be on an $IgG_{2a}$ molecule. Similarly, a DBA/2 slow-moving $\gamma$-globulin fraction was maximally precipitated (about 80 %) by alloantisera specific for either Ig1.2 or Ig1.3. Since Ig1.2 has previously been shown to be on $IgG_{2a}$ molecules and since specificities 1.2 and 1.3 must be on the same molecule on DBA/2 mice, this defines Ig1.3 as being an $IgG_{2a}$ specificity. Similarly, Ig1.11 was shown to be on $IgG_{2a}$ globulin. In the studies by Lieberman and Potter[207,294,295] only four antigenic determinants could definitely be assigned to the $IgG_{2a}$ class, since myeloma proteins were not available in any strain other than BALB/c mice. This left five unassigned antigenic determinants. All of these five determinants were presumed to be 7S immunoglobulin determinants, since in immunoelectrophoretic plates the precipitin arcs have an electrophoretic mobility characteristic of 7S immunoglobulins. Determinants 1–5 were all shown to be controlled by five allelic chromosome regions.[121,204] Comparison of the strain distribution of these specificities with specificities defined by Herzenberg and Warner suggest a probable equivalence for all but two of the specificities (Table IV).

The submolecular localization of several of these specificities has been analyzed. Mishell and Fahey[243] studied a pair of isoantigens at the same locus, and showed that they were present on $IgG_{2a}$ globulins, and, furthermore, that they were present only on the Fc part of the molecule. Subsequently Dray and Young[62] also showed that the specific determinants on $IgG_{2a}$ and $IgG_{2b}$ were localized to the Fc fragment, using alloantisera prepared in LP mice immunized with a BALB/c $IgG_{2a}$ myeloma. Potter also showed that the allotypic specificity detected by this antiserum was located on the Fc fragment. Analysis by Warner and Herzenberg (unpublished observations) has shown that specificity Ig1.5, which is present on an NZB $IgG_{2a}$ myeloma, is also located on the Fc fragment.

The Fc papain fragments from several myeloma proteins from the $IgG_{2a}$ class have been shown to give virtually identical tryptic peptide maps.[295] It will be of interest to determine whether multiple differences will be found by this chemical method, since several antigenic differences exist between the $IgG_{2a}$ H chains of these two alleles.

## Ig-2 Locus

Several anti-DBA/2 alloantisera were shown to form two lines of precipitation on Ouchterlouny tests with DBA/2 serum.[151] One band is due to a reaction with the Ig1.3 determinant present on $IgG_{2a}$ globulin, the second to a reaction of a serum protein with the following properties: electrophoretic mobility on agar gel and starch block identical to IgA heterogeneous sedimentation in sucrose density gradients partly in the $7S$ region, but extending almost to the $19S$ region; absence in newborn serum; and, finally, complete precipitation of this protein by specific rabbit anti-mouse IgA. This constituted the first description of an allotype on IgA globulin. A second serum was then found to recognize an IgA alloantigen in the C3H strain. Michell and Fahey[151] also showed that these Ig2 antigens were located to the Fc fragment of IgA molecules.

Three IgA allotypic specificities have been defined by Lieberman and Potter,[207] and were shown to be on the Fc fragment of the IgA myeloma. Several plasma cell tumors in BALB/c mice produce $3.9S$ IgA protein that appears in the urine. This protein contains one $\kappa$-type light chain and one $\alpha$ chain.[293] It has been called an IgA halfmer molecule. Homologous antisera prepared against several of these halfmers do not precipitate with normal sera from many inbred strains, but do precipitate the halfmers from several BALB/c plasma cell tumors, irrespective of the halfmers used to prepare the homologous antisera. None of the halfmers were precipitated by the alloantisera that defined the IgA allotypic specificities of Lieberman and Potter. It would therefore appear that these IgA allotypic specificities are dependent on the quaternary structure of the IgA molecule. It has been pointed out by Potter and Lieberman[300] that the IgA immunoglobulins of several strains lose their antigenicity during storage and repeated freezing and thawing. Preliminary studies by Abel and Grey (unpublished observations) have suggested that mouse IgA is like human IgA of the minor sub-class,[94,195,360] that is, the chains separate in starch urea gels without prior reduction. These latter two observations may be relevant to each other in again suggesting that the allotypic specificities of IgA are dependent upon the quaternary structure of the molecule.

## Ig-3 Locus

Lieberman *et al.*[206] identified allotypic specificities on two different myeloma proteins and the corresponding normal IgG globulins of BALB/c mice. Further studies[61,295] showed that these alloantibodies corresponded to antigenic determinants on either the $IgG_{2a}$ or $IgG_{2b}$ immunoglobulin class. The $IgG_{2b}$ determinants were also localized on the Fc fragment. It should be pointed out that all studies with allotypic specificities of the $IgG_{2b}$ globulins have been hampered by the great difficulty experienced in the production of appropriate alloantisera. In many cases, although many mice are immunized with an identical procedure, only one mouse out of a large number produces alloantibodies specific for the $IgG_{2b}$ globulins, and, furthermore, on repeated immunization these alloantibodies may disappear. Another difficulty arises in that in most cases of immunization with antibodies derived from normal mice (as against immunization with myeloma proteins) the alloantisera contain antibodies directed to both $IgG_{2a}$ and $IgG_{2b}$ allotypic antigens. Appropriate absorptions of these sera with myeloma proteins of either type are often useful in the production of specific sera which will react to the allotypic antigens of only one immunoglobulin class.[153,370] Immunization of strain A/He or AL mice with BALB/c $IgG_{2b}$ myeloma proteins has been shown to produce antisera specific for $IgG_{2b}$ allotypic specificities.[295] One as yet unexplained result obtained from these sera has been that after absorption of antisera with normal BALB/c serum (which would be expected to remove all alloantibodies to BALB/c-type $IgG_{2b}$ globulin) the sera still possess an unexpected capacity to precipitate $IgG_{2b}$ myeloma immunoglobulins from BALB/c mice *and* normal $IgG_{2b}$ immunoglobulins from the serum of eight strains carrying another unassigned determinant. This finding would seem to suggest similarity between BALB/c $IgG_{2b}$ myeloma proteins and the normal $IgG_{2b}$ protein in genetically different strains. Further studies are clearly necessary to explain this unusual phenomenon. In independent studies six allotypic determinants of $IgG_{2b}$ globulins were described by Warner *et al.*[153,369,370] Specific localization to the $IgG_{2b}$ class could again be positively assigned to all of these determinants, since (using myeloma proteins) five were present in BALB/c mice and the remaining one was present in A/J mice.

## Ig-4 Locus

The Ig-4 locus responsible for the coding of $IgG_1$ heavy chain was defined by Herzenberg *et al.*[152,242] on the basis of specific electrophoretic mobility of the Fc fragment of $IgG_1$ globulins in different mouse strains. The segregation of this $IgG_1$ heavy-chain locus was followed through an intercross and found to be tightly linked to the other heavy-chain gene loci. No allotypic specificities at this locus were detected with alloantisera by Herzenberg's group.[153] In studies by Potter and Lieberman[294] the $IgG_1$ immunoglobulins were also not shown to possess a unique polymorphism as detected by specific allotypic antigens. However, Dray *et al.*[61] did report that several antisera prepared with normal immunoglobulins precipitated very weakly with $IgG_1$ myeloma proteins, although very strongly with $IgG_{2a}$ proteins. Initially it was assumed that the $IgG_1$ myeloma protein was contaminated with $IgG_{2a}$ globulin. Further analysis with these antisera was then made by Potter and Lieberman.[294] The same antisera were tested against a purified Fc fragment from two different $IgG_1$ myeloma proteins. The data obtained indicated that the myeloma MOPC-21 and $IgG_{2a}$ proteins shared common antigenic determinants present on the Fc fragment. The determinants were designated G8 and F8, and showed the same distribution among mouse inbred strains. Direct immunization of LP mice with the $IgG_1$ myeloma protein MOPC-21 gave antisera which identify determinant 8. The unexpected finding in this system was that this antiserum, which reacted with the MOPC-21 Fc fragment, did not precipitate the Fc fragment of another $IgG_1$ myeloma (MOPC-31). The tryptic peptides in the Fc fragments of these two $IgG_1$ myeloma proteins were quite similar. The possibility must exist, however, that these do belong to different $IgG_1$ subgroups. If this were the case, it would suggest the sharing of an allotypic antigen between one of these $IgG_1$ groups and $IgG_{2a}$ globulin.

## Shared Allotypic Specificities

In all the preceding studies the allotypic specificities defined were shown to be present on only a single immunoglobulin-class heavy chain. This situation is completely compatible with the Gm system in man, where each allotypic specificity is located on a given IgG subgroup. Three allotypic specificities detected by Warner and Herzenberg[369] were, however, found to show an anomolous distribution in myeloma proteins. These specificities had originally been designated Ig1.9, Ig3.5, and Ig3.6, as they were, respectively, first found on $IgG_{2a}$ or $IgG_{2b}$ globulins. Extensive analysis with the antisera and antigens used to define these specificities showed, however, that all three of these allotypic determinants were present on both $IgG_{2a}$ and $IgG_{2b}$ myeloma proteins of BALB/c mice. Since several myeloma proteins were involved and the allotypic antigens were not detected on IgA, IgM, or $IgG_1$ myelomas, it is unlikely that they are located on the L chains on the $IgG_2$ molecules, but rather on the H chains. Submolecular localization of these common allotypic antigens is of considerable importance, since the only other H-chain allotypic specificities thus far found to be present in more than one immunoglobulin class are those of the a locus in rabbits, and these are present in the Fd portion of the H chain. In view of the close linkage of the Ig-1 and Ig-3 loci and the many physicochemical and antigenic similarities of their respective polypeptides, it is very probable that a gene duplication was responsible for the development of these three loci (see later section). Whether the duplication was followed by or preceded by the mutational changes giving rise to the common allotypic specificities, or, indeed, whether an entirely different immune mechanism was responsible for their production, will require further elucidation.

One myeloma protein produced by a plasma cell tumor arising in a (NZB $\times$ BALB/c)$F_1$ hybrid mouse has been found to have a most abnormal distribution of both class-defining and allotypic specificities. Antigenic studies on this myeloma protein, termed GPC-5,[153,370] showed that it carried the class-defining specificity of $IgG_{2b}$ globulin and one of the two $IgG_{2a}$ class-defining specificities. Analysis with mouse alloantisera showed that it carried specificities 1.5 and 3.3. This was therefore the first analyzed mouse myeloma protein not carrying the entire set of allotypic specificities normal to its class and allotype. It is also the first myeloma protein in either man or mouse shown to carry the allotypic specificity, and, inferentially, part of the amino acid sequences of two different immunoglobulin classes, i.e., the gene product of two loci. It was suggested that the participation of parts of two genetic loci in the determination of the heavy chain of GPC-5 may resemble the genetic determination of the Lepore type hemoglobin. These hemoglobins were shown by Baglioni[14] to contain the N-terminal part of the $\delta$ chain joined to the C-terminal part of the $\beta$ chain of hemoglobin. It is postulated that the formation of the hemoglobin Lepore gene is the result of nonhomologous crossing over between corresponding points of the $\beta$ and $\delta$ genes. As the allotypic specificities controlled by the two loci involved in the GPC-5 protein are both of NZB specific type, the recombinational event for GPC-5 must have been intrachromosomal, that is, sister chromatid rather than involving the two homologous chromosomes. Regardless of the genetic mechanism involved, the origin of the GPC-5 gene may have occurred during the development of the tumor, or may have occurred during evolution of the NZB genome, or, finally, be the result of a regular somatic event occurring in plasma-cell differentiation. If either of these latter two are correct, then this myeloma protein could be considered to be the expression of a normal immunoglobulin in NZB serum. Several more $IgG_{2b}$ myeloma proteins have now been produced in $(BALB/c \times NZB)F_1$ hybrid mice. Analysis of their antigenic constitution is proceeding.[367b]

## Rabbit

### a1 Locus

The IgG immunoglobulins of one rabbit may differ from those of another in allotypic antigenic determinants controlled by either the *a* or *b* loci. The allotypic specificities of the a locus have been associated with the heavy polypeptide chains of IgG immunoglobulins.[93,336] Earlier studies had shown that papain digestion of rabbit IgG, which separates the Fc piece of the heavy chain from the Fab piece, leaves all the allotypic determinants in the Fab piece; none are detectable in the Fc piece.[183,226] These results therefore localized the *a*-locus determinants to the Fd portion of the heavy chain of rabbit IgG immunoglobulin. Since the class-defining specificities which distinguish the different immunoglobulin heavy-chain classes are localized on the Fc fragment rather than on the Fd, and since common antigenic determinants had been previously shown on the Fd fragments of $IgG_1$ and $IgG_2$ globulins in guinea pigs,[254] it is pertinent to examine the distribution of the *a*-locus alleles in the different immunoglobulin classes. In the first description of IgA immunoglobulin in the rabbit by Feinstein[92] allotypic specificities As1, As2, and As3 were shown to be present on the IgA globulin. However, in a following study[36] As1 and As2 specificities could not be found on the IgA immunoglobulin isolated from colostrum. It was suggested[316] that the *a*-locus determinants may have been missed if antisera of insufficient strength were used, since in another study on rabbit colostrum IgA the allotypic specificities controlled by the *a* locus were again positively identified to be present on the IgA immunoglobulin.[203,316]

In 1963 Todd[354] presented evidence that the allotypic specificities of the *a* locus are present on the IgM molecule as well as on IgG. Stemke and Fischer[338] also demonstrated this association in showing that the neutralizing activity of antisera against bacteriophage T4 obtained eight days after primary immunization is due to IgM antibody and that this neutralizing activity could be partially inhibited by treatment of antiserum directed against the group-*a* allotypic specificity carried by the whole rabbit serum. The extent to which the allotypes present on the heavy chains are duplicated on the two immunoglobulins IgM and IgG has been investigated by inhibition of phage neutralization and by radiotracer technique.[355] The inhibition by antiallotype sera of phage neutralization by IgM antibody was shown to be essentially completely removed by prior absorption of the antiallotype sera with IgG of the same heavy-chain allotype. However, a preparation of IgM containing allotype As1 exhausted extensively but not completely the precipitating ability of the anti-As1 serum for an As1 IgG preparation labeled with [125]I. It was concluded that in the allotype sera investigated all of the antibodies directed against the allotypic sites present on the heavy chain of IgM react with IgG, but not all the antibodies directed against the heavy-chain allotypic sites present on IgG are capable of reacting with IgM.

These facts therefore demonstrate that the antigenic site responsible for the allotypic specificity present on the H chain of IgG is structurally related to its counterpart on the H chain of IgM. Several possibilities could be invoked to explain the antigenic deficiency of IgM with respect to IgG. Some of the sites on IgM might be hidden by association of the molecular subunits. Alternatively, the alloantisera which are produced against IgG immunoglobulin may recognize configurations arising from interaction at such sites, and which are not completely reproduced in the IgM molecule.

Several studies have indicated that the allotypic specificities of the heavy chain in rabbit IgG are determined by amino acid sequence differences, rather than by a prosthetic group such as carbohydrate. Tryptic peptide maps of the heavy polypeptide chains derived from rabbits of different genotypes have shown practically identical fingerprints.[333] However the patterns of heavy polypeptide chains carrying the As2 allotypic specificity can be distinguished from those carrying either As1 or As3 by the presence of a yellow spot and the absence of a brown spot. These distinguishing spots are absent from the peptide map of the corresponding Fc fragment. It should be noted, however, that a significant portion of the Fd fragment appears to be too heterogeneous to be examined by the fingerprint method, since only a few additional spots are found in the intact heavy chain as compared to the map of the Fc fragment.

Detailed amino acid compositions of purified rabbit antibodies to hapten antigens prepared in rabbits of different allotypes of the $a$ locus have shown that there are many differences in composition between antibodies $a^1$, $a^2$, and $a^3$ of homozygous rabbits. They involve at least 12 residues, involving six amino acids, and may therefore extend over a lengthy portion of the Fd fragment.[187] Independent studies have also shown that the amino acid composition is significantly different for the three allotypes As1, As2, and As3 with respect to seven amino acids and possibly four others. A minimum of 4–9 positions on the Fd fragment are involved when any two allotypes are compared.[172] Previous studies, based on the finding of characteristic differences in the average amino acid composition of five purified antibodies,[189] have shown that the specificity of antibodies is determined by differences in their primary structure. These differences were shown to be independent of those associated with the allotypic differences and also independent of the charge on the determinant group of the antigen employed.[187] It therefore appears from both of these studies that multiple amino acid differences are involved in the allotypic variation between the $a^1$, $a^2$, and $a^3$ alleles. This is in contrast to the single amino acid substitution reported to be responsible for alleles at the Inv locus. To determine more precisely the location of these amino acid differences, Fd fragments of purified antibodies obtained from rabbits of different allotypes were cleaved with cyanogen bromide. Studies of the amino acid compositions of the peptides produced by this cleavage revealed that the changes associated with antibody specificity were distributed over a considerable sequence which extends close to the C-terminal end of the Fd fragment. The distribution of amino acid changes associated with the allotypic markers also overlapped those involved in antibody specificity, indicating that allotypic antigens were controlled by variations in several nonconsecutive segments of the Fd sequence.[188] Preliminary sequence studies of the heavy chain of rabbit immunoglobulin G has been reported by Porter.[285] In one position a correlation with allotype was evident; arginine was found to be missing in a peptide from As3 rabbits, but present in rabbits of As1 and As2. Preliminary studies, in fact, suggested that positions near the beginning of Fd and at the beginning of the Fc sections were both under the control of the same gene, suggesting that the whole chain in fact is coded for by one gene.

## a2 Locus

The $a2$ gene was defined by Hamers et al.[142] as the gene corresponding to the immunoglobulin class termed $IgG_2$ which carries the allotypic specificity As8. This allotypic specificity has not been found to be present on either rabbit IgM, IgA, or $IgG_1$ molecules. Analysis of papain fragments of rabbit IgG globulins which include $IgG_1$ and $IgG_2$ confirmed previous observations in showing that the As1 specificity was present in the Fab fragment, but Hamers further demonstrated the distinction of the $IgG_2$ class in that the specificity As8 was present in the Fc fragment of the molecule.[139]

## Ms Locus

The allotypic specificity Ms1 was detected by Kelus and Gell[181] using a typing serum raised by immunization of an As3, 4, and 5 rabbit with anti-

*Proteus* antibody from an As3, 4 donor. The specificity detected appeared to localize on the IgM as judged by immunodiffusion, ultracentrifugation, and gel-filtration analysis. It was not present on IgG globulins. A second specificity (probably allelic) demonstrated by Sell[315] was also shown to be present on macroglobulin. Submolecular localization of these specificities has not yet been described. One recent study has shown a most unusual association of two of the Ms determinants.[179] In tests for the occurrence of As3 and Ms1 determinants in individual serums samples possessing Ms1 were never found in an animal lacking As3. Similarly, individuals having Ms2 and lacking As4 were never observed. As3 is located on the H chain and As4 on the L chain, and the *a* and *b* genes appear to be unlinked, thus this observed interrelationship between the Ms and As specificities cannot be easily explained. At the present time it is not known if the As and Ms allotypic specificities are located on the same or different IgM molecules. Preliminary experiments suggest that they occur separately.[179]

## B Locus

Specificities As4, 5, and 6 are controlled by alleles at the second locus *b*. Studies with IgG chain separation showed that the light chain contains the *b*-locus determinants.[93] However, in the heavy chain both *a*- and *b*-locus determinants were detected by the qualitative methods of testing used. Stemke[336] showed evidence which suggested that such results were in fact due to contamination of the heavy chain with light chain. Using highly purified rabbit H chains Wilheim and Lamm[373] were in fact able to show complete absence of As4 determinants from purified H chains. The specificities of the *b* locus are therefore restricted solely to rabbit light chains. The specificity As9 appears to be related to the *b* locus, since in heterozygous rabbits As9 is associated with only one other specificity of the *b* group, whereas rabbits homozygous for As9 do not have allotypic specificities As4, 5, or 6. An evaluation was made of the number of As4 allotypic determinants of rabbit IgG immunoglobulins using double-labeled techniques with univalent antibody fragments.[219] Antibody–antigen molar ratios in the soluble complexes of univalent anti-As4 Fab fragments reacting with IgG immunoglobulin from As4 homozygous rabbits implied that some of the IgG immunoglobulin molecules had a minimum of two or three As4 determinants per light polypeptide chain. As previously described, confirmatory evidence was also obtained for the lack of As4 specificity from some IgG molecules.

Differences in amino acid composition of light polypeptide chains of rabbit IgG were studied by Reisfeld *et al.*[305] Light chains carrying As4 differed from those carrying As5 by an average of 15 residues per chain, involving seven amino acids. In studies with L chains by the method of starch urea electrophoresis not correlation was found between the allotype and the band pattern. However, peptide maps of purified rabbit L chains isolated from homozygous As4 and As5 rabbits showed detectable differences, correlating with the allotype in at least three peptides giving strong spots, and hence likely to derive from the constant portion in the polypeptide chain.[322] This again contrasts with the single difference found in human light-chain allotypes, but does agree with the study of Mage et al.[219] in showing multiple antigenic determinants on the light chain.

### Human

### Molecular and Submolecular Localization of the Genetic Factors

Generalizations regarding genetic control of the synthesis of a variety of well-studied proteins have been derived from experiments with unicellular microorganisms and with other vertebrate proteins, such as the hemoglobins, cytochromes, and haptoglobins.[34] While it appears likely that many of the conclusions derived from such studies will also be applicable to the immunoglobulins, some question remains, in view of the unique variability in structure required by the immunoglobulins for their proper function. Since this variability is greater than that encountered in any other protein, the possibility exists that additional, hitherto unrecognized genetic mechanisms may operate in the control of immunoglobulin synthesis. However, recent studies of the synthesis of light and heavy chains in mouse and rabbit lymphoid tissue have clearly demonstrated that the assembly of these chains appears to be similar to that of all other proteins studied to date.[11,21,318]

While the control of the synthesis of the variable regions of the antibody molecules is difficult to explain at this time, it would appear that synthesis of the constant region follows the classical rules of inheritance worked out in these other systems. Thus, as already demonstrated with many complex proteins, one genetic locus controls the synthesis of a single type of polypeptide chain; consequently, genetic factors controlled at any one locus express themselves on only a single type of chain.[105,110,113,147,227,228,348]

The early studies clearly demonstrated that Gm activity was associated only with the IgG globulin;[226] in contrast, Inv activity was associated with normal and "pathological" IgG, IgM, and IgA globulins, as well as the Bence-Jones proteins.[105,144] ($\gamma_E$ and $\gamma_D$ have not been tested; however, it seems likely that they too will have Inv activity.) Since Inv activity was found in the Fab fragment of IgG,[105,147] and, more specifically, in the light chains, and since light chains are common to all immunoglobulins, Inv activity must, of necessity, be associated with all immunoglobulin types* (Inv activity appears, however, to be restricted to type-$\kappa$ light chain).

The reason for the restriction of the Gm factors to IgG globulin became obvious when Gm(1), (2), and (5) ($a$, $x$, and $b$) [and, more recently, Gm(22)($y$)] were located on the Fc fragment of the $\gamma$-chain, the structural unit unique to the IgG globulins.[105,147] All the Gm factors found to date have been located on the (heavy) chain of IgG; however, two of them, Gm(3, 4)† and (17), were subsequently found to be located in the Fab fragment, presumably the piece.[127,190,209,210,283] Of particular interest is the finding that these factors are not detectable on either the isolated light or heavy chain, but require the presence of both in a reconstituted form. Since in these studies the specificity depended on the Gm type of the heavy chain, while any $\lambda$ or $\kappa$ light chain regardless of its origin or Inv type could restore activity to the proper heavy chain, it would appear that the serologic specificity resides in the heavy chain, while the light chain may simply provide the proper quaternary structures necessary for the expression of the Gm specificity in the serological assay.[283]

Recent correlative studies of the $\gamma$-chain subgroups and the Gm factors have provided a number of provocative and interesting findings which have resulted in a revaluation of the probable mode of inheritance of these factors. The localization of Gm(1), (2), (3), (4), (17), and (22) only on molecules of the IgG$_1$ class, Gm(5) and (21) on molecules of the IgG$_3$ class,[194,228] and, more recently, Gm($n$) on molecules of the IgG$_2$ class has raised the possibility that there are at least three closely linked loci, each controlling the synthesis of a single polypeptide chain, instead of a single locus with multiple alleles. The finding that Gm(5) and (21) are localized to the IgG$_3$ class also explains their relative greater lability on papain digestion, since the Fc fragments of this subgroup are rapidly destroyed by papain.[298,345]

It should be noted that studies with homogeneous myeloma proteins and Bence-Jones proteins have been particularly useful in elucidating the possible molecular distribution of Gm and Inv activity in the molecules of a heterozygous subject. While a few IgG$_1$ myeloma proteins from Chinese individuals were both (1+) and (4+), all Caucasian and Negro myeloma proteins have been shown to carry no more than one of the four major genetic factors studied to date [Gm(1), (5), (4), or (21)].[194,228] Similarly, Bence-Jones proteins and myeloma proteins possess, at most, one of the known Inv factors on their light chains.

In the case of IgG$_1$ myeloma proteins additional complexity has been

---

* An as yet unexplained finding is the observation that 12 myeloma proteins with $\kappa$ light chains belonging to the IgG$_2$ apd IgG$_4$ subtypes were Inv-negative.[358] To date only the intact proteins have been studied, and the isolated light chains of these proteins have not yet been tested for Inv activity (Steinberg, personal communication, Dec. 1966).

† Gm(3) and (4) appear to be identical.

introduced by the recognition of two major sets of Gm factors. Two of these, Gm(1)(*a*) and (22)(*y*), are always found on the Fc fragment; the other two, Gm(4)(*f*) and (17)(*z*), are on the Fd fragment. Since all Caucasian and Negro myeloma proteins studied to date are Gm(1+), (17+)(*a*+*z*+), or Gm(4+)(*f*+*y*+), these two parts of the heavy chain appear to be under the control of a single locus.[193,209,210] The finding of seral myeloma proteins which were Gm(1+22+4+)(*a*, *y*, *f*) from Chinese patients can best be explained by a process of intragenic crossing over. The existence of both Gm(1)(*a*) and (22)(*y*) in the same Fc fragment clearly indicates that they cannot be homologous.

The studies of myeloma proteins suggest strongly that the $\gamma$-globulin of heterozygous subjects contains a mixture of molecules, some carrying the factor(s) determined by one allele and some by the other, rather than mixed molecules bearing the products of both alleles at each locus.

Similar studies with antibodies to Rh antigens,[6,104,144,228] blood-group substances,[6,380] malaria parasites,[51] and certain simple haptens[6] from a single heterozygous subject have also been informative, but not nearly as definitive as those obtained with paraproteins, presumably because a purified antibody, even to an apparently simple haptenic determinant, is not a homogeneous protein, but rather a mixture of molecules with different binding constants, which are presumably synthesized by a number of different clones of cells. Studies of the distribution of Gm factors in such antibodies produced by heterozygous subjects have shown that in general the number of molecules bearing each of the possible Gm or Inv factors deviated from that in the subject's normal serum, and occasionally one or another Gm factor was completely deleted.[6,51,104,144,228,380] Occasionally, purified antibodies bearing only one of the two possible alleles may be produced by chance. It seems possible that a very simple haptene may eventually induce the production of an antibody that may be as homogeneous as a myeloma protein. It is of some interest that in none of the studies was there any correlation between the specificity of antibodies in different subjects and the Gm type of the isolated antibody, so that the genotype of the cell does not limit the type of antibody produced. The observation that antibodies to a complex antigen, like the malaria parasite, may show genetic deletions suggests that this phenomenon may simply reflect the genetic potential of the clone of cells originally stimulated, and that this may initially have involved only a small number of cells.

In addition to genetic factors already cited, other genetic factors undoubtedly exist, but have not yet been defined in man by the current assay system. Thus, it seems probable that a series of genetic factors, under the control of several other loci, exist for the $\mu$, $\alpha$, $\delta$, and $\epsilon$ chains.

## Molecular Basis of Gm Specificities

Studies aimed at an understanding of the chemical basis of Gm specificity have been progressing rapidly in the past few years. Surprisingly enough, significant data were first obtained from studies of the $\gamma$ chains, and only during the past two years has it been possible to elucidate the differences in light chains differing in their Inv type. Since structural studies of light chains have now progressed further, the differences related to Inv type are well understood. Because of their complexity, the presumed existence of multiple Gm loci, and the apparent existence of multiple differences between closely related Gm factors, our knowledge of the genetic factors associated with the heavy chains is not nearly as far advanced, nor as definitive. Nevertheless, it is quite apparent that the various Gm and Inv determinants reflect differences in the primary structure of the respective polypeptide chains, rather than in the carbohydrate or other prosthetic groups.[15,99,162,234,352] Much of the information has been derived from studies of myeloma proteins and Bence-Jones proteins.

$\kappa$ **Light Chains—Inv(2) and (3).** Studies of peptide maps and of amino acid sequences have clearly demonstrated that $\kappa$ and $\lambda$ chains differ strikingly in their primary structure and that they are probably under separate genetic control. Initial attempts by the techniques of peptide mapping failed to detect any differences in the fingerprints of Bence-Jones proteins of the $\kappa$ type that could be related to the Inv type. More recently similar studies of amino-ethylated proteins, a procedure which makes additional cysteine bonds which are susceptible to the action of trypsin, have revealed the existence of a peptide which assumes a different position in maps from proteins that are Inv(2+) as compared to molecules that are Inv(3+). Isolation of the relevant peptides and amino acid analysis revealed the presence of N-terminal leucine in the Inv(2+) peptide and valine in the peptide from Inv(3+) molecules.[15] The same information was also obtained from the almost complete elucidation of the amino acid sequence of three Bence-Jones proteins, and partial analysis of a number of others, some of which were Inv(2+) and some of which were Inv(3+).[162] These studies revealed that amino acid residues 106–214 were identical in all proteins, with the exception of residue 189, which was leucine in Inv(2+) and valine in Inv(3+) proteins. This type of interchange can be readily explained by a mutation of a single base pair. So far, serologic activity has not been recovered either with the characteristic peptide or with the whole trypsin digest.[15]

$\gamma$ **Chains (Gm).** Structural characteristics related to Gm specificity were first noted in studies of Fc fragments and heavy chains of normal $\gamma$-globulins from Caucasian subjects who were Gm(1+5−), Gm(1−5+), and Gm(1+5+).[234] One peptide was noted to be consistently present in molecules from Gm(1+5−) subjects, which was always absent in those who were Gm(1−5+), while another peptide was present in those who were Gm(1−5+) and absent in proteins of Gm(1+5−) subjects. Both peptides were present in γ-globulin from the heterozygous subjects. With the discovery of other Gm factors, especially Gm(4), which in Caucasians is invariably associated with Gm(5), and the recognition of the existence of several antigenically distinguishable γ-chain subgroups, it became essential to study myeloma proteins, since, as previously stated, such proteins are far more antigenically and genetically homogeneous than the γ-globulin of normal subjects. These studies of myeloma proteins have confirmed the finding in normal subjects of a peptide, termed the "$a$" peptide, which is present only in Fc fragments and heavy chains from Gm(1+) subjects and absent in Gm(1−) proteins.[99,351] The peptide, originally noted to be associated with Gm(5)($b$) and known as the "$b$" spot, has, however, been found in peptide maps from all Gm(1−) [i.e., Gm($a$−)] myeloma proteins belonging to the IgG$_1$, IgG$_2$, and IgG$_3$.[99] Some of these proteins were positive for Gm(4)($f$), others were either Gm(5+)($b$+) or Gm(21+)($g$+), and others negative for all four of these factors. Since the one finding common to all these proteins was the absence of Gm(1) activity, this peptide has how been termed the "non-$a$" peptide. In view of these findings, it is obvious that the "non-$a$" peptide *per se* cannot have serologic specificity. In addition to the presence or absence of the "$a$" and "non-$a$" peptides, the molecules belonging to these three classes differ in a few other peptides, usually in the basic region of the map.[99] It seems possible that some of these may be directly related to the various "non-$a$" serological specificities.

These differences are perhaps relevant to the current controversy as to whether the Gm factors are elaborated by genes at one locus or by genes at several (presumably closely linked) loci. Since IgG$_1$, IgG$_2$, and IgG$_3$ Fc fragments differ from each other by at least several peptides, it would appear that these fragments are constituents of different polypeptide chains. The fourth subgroup IgG$_4$ differs from the other three in lacking both the Gm($a$) and (non-$a$) peptides, and also lacks three other peptides in other regions of the map.[99] All attempts to recover serologic activity from the trypsin digest or the isolated peptides have been unsuccessful to date.

Two recent reports[99,351] provide more-detailed information about the two peptides in question.[99] One of them compared the amino acid analysis of the "$a$" spot with the "non-$a$" spot from Gm(5+), (4+), and Gm(−) proteins. The amino acid composition of all the "non-$a$" spots proved to be identical. Both peptides were pentapeptides. The "$a$" spot consisted of one residue of lysine, aspartic acid, threonine, leucine, and glutamic acid, while the "non-$a$" spot contained three of the same amino acid residues (lysine, threonine, and glutamic acid) and differed in two (glutamic acid and methionine sulfone). Sequence studies by Thorpe and Deutsch[351] have shown that the "*a*" peptide has the sequence: aspartic acid, glutamic acid, leucine, threonine, lysine; while the non-*a*" peptide from a Gm(4+) subject can be written as: methionine, glutamic acid, glutamic acid, threonine, lysine.* Both are part of an undecapeptide which has the structure threonine, leucine, proline, proline, serine, and arginine in the amino-terminal half, and therefore appears to be derived from the same region of the heavy chain.

The precise relationship of these two peptides to each other and their development in evolution remain to be determined.

Sufficient data are not yet available to permit detailed interpretations of the observed structural differences related to the Gm factors. Comparison of the amino acid composition and sequence of the "*a*" spot with that of "non-*a*" spots shows similarities in three of the amino acids (lysine, threonine, and one residue of glutamic acid), and the replacement of an aspartic acid or asparagine and a leucine residue in the "*a*" spot by a glutamic acid residue and a methionine residue in the "non-*a*" spots. The possibility exists that these changes may be the result of point mutations of a structural gene, as is the case for hemoglobins.[171] However, in the absence of definitive proof for such a mechanism alternative possibilities must be considered. Among these is the possibility that the two peptides are derived from each other by other mechanisms recently thought to account for the variability in antibody structure, e.g., nonhomologous crossing-over, unequal homologous crossing-over, interchromatid inversion with reversed complementarity,[324,325] insertion of inactive DNA,[65] and possibly other mechanisms. Another possibility which may explain the existence of at least two nucleotide substitutions is the possibility that the "*a*" and "non-*a*" peptides are not directly related, but have evolved from each other through a number of intermediate stages which remain to be identified. Further speculation seems unwarranted until the amino acid sequence of the pertinent peptides is known and the precise mode of inheritance of these factors is fully elucidated. The delineation of structural difference between Gm(z+)(17+) and Gm(f+)(4+) Fd fragments has been made extremely difficult by the great variability in composition of this part of the molecule; thus, no structural studies are available at this time.

## III. EVOLUTIONARY ASPECTS OF ANTIGENIC DETERMINANTS

Despite the clear-cut distinction of the different immunoglobulins into classes with different properties, many chemical and genetic studies have

---

* Subsequent work (A. C. Wang and H. Fudenberg, *J. Mol. Biol.*, in press) demonstrated that the sequence of the "non-*a*" peptide is Glu-Glu-Met-Thr-Lys.

indicated substantial similarities in structure and genetic control. Studies of the physicochemical nature of humoral antibodies produced in different vertebrate species have shown that a molecule resembling IgG appears in dogfish,[223,225] and by the level of the bullfrog an IgG species evolved.[224] Ontogenically, a similar pattern occurs, in that IgM synthesis precedes IgG synthesis in the developing embryo or fetus.[130,350] These and other studies have led to the concept of an evolution of the immunoglobulin polypeptide chain from a common ancestral gene.

## Within Species

Peptide maps of H chains or Fc fragments of several myeloma proteins in BALB/c mice have shown several notable features: (1) the Fc fragment of different myelomas of the same class are identical; (2) the Fd fragments of different myelomas of the same class are all unique; (3) the Fc fragment of myelomas of different groups either show little similarity at all (IgG$_1$ *versus* IgG$_2$), or show a combination of identity and distinction (IgG$_{2a}$ *versus* IgG$_{2b}$). Furthermore, it has been clearly shown that IgG$_{2a}$ is linked to IgG$_{2b}$, IgA to IgG$_{2a}$, and IgG$_1$ to IgG$_{2a}$. Out of many thousands of mice no recombination has to date been detected between these genetic loci. These results can be interpreted in two ways: (1) the four heavy chain genes for IgG$_{2a}$, IgG$_{2b}$, IgA, and IgG$_1$ (and probably the as yet undetected IgM gene) are very closely linked, and some unusual mechanism for explaining diversity in the Fd region exists, or (2) many genes are present within the region of each H-chain type, but with accumulation of mutations representing different antibody specificities. The latter concept of a highly redundant region is unlikely, since (1) no mutation can have occurred in the Fc region of the different genes of a given class (on the basis of the proteins so far examined), and (2) evidence of recombination would be expected in such a long repetitive region, but has not been found. The close structural relationship between the IgG$_{2a}$ and IgG$_{2b}$ heavy chains suggest that these originated from a relatively recent duplication in evolution of *Mus musculus*. The proximity of Ig1 and Ig3 loci is further inferred from the studies of the GPC-5 myeloma, which was suggested to have arisen from a nonhomologous cross-over between adjacent Ig-1 and Ig-3 loci. Analysis of the allotypic specificities also suggests a multigenic nature in that class to be unlikely, since matations affecting allotypic specificities would have to be identical in all genes within the region. Furthermore, several other strains which fall into the same allelic group may, in fact, have had a common ancestral origin.[154,294] The finding of common allotypic specificities present on IgG$_{2a}$ and IgG$_{2b}$ but not on the other mouse immunoglobulins may parallel the results in rabbits. These specificities may have arisen prior to gene duplication into the IgG$_{2a}$ and IgG$_{2b}$ classes; this, however, would have necessitated an identical series of mutations in each chromosomal type in order for identical IgG$_{2a}$ and IgG$_{2b}$ specificities to occur in all types.

The macroglobulin $\mu$ chain apparently preceded the $\gamma$ chain in evolution.[223,224,225] Accordingly, it was suggested[320] that the $\mu$-chain gene in turn was evolved by duplication from the L-chain gene. Analysis of the C-terminal end-groups of human $\mu$ chains[56] indicates that a half-cystyl residue is at or near the C terminus, just as in $\kappa$ and $\lambda$, but not in $\gamma$ chains. This would suggest an origin of the $\mu$ chain from the L chain. Since the light- and heavy-chain gene loci are unlinked (shown in rabbits), an early separation of the resulting light- and heavy-chain genes must have occurred. This process may then have been followed by repeated gene duplication, separately, of the light- and heavy-chain genes to give the light-chain region and the heavy region. It has been speculated[242] that the light- and heavy-chain genes remain unlinked and that the heavy-chain gene loci remain linked to each other because of some facilitation of the genetic control mechanism.

Todd and Inman[355] have shown that IgM and IgG heavy chains in the rabbit both seem to react with the same antiallotype sera, and other studies show that IgA reacts as well. It could be presumed that if multiple genes were responsible for allotypic specificities on the H chains of these immunoglobulins (and hence typing sera would be multispecific), they must be very closely linked, since segregation would ultimately lead to individual rabbits carrying all the $a$-locus specificities. Todd and Inman[355] have shown that this is not the case, since rabbit IgG can absorb out all the anti-$a$ alloantibody that will react with IgM. Hence, a structural relationship does exist between the H chains of IgM and IgG (and, presumably, IgA). This would imply a common genetic origin. Furthermore, it appears at present that a single gene is responsible for coding the entire H chain (rather than one for the Fd fragment and one for the Fc fragment). If the allotypic variation of this rabbit H-chain gene had occurred prior to the duplication giving rise to $\mu$, $\alpha$, and $\gamma$, then a separate (independent) origin of the classes must have occurred for each of the presently known chromosomal types of the heavy chain. This would seem to be rather unlikely. However, the alternative is equally unfavorable, as it would imply that each of the duplicated H-chain-gene loci (which then independently mutated to give the class-defining specificity on the Fc fragment) also went through the same mutations in the Fd region to give the A specificities. Further studies are clearly needed to resolve this problem. An independent origin of the IgA and IgG heavy chains by separate duplication from the light chain rather than from duplication of the new chain must also be considered.[178]

## Between Species

Extensive data obtained on many amino acid sequence analyses of the light chains of immunoglobulins (usually of Bence-Jones proteins) in man or mouse have recently become available.[161,166,299] Comparison of the amino acid sequences of human $\kappa$ and $\lambda$ and mouse $\kappa$ and $\lambda$ show several basic findings: (1) all the light chains must have the same general conformation, because they exhibit the same twofold symmetry owing to a similar location of the two intrachain disulphide bridges and because of similar length; (2) the $\kappa$ chains of the two species are more closely related than the $\kappa$ and $\lambda$ of man. Preliminary studies show a similarity between mouse $\kappa$ and $\lambda$ perhaps to a greater degree than human $\kappa$ and $\lambda$.

The preliminary data do not, however, show much similarity between mouse and human $\lambda$. Thus, the interspecies homology of $\kappa$ chains is greater than the intraspecies homology of human $\kappa$ and $\lambda$. For example, in the carboxyl half of mouse and human $\kappa$ chains 64 identical positions exist; in other words, 60 % homology of the constant half of the chain. Including gaps and insertions, there are 61 positions in the carboxyl half of the light chain where human $\lambda$ differs from both mouse and human $\kappa$ chains; in almost half of the latter cases the same amino acid is substituted in both $\kappa$ chains for the one in $\lambda$. This is even further evidence for an early evolutionary diversion of the genes for $\kappa$ and $\lambda$.

Recent studies have led to the near completion of a complete amino acid sequence of the Fc fragment of rabbit IgG heavy chain. On the basis of comparisons of amino acid sequence of this Fc fragment with human $\kappa$-type Bence-Jones proteins a mechanism for the evolution of immunoglobulin was proposed.[158,159] When the sequences of the Fc fragment and the $\kappa$-type Bence-Jones protein are aligned from their carboxyl terminus significant stretches of sequence homology are observed. The two halves of the Fc fragment exhibit significant stretches of sequence homology, as do the variant and invariant halves of the $\kappa$-type Bence-Jones protein. Finally, when the two halves of Bence-Jones proteins and the two halves of the Fc fragment are correctly aligned, a significant degree of homology is shown. It was therefore concluded that the light and heavy chains of immunoglobulins were derived from a common ancestral gene that determines the sequence of a protein containing about 110 residues.[158,159] This ancestral gene first showed contiguous duplication, giving rise to a primitive light-chain gene. Contiguous duplication led to heavy chain and complete duplication led to the $\kappa$ and $\lambda$ types. The heavy-chain gene, in turn, yielded, by a series of complete duplications each of the major types of heavy chains, and, by further duplications, the subclasses of the major heavy-chain genes. One might speculate that the light chains would also continue to give complete duplication, perhaps leading to light-chain subclasses. Several studies have indeed indicated variations of human $\lambda$-type chains,[300] and preliminary investigations have indicated a subtype of the human $\kappa$ chain.[250] A detailed discussion of the sequence studies of immunoglobulins as relating to the evolution is found in the Nobel symposium III on $\gamma$-globulins.[185]

## IV. EXPRESSION OF IMMUNOGLOBULINS

### Expression of Immunoglobulin Genes on Individual Molecules

A given molecule in a rabbit heterozygous at both $a$ and $b$ loci will carry either allele at each locus, but never both alleles in the same molecule. For example, if the rabbit carries allotypic specificities As1,2/4,5, the serum will contain molecules of As1/4, 1/5, 2/4, and 2/5. All molecules are symmetrical, in that no single molecule carries one H chain of As1 type and the other H chain of As2 type. A similar restriction applies to the light chain. There is no restriction, however, about association of light chains with heavy chains, and because of this, molecules can arise which are not present in either parent. The molecules are themselves completely symmetrical, both heavy chains carrying the allotypic specificities.[124] Similar studies in mice (N. L. Warner, unpublished observations) have shown that the $IgG_{2a}$ globulins in mice heterozygous at the Ig-1 locus all carry one of the parental allelic types, but never both. This has been demonstrated by showing that an [125]I-labeled $IgG_2$ preparation from (C57BI $\times$ A/J)F1 hybrid mice is partially precipitated by alloantisera specific for either the C57 or A/J allelic type. If these two alloantisera are made in a strain of third allelic type, for example, in BALB/c, the two sera can be mixed and will result in complete precipitation of all of the labeled $\gamma$-globulin, indicating that the Ig-1$b$ and Ig-1$e$ allelic globulins are present on different molecules. It has been shown that hybrid molecules can be readily produced in vitro by the recombination of artificially-split half-molecules; hence, no physicochemical bar exists to the association of different allelic determinants in one molecule.[222,317]

### Expression of Immunoglobulin Classes in the Immune Response

It has been previously mentioned that IgM synthesis precedes IgG synthesis in the developing embryo. Indeed, this sequential synthesis of IgM followed by IgG antibodies had in past years also been considered to be an almost invariant feature of the immune response. The timing of the initial IgM versus IgG antibody appearance in serum during an immune response is a matter of considerable theoretical interest, since it is central in establishing whether a single cell during differentiation synthesizes first IgM and then IgG antibody in the same cell, or whether IgM and IgG are instead synthesized by separate cell lines. Earlier results[20,335,338] showing that IgM antibody preceded IgG antibody in an immune response may have been due in part to the greater sensitivity of detection of the IgM antibody with the method used. Recent techniques (e.g., radioimmunoelectrophoresis) capable of detecting similar amounts of IgM or IgG antibodies indicate that IgG antibody can be found much earlier in the primary response than was previously recognized. Indeed, several groups have reported[45,109,378] a simultaneous appearance of IgM and IgG antibodies after primary immunization. Further, many variables can affect the expression of different immunoglobulin classes in the immune response.[10,43,70,372] These variables include route of immunization, dose of antigen, presence or absence of adjuvant, and, when present, type of adjuvant used, and even the genotype of the recipient animal. It appears likely that if variables such as these can affect the expression of different immunoglobulin H-chain genes in an immune response, they do so by determining which cell type will be triggered in the immune response, rather than by affecting an intracellular differentiation of sequential expression of IgM into IgG. Further circumstantial evidence against IgM-to-IgG conversion has been obtained by studies[38,176,278] of the transfer of unprimed cells to irradiated mice, immunization with sheep red cells, and assay for antibody-producing cells by the Jerne plaque technique.[233] The results show that both IgM and IgG plaque-forming cells have a clonal distribution in spleen colonies. A variable degree of association of IgM and IgG colonies is found, and numerous pure clones of cells of one or another type are present. Thus, it is unlikely that a complete transition of a clone from all-IgM production to all- or prevalent-IgG production has occurred.

Individual immunoglobulin-producing cells can be shown by immunofluorescence and other methods to produce only one variant of immunoglobulin; that is, $\alpha$, $\mu$, and $\gamma$ chains in both rabbit and man have been shown by direct tests to be produced in different cells.[26,233,279] It should be borne in mined, however, that this type of examination is of a static nature only, since it examines the expression of a given cell at a single moment in time. It is quite conceivable that all cells synthesizing $\mu$ chain at the time of examination may then go on to produce $\gamma$ chain, and, conversely, all cells found to contain $\gamma$ chain may at an earlier stage have been synthesizing $\mu$ chains. Accordingly, it would have to be assumed that the switch-over period was very rapid, in that both $\mu$ and $\gamma$ chains would not be present together for any appreciable time. In order to answer this question conclusively, a clone of antibody-forming cells specifically synthesizing a single antibody must be followed throughout the development of the immune response from the very initiation of the immune response. At the present time only one published report[252] has undertaken an examination of this question. This study did, in fact, show that at a time immediately prior to the appearance in serum of IgG antibodies a high proportion of cells which were directly shown to be producing the antibodies in question contained both IgM and IgG classes of antibodies. However, the distinction of IgM and IgG antibodies was partially based on the use of mercaptoethanol treatment as a discriminating agent, and since several recent studies[1,2,74,372] have shown that mercaptoenthanol-sensitive 7S (IgG) antibodies exist, this question must remain open. However, it can presently be stated that most of the cells most of the time are in fact expressing the product of only one immunoglobulin heavy-chain gene and one immunoglobulin light-chain gene.

### Cellular Expression of Alleles of the Immunoglobulin Loci

The expression of alleles at immunoglobulin loci in heterozygous animals has invariably shown that a single immunoglobulin-synthesizing cell is expressing not only one immunoglobulin locus, but only one allele at that particular locus. It has been generally assumed in the past for all systems that both alleles function at all loci, with the notable exception described by Lyon[213] for some X-linked genes. The immunoglobulin loci which are not X-linked constitute the first autosomal exception to this rule in vertebrates. Since only one allelic type of light or heavy chain is synthesized per cell, the absence of hybrid immunoglobulin molecules in heterozygous individuals is not surprising. A single cell synthesized only one light-chain and one heavy-chain type, and since light and heavy chain combination has been shown to take place prior to release of the intact molecule from the cell,[12,133,200,314] one would expect to find only homozygous molecules in the serum of heterozygous individuals. This obviates the necessity of invoking preferential association of chains during synthesis within the cell. It is tempting to speculate that this outstanding exception of immunoglobulin-producing cells in having only one allele functioning (allelic exclusion) is of importance in antibody synthesis.

The evidence for allele exclusion within the immune system comes from three main sources. (1) The restrictions on the genetic markers of myeloma-globulins in man and mouse as compared with the genotype of the individual in whom the myeloma arises. For example, the myeloma protein of $IgG_1$ class in an individual who is heterozygous Gm(1, 4) will contain either Gm(1) or Gm(4), but not both. (2) The distribution of cells bearing or secreting immunoglobulin of one genetic type has been studied by immuno-fluorescence in both man and rabbit. These studies[35,52,53,280] have shown that virtually all cells carry or secrete immunoglobulin of only one genetic type. (3) Since myeloma cells frequently show chromosomal abnormality,[49,123,168,370b] one might doubt the value of extrapolation from myeloma to the normal state. It should therefore be stressed that allelic exclusion has been shown to hold for antibody in normal immune responses. For example, in man, in Rh sensitization the anti-Rh antibody may well be predominantly of one Gm type.[104,144,228] This has also been shown to be the case for antibodies to polysaccharide antigens.[6,380] In hetrozygous mice developing autoimmune haemolytic anaemia individual mice will express the autoantibodies of either parental type but rarely both parental types in one mouse (N. L. Warner, unpublished observations).

Several hypotheses have been advanced to explain allelic exclusion. Two basic types of hypotheses can be considered. One assumes that the immunoglobulin-synthesizing cell in the heterozygous animal is indeed heterozygous, and attributes the above findings to the turning on or off of genes or chromosomes. The second basic hypothesis states that the immuno-globulin-synthesizing cell even in a heterozygous individual is homozygous for the immunoglobulin genes. Several examples of somatic crossing-over or chromosome reassortment have recently been described.[19,122,139] One example of a chromosome polymorphism in the deer mouse has in fact directly demonstrated homozygosity in a clone of cells for this particular chromosome in a heterozygous mouse.[258] It was speculated by Ohno et al. in this paper[258] that a similar occurrence may indeed occur for the chromosome carrying the immunoglobulin genes. Preliminary studies on the chromosomes of human lymphoid cells in vitro[122] and of mouse myeloma-producing cells[370b] have occasionally shown examples of chromosome rearrangements and possible somatic crossing-over. In the absence of any direct data bearing on this question most theories have concentrated on the first hypothesis, namely, the turning on or off of genes or chromosomes. On the basis of studies by Nanney[247] in the ciliated protozoan Tetrahymena pyriformis a hypothetical scheme for allelic exclusion has been developed.[136] It is based on the concept that a cluster of cistrons exists which are of sufficiently similar complementarity that the messenger RNA made on the template of one DNA segment might conceivably hybridize with DNA in an adjacent, i.e., linked, cistron or on the allelic cistron. Such hybridization might conceivably prevent messenger RNA formation by these other allelic or adjacent cistrons. An objection to this has been raised by Cohn,[48] in that one would wonder why the messenger RNA of the original gene was not itself repressed. It has been shown in rabbits and man that the light- and heavy-chain immunoglobulin loci are unlinked. It is not known, however, whether the two loci are on different chromosomes or on extreme positions (perhaps on opposite sides of the centromere) on a single chromosome. If chromosome inactivation in some way were to be considered, it would seem more reasonable if the light- and heavy-chain loci were in fact on the same chromosome. The mechanism of allele exclusion might in some manner invoke the activation of one cristron each for the light and heavy chains randomly. In this case allelic exclusion, as well as expression of a given immunoglobulin class, are explained. It was emphasized, however, that this was not different in principle from the turning on or off of any gene during differentiation, whereas allelic exclusion is unique to the immunoglobulin system. There are only two well-established mechanisms in which a single diploid cell expresses one of two alleles. These are sex-chromosome inactivation[213] and cisdominant operator constitutive mutation in bacteria.[374] A detailed discussion of the possible relation of this latter theory to allelic exclusion in immunoglobulin-synthesizing systems has recently been presented.[49] Further studies, perhaps perticularly emphasizing analysis of chromosomes in various lines and sublines of mouse myeloma tumors, will be pertinent to the resolution of this most-intriguing question in immunogenetics.

The effects of antiallotype antibodies on fetal and neonatal production of $\gamma$-globulin is another biologic facet meriting further exploration. The production of maternal antibodies to fetal Gm determinants in humans has already been cited.[115] It seems possible that interaction of maternal antibody with fetal cells responsible for synthesis of the $\gamma$-globulin might result in deleterious consequences to the fetus. Fortunately, the vast majority of the anti-Gm's formed, at least in humans, are IgM globulins, which do not cross the placenta.[107] However, about 10% of the anti-Gm's are of the IgG type, and thus can cross the placenta. Such IgG antibodies may be important in the etiology of the disease known as transitional hypogammaglobulinemia of infancy, which is charatcerized by a marked delay in onset of antibody formation by the neonate, and hence repeated infection during the first two years of life. Presumably, IgG anti-Gm antibodies in the mother crossing the placenta could bind to the immunologically competent cells in the fetus, hampering mitosis of these cells, and thus antibody formation.[115] In mice[155,156,205] and in rabbits[59,218] transplacental passage of maternal antibody directed toward fetal genetically determined antigens in fetal $\gamma$-globulin subsequently causes significant depression in the newborn of production of $\gamma$-globulins bearing the specific determinants and a compensatory increase in heterozygoses of $\gamma$-globulin molecules carrying the other determinants.[218]

This effect is still present in rabbits three years after birth.[218] This phenomenon of allotype "suppression" and associated "compensation" is interwoven with those of immunological tolerance, protein synthesis, and antibody formation. Experiments devised to examine these phenomena are now in progress in several laboratories.

# BIBLIOGRAPHY

1. Adler, F. L., Studies on mouse antibodies. I. The response to sheep red cells, *J. Immunol.* **95**:26 (1965).
2. Adler, F. L., Studies on mouse antibodies. II. Mercaptoethanol-sensitive 7S antibodies in mouse antisera to protein antigen, *J. Immunol.* **95**:39 (1965).
3. Alepa, F. P., and A. G. Steinberg, The production of anti-Gm reagents by rhesus monkeys immunized with pooled human gamma globulin, *Vox Sang.* **9**:333 (1964).
4. Allen J. C. and H. G. Kunkel, Antobodies to genetic types of gamma globulin after multiple transfusions, *Science* **139**:4, 8 (1963).
5. Allen, J. C., and H. G. Kunkel, Hidden rheumatoid factors with specificity for native gamma globulin, *Arth. Rheum.* **9**:758 (1966).
6. Allen, J. C., H. G. Kunkel, and E. A. Kabat, Studies on human antibodies. II. Distribution of genetic factors, *J. Exp. Med.* **119**:453 (1964).
7. Appella, E., and D. Ein, Two types of lambda polypeptide chains in human immunoglobulins based on amino acid substitution at position 190, *Proc. Natl. Acad. Sci. U.S.* **57**:1449 (1967).
8. Appella, E., K. R. McIntyre, and R. N. Perham, Lambda Bence-Jones proteins of the mouse: Chemical and immunological characterization, *J. Mol. Biol.* **27**:391 (1967).
9. Arnason, B. G., C. de Vaux-St. Cyr, and J. B. Shaffner, A comparison of immunoglobulins and antibody production in the normal and thymectomized mouse, *J. Immunol.* **93**:915 (1964).
10. Asherson, G. L., and S. H. Stone, Slective and specific inhibition of 24 hour skin reactions in the guinea pig. I. Immune deviation: description of the phenomenon and the effect of splenectomy, *Immunology* **9**:205 (1965).
11. Askonas, B. A., and A. R. Williamson, Biosynthesis of immunoglobulins: Free light chain as an intermediate in the assembly of gamma-G-molecules, *Nature* **211**:369 (1966).
12. Askonas, B. A., and A. R. Williamson, Biosynthesis of immunoglobulins on polyribosomes and assembly of the IgG molecule, *Proc. Roy. Soc. B* **166**:232 (1966).
13. Audran, R., C. Matte, and M. Steinbuch, Determination des facteurs Gm(a), Gm(b) et Gm(x) à l'aide de SNagg (sérums normaux agglutinants) par une réaction d'hemagglutination passive, *Rev. Franc. Etud. Clin Biol.* **11**:197 (1966).
14. Baglioni, C., The fusion of two peptide chains in hemoglobin Lepore and its interpretation as a genetic deletion, *Proc. Natl. Acad. Sci. U.S.* **48**:1880 (1962).
15. Baglioni, C., and D. A. Cioli, A study of immunoglobulin structure. II. The comparison of Bence Jones proteins by peptide mapping, *J. Exp. Med.* **124**:307 (1966).
16. Ball, J., R. DeGraaf, H. A. Valkenberg, and F. Westendorp-Boerma, Comparative studies of serologic tests for rheumatoid disease. I. A comparison of a latex test and two erythrocyte agglutination tests in a random population sample, *Arth. Rheum.* **5**:55 (1962).
17. Bartfeld, H., Incidence and significance of seropositive test for rheumatoid factor in nonrheumatoid diseases, *Ann. Intern. Med.* **52**:1059 (1966).
18. Barth, W. S., and J. L. Fahey, Heterologous and homologous skin-sensitizing activity of mouse 7S $\gamma_1$- and 7S $\gamma_2$-globulins, *Nature* **206**:730 (1965).
19. Bateman, A. J., A probable case of mitotic crossing-over in the mouse, *Genet. Res.* **9**:375 (1967).
20. Bauer, D. C., M. J. Mathies, and A. B. Stavitsky, Sequences of synthesis of $\gamma$-1 macroglobulin and $\gamma$-2-globulin antibodies during primary and secondary responses to proteins, salmonella, and phage, *J. Exp. Med.* **117**:889 (1963).

21. Becker, M. J., and A. Rich, Polyribosomes of tissues producing antibodies, *Nature* **212**:142 (1966).
22. Benacerraf, B., *in* "IIIrd International Pharmacological Congress, Sao Paulo, Brazil" (1966).
23. Benacerraf, B., Z. Ovary, K. J. Bloch, and E. C. Franklin, Properties of guinea pig 7S antibodies. I. Electrophoretic separation of two types of guinea pig 7S antibodies, *J. Exp. Med.* **117**:937 (1963).
24. Bence Jones, H., "Dr. Bence Jones on Chemical Pathology," Gulstonian Lecture III, *Lancet* **ii**:88 (1847).
25. Bennet, J. C., L. E. Hood, W. I. Dreyer, and M. Potter, Evidence for amino acid sequence differences among proteins resembling the L-chain subunits of immunoglobulins, *J. Mol. Biol.* **12**:81 (1965).
26. Bernier, G. M., and J. J. Cebra, Frequency distribution of alpha, gamma, kappa, and lambda polypeptide chains in human lymphoid tissues, *J. Immunol.* **95**:246 (1965).
27. Binaghi, R., B. Benacerraf, K. Bloch, and S. Kourilsky, Properties of rat anaphylactic antibody, *J. Immunol.* **92**:927 (1964).
28. Bloch, K. J., The anaphylactic antibodies of mammals including man, *Prog. Allergy* **10**:84 (1967).
29. Bloch, K. J., S. M. Kourilsky, Z. Ovary, and B. Benacerraf, Properties of guinea pig 7S antibodies. III. Identification of antibodies involved in complement fixation and hemolysis, *J. Exp. Med.* **117**:965 (1963).
30. Bloch, K. J., Z. Ovary, S. M. Kourilsky, and B. Benacerraf, Properties of guinea pig 7S antibodies. VI. Transmission of antibodies from maternal to fetal circulation, *Proc. Soc. Exp. Biol. Med.* **114**:79 (1963).
31. Bornstein, P., and J. Oudin, A study of rabbit gamma globulin allotypy by means of hetero-immunizations, *J. Exp. Med.* **120**:655 (1964).
32. Brambell, F. W. R., The passive immunity of the young mammal, *Biol. Rev.* **33**:488 (1958).
33. Brandtzaeg, B., H. H. Fudenberg, and J. Mohr, The Gm(r) serum group, *Acta Genetica* **11**:170 (1961).
34. Bryson, V., and H. J. Vogel (eds.), "Evolving Genes and Proteins," Academic Press, New York (1965).
35. Cebra, J. J., J. D. Colberg, and S. Dray, Rabbit lymphoid cells differentiated with respect to alpha-, gamma-, and mu-heavy polypeptide chains and to allotypic markers Aa1 and Aa2, *J. Exp. Med.* **123**:547 (1966).
36. Cebra, J. J., and J. B. Robinns, Gamma-A-immunoglobulin from rabbit colostrum, *J. Immunol.* **97**:12 (1966).
37. Cebra, J. J., and P. A. Small, Polypeptide chain structure of rabbit immunoglobulins. 3. Secretory gamma-A-immunoglobulin from colostrum, *Biochemistry* **6**:503 (1967).
38. Celada, F., and H. Wigzell, Immune responses in spleen colonies. II. Clonal assortment of 19S- and 7S-producing cells in mice reacting against two antigens, *Immunology* **11**:453 (1966).
39. Clausen, J., and J. Heremans, An immunologic and chemical study of the similarities between mouse and human serum proteins, *J. Immunol.* **84**:128 (1960).
40. Clausen, J., J. Heremans, M. Th. Heremans, and R. Rask-Nielsen, Immunoelectrophoretic studies of serums from mice carrying two transplantable plasma-cell leukemias, *J. Natl. Cancer Inst.* **22**:57 (1959).
41. Cobau, C. D., and D. R. Korst, Alterations of gamma globulin with plasma cell neoplasm in mice, *Proc. Soc. Exp. Biol. Med.* **101**:356 (1959).
42. Coe, J. E., Strain variations of mouse 7S γ1 globulins, *Immunochemistry* **3**:427 (1966).

43. Coe, J. E., 7*S* gamma-1 and 7*S* gamma-2 antibody response in the mouse, I. Influence of strain, antigen, and adjuvant, *J. Immunol.* **96**:744 (1966).
44. Coe, J. E., Mouse immunoglobulin allotypes: detection with rabbit antiserums, *Science* **155**:562 (1967).
45. Cohen, I. R., and L. C. Norins, Natural human antibodies to Gram-negative bacteria: immunoglobulins G, A, and M, *Science* **152**:1257 (1966).
46. Cohen, S., and C. Milstein, Structure and biological properties of immunoglobulins, *Adv. in Immunology* **7**:1 (1967).
47. Cohen, S., and R. R. Porter, Structure and biological activity of immunoglobulins, *Adv. Immunology* **4**:287 (1964).
48. Cohn, M., *in* "Nobel Symposium 3, Gamma Globulins," (J. Killander, ed.), p. 311, Almquist and Wiksell, Stockholm (1967).
49. Cohn, M., *in* "Symposia on Differentiation and Immunology of the International Society for Cell Biology, Gatlinburg, Tennessee, 1967," Vol. 7, in press.
50. Cummings, N. A., and E. C. Franklin, A typical $\gamma$-1-A-globulin with the electrophoretic properties of an $\alpha$-2-globulin occurring in a multiple myeloma, *J. Lab. Clin. Med.* **65**:8 (1965).
51. Curtain, C. C., and A. Baumgarten, The distribution of genetic factors in malaria antibodies as determined by a fluorescent antibody test, *Australian J. Exp. Biol. Med. Sci.* **43**:351 (1965).
52. Curtain, C. C., and A. Baumgarten, Immunocytochemical localization of the immunoglobulin factors Gm(a), Gm(b), and Inv(a) in human lymphoid tissue, *Immunology* **10**:499 (1966).
53. Curtain, C. C., and T. Golab, Localization of the immunoglobulin factors Gm(a), Gm(b), and Gm(x) in lymphoid tissue obtained from an individual of $Gm^{ax/ab}$ genotype, *Australian J. Exp. Biol. Med. Sci.* **44**:589 (1966).
54. Deutsch, H. F., and J. I. Morton, Human serum macroglobulins and dissociation units. I. Physicochemical properties, *J. Biol. Chem.* **231**:1107 (1958).
55. Doolittle, R. F., and K. H. Astrin, Light chains of rabbit immunoglobulin: assignment to the kappa class, *Science* **156**:1755 (1967).
56. Doolittle, R. F., S. J. Singer, and M. Metzgar, Evolution of immunoglobulin polypeptide chains: carboxy-terminal of an IgM heavy chain, *Science* **154**:1561 (1966).
57. Dray, S., Three $\gamma$-globulins in normal human serum revealed by monkey precipitins, *Science* **132**:1313 (1960).
58. Dray, S., Effect of maternal isoantibodies of the quantitative expression of two allelic genes controlling gamma-globulin allotypic specificities, *Nature* **195**:677 (1962).
59. Dray, S., R. Lieberman, and H. A. Hoffman, Two murine $\gamma$-globulin allotypic specificities identified by ascitic fluid isoprecipitins and determined by allelic genes, *Proc. Soc. Exp. Biol. Med.* **113**:509 (1963).
60. Dray, S., and A. Nisonoff, Contribution of allelic genes Ab[4] and Ab[5] to formation of rabbit 7*S* $\gamma$-globulins, *Proc. Soc. Exp. Biol. Med.* **113**:20 (1963).
61. Dray, S., M. Potter, and R. Lieberman, Immunochemical and genetic studies of two distinct gamma-G-immunoglobulins in BALB-c mice, *J. Immunol.* **95**:832 (1965).
62. Dray, S., and G. O. Young, Genetic control of two $\gamma$-globulin isoantigenic sites in domestic rabbits, *Science* **131**:738 (1960).
63. Dray, S., G. O. Young, and L. Gerald, Immunochemical identification and genetics of rabbit gamma-globulin allotypes, *J. Immunol.* **91**:403 (1963).
64. Dray, S., G. O. Young, and A. Nisonoff, Distribution of allotypic specificities among rabbit gamma-globulin molecules, *Nature* **199**:52 (1963).

65. Dreyer, W. J., and J. C. Bennet, The molecular basis of antibody formation: a paradox, *Proc. Natl. Acad. Sci. U.S.* **54**:864 (1965).
66. Dubiski, S., and D. Cinader, A new allotypic specificity in the mouse (MuA2), *Can. J. Biochem. Physiol.* **41**:1311 (1963).
67. Dubiski, S., and P. J. Muller, A "new" allotypic specificity (A9) of rabbit immuno-globulin, *Nature* **214**:696 (1967).
68. Dubiski, S., J. Rapacz, and A. Dubiska, Heredity of rabbit gamma-globulin iso-antigens, *Acta Genetica* **12**:136 (1962).
69. Dunn, T. B., Plasma-cell neoplasms beginning in the ileocecal area in strain C3H mice, *J. Natl. Cancer Inst.* **19**:371 (1957).
70. Dvorak, H. F., J. B. Billote, J. S. McCarthy, and M. H. Flax, Immunologic un-responsiveness in the adult guinea pig. I. Suppression of delayed hypersensitivity and antibody formation to protein antigens, *J. Immunol.* **94**:966 (1965).
71. Edelman, G. M., and J. A. Gally, The nature of Bence-Jones proteins. Chemical similarities to polypeptide chains of myeloma globulins and normal $\gamma$-globulins, *J. Exp. Med.* **116**:207 (1962).
72. Edelman, G. M., and M. D. Poulik, Studies on structural units of $\gamma$-globulins, *J. Exp. Med.* **113**:861 (1961).
73. Eidinger, D., and H. F. Pross, The immune response to sheep erythrocytes in the mouse. I. A study of the immunological events utilizing the plaque technique, *J. Exp. Med.* **126**:15 (1967).
74. Epstein, W. V., and H. H. Fudenberg, Demonstration of Gm 1(a) and anti-Gm 1(a) specificities by tanned cells coated with individual $\gamma$-globulins, *J. Immunol.* **89**:293 (1962).
75. Fahey, J. L., Immunochemical studies of twenty mouse myeloma proteins: evidence for two groups of proteins similar to gamma and beta-2A globulins in man, *J. Exp. Med.* **114**:385 (1961).
76. Fahey, J. L., Physicochemical characterization of mouse myeloma proteins: demon-stration of heterogeneity for each myeloma globulin, *J. Exp. Med.* **114**:399 (1961).
77. Fahey, J. L., Heterogeneity of $\gamma$-globulins, *Adv. Immunol.* **2**:41 (1962).
78. Fahey, J. L., Heterogeneity of myeloma proteins, *J. Clin. Invest.* **42**:111 (1963).
79. Fahey, J. L., Studies of gamma- and beta-2-A-globulins. Comparison of immuno-chemical properties of S and F (papain) fragments of myeloma proteins from inbred mice, *J. Immunol.* **90**:576 (1963).
80. Fahey, J. L., and W. F. Barth, The immunoglobulins of mice. 4. Serum immuno-globulin changes following kirth, *Proc. Soc. Exp. Biol. Med.* **118**:596 (1965).
81. Fahey, J. L., W. F. Barth, and L. W. Law, Normal immunoglobulins and antibody response in neonatally thymectomized mice, *J. Natl. Cancer Inst.* **35**:663 (1965).
82. Fahey, J. L., W. F. Barth, and Z. Ovary, Differences in the electrophoretic mobility of antibody from inbred strains of mice, *J. Immunol.* **94**:819 (1965).
83. Fahey, J. L., and J. H. Humphrey, Antibodies with differing molecular sizes in mice, *Immunology* **5**:104 (1962).
84. Fahey, J. L., and M. E. Lawrence, Antibody differences in several strains of mice, *Fed. Proc.* **21**:19 (1962).
85. Fahey, J. L., and E. M. McKelvey, Quantitative determination of serum immuno-globulins in antibody-agar plates, *J. Immunol.* **94**:84 (1965).
86. Fahey, J. L., and M. Potter, Bence-Jones proteinuria associated with a transplantable mouse plasma cell neoplasm, *Nature* **184**:654 (1959).
87. Fahey, J. L., and S. Sell, The immunoglobulins of mice. V. The metabolic (catabolic) properties of five immunoglobulin classes, *J. Exp. Med.* **122**:41 (1965).

88. Fahey, J. L., and A. Solomon, Two types of $\gamma$-myeloma proteins, $\beta$2A-myeloma proteins, $\gamma_1$-macroglobulins, and Bence-Jones proteins identified by two groups of common antigenic determinants, *J. Clin. Invest.* **42**:811 (1963).
89. Fahey, J. L., Barth, W. F., and Law, L. W., Normal immunoglobulins and antibody response in neonatally thymectomized mice, *J. Nat'l. Cancer Inst.* **35**:663 (1965).
90. Fahey, J. L., J. Wunderlich, and R. Mishell, The immunoglobulins of mice. I. Four major classes of immunoglobulins: 7S $\gamma$-2-, 7S $\gamma$-1-, $\gamma$-1A($\beta$-2A)-, and 18S $\gamma$-1M-globulins, *J. Exp. Med.* **120**:223 (1964).
91. Fahey, J. L., J. Wunderlich, and R. Mishell, The immunoglobulins of mice. II. Two subclasses of mouse 7S $\gamma$-2-globulins: $\gamma$-2a- and $\gamma$-2b-globulins, *J. Exp. Med.* **120**:243 (1964).
92. Feinstein, A., Character and allotypy of an immune globulin in rabbit colostrum, *Nature* **199**:1197 (1963).
93. Feinstein, A., P. G. H. Gell, and A. H. Kelus, Immunochemical analysis of rabbit gamma-globulin allotypes, *Nature* **200**:653 (1963).
94. Feinstein, D., and E. C. Franklin, Two antigenetically distinguishable subclasses of human A myeloma proteins differing in their heavy chains, *Nature* **212**:1496 (1966).
95. Fleischman, J. B., Immunoglobulins, *Ann. Rev. Biochem.* **35**:835 (1966).
96. Fleischman, J. B., R. R. Porter, and E. M. Press, The arrangement of the peptide chains in $\gamma$-globulin, *Biochem. J.* **88**:220 (1963).
97. Fougereau, M., and G. M. Edelman, Corroboration of recent models of the $\gamma$G immunoglobulin molecule, *J. Exp. Med.* **121**:373 (1965).
98. Frangione, B., and E. C. Franklin, Structural studies of human immunoglobulins. Differences in the Fd fragments of the heavy chains of G myeloma proteins, *J. Exp. Med.* **122**:1 (1965).
99. Frangione, B., E. C. Franklin, H. H. Fudenberg, and M. E. Koshland, Structural studies of human gamma-G-myeloma proteins of different antigenic subgroups and genetic specificities, *J. Exp. Med.* **124**:715 (1966).
100. Frangione, B., F. Prelli, and E. C. Franklin, *Immunochemistry*, in press.
101. Franklin, E. C., The immune globulins—Their structure and function, and some techniques for their isolation, *Prog. Allergy* **8**:58 (1964).
102. Franklin, E. C., G. M. Edelman, and H. G. Kunkel, *in* "Symposium on Immunology," (V. Najaar, ed.), pp. 92–97, John Wiley and Sons, New York (1959).
103. Franklin, E. C., and B. Frangione, Two serologically distinguishable subclasses of $\mu$-chains of human macroglobulins, *J. Immunol.* **99**:810 (1967).
104. Franklin, E. C., and H. H. Fudenberg, Antigenic heterogeneity of human Rh antibodies, rheumatoid factors, and cold agglutinins, *Arch. Biochem.* **104**:433 (1964).
105. Franklin, E. C., H. H. Fudenberg, H. Meltzer, and D. R. Stanworth, The structural basis for genetic variations of normal and human $\gamma$-globulins, *Proc. Natl. Acad. Sci. U.S.* **48**:914 (1964).
106. Franklin, E. C., H. R. Holman, H. J. Muller-Eberhard, and H. G. Kunkel, An unusual protein component of high molecular weight in the serum of certain patients with rheumatoid arthritis, *J. Exp. Med.* **105**:425 (1957).
107. Franklin, E. C., and H. G. Kunkel, Comparative levels of high molecular weight (19S) gamma globulin in maternal and umbilical cord sera, *J. Lab. Clin. Med.* **52**:724 (1958).
108. Franklin, E. C., J. Lowenstein, B. Bigelow, and M. Meltzer, Heavy chain disease—A new disorder of serum gamma globulins: report of the first case, *Am. J. Med.* **37**:332 (1964).
109. Freeman, M. J., and A. B. Stavitsky, Radioimmunoelectrophoretic study of rabbit anti-protein antibodies during the primary response, *J. Immunol.* **95**:981 (1966).

110. Fudenberg, H. H., The hereditary gamma globulin (Gm) groups: interpretations and extensions, *Prog. Allergy* **7**:1 (1963).
111. Fudenberg, H. H., The immune globulins, *Ann. Rev. Microbiol.* **19**:301 (1965).
112. Fudenberg, H. H., Compleat immunology: science or septophrenia? *Clin. Exp. Immunol.* **2**:1 (1967).
113. Fudenberg, H. H., D. Feinstein, W. McGehee, and E. C. Franklin, Molecular localization of Gm(a) and Gm(b) factors in Negroes, *Vox Sang.* **11**:45 (1966).
114. Fudenberg, H. H., and E. C. Franklin, Rheumatoid factors and the etiology of rheumatoid arthritis, *Ann. N.Y. Acad. Sci.* **124**:(Part II), 884 (1965).
115. Fudenberg, H. H., and B. R. Fudenberg, Antibody to hereditary human gamma-globulin (Gm) factor resulting from maternal–fetal incompatibility, *Science* **145**:170 (1964).
116. Fudenberg, H. H., and H. G. Kunkel, Physical properties of the red cell agglutinins in acquired hemolytic anemia, *J. Exp. Med.* **106**:689 (1957).
117. Fudenberg, H. H., and L. Martensson, The Gm and Inv, and the rheumatoid factors: interrelations, interpretations and implications, *Bull. Rheum. Dis.* **13**:313 (1963).
118. Fudenberg, H. H., E. R. Steihm, E. C. Franklin, M. Meltzer, and B. Frangione, Antigenicity of hereditary gamma-globulin (Gm) factors—biological and biochemical aspects, *Cold Spring Harbor Symp. Quant. Biol.* **29**:463 (1964).
119. Furth, R. van, H. R. Schuit, and W. Hijmans, The immunological development of the human fetus, *J. Exp. Med.* **122**:1173 (1965).
120 Gell, P. G. H., and A. S. Kelus, Lack of natural tolerance to allotypic gamma globulins in rabbits, *Nature* **211**:766 (1966).
121. Gengozian, N., and G. Doria, Allotypic specificities in four strains of inbred mice as revealed by reciprocal immunizations, *J. Immunol.* **93**:426 (1964).
122. German, J., Cytological evidence for crossing-over *in vitro* in human lymphoid cells, *Science* **144**:298 (1964).
123. German, J., C. E. Biro, and A. G. Bearn, Chromosomal abnormalities in Waldenström's macroglobulinemia, *Lancet* **ii**:48 (1961).
124. Gilman, A. M., A. Nisonoff, and S. Dray, Symmetrical distribution of genetic markers in individual rabbit γ-globulin molecules, *Immunochemistry* **1**:109 (1964).
125. Gitlin, D., J. Kumate, J. Urrusti, and C. Morales, The selectivity of the human placenta in the transfer of plasma proteins from mother to fetus, *J. Clin. Invest.* **43**:1938 (1964).
126. Gold, E. R., Spezifitat von antisera gegen menschlikes G-immunoglobulin, *Z. immunostats forschung allergie und klinische immunologie* **132**:125 (1967).
127. Gold, E. R., W. J. Mandy, and H. H. Fudenberg, Relation between Gm(f) and the structure of the γ-globulin molecule, *Nature* **207**:1099 (1965).
128. Gold, E. R., L. Martensson, L. Ropartz, C. Rivat, and P. Y. Rousseau, Gm(f)—A determinant of human gamma-globulin, *Vox Sang.* **10**:299 (1965).
129. Goldstein, G., N. L. Warner, and M. C. Holmes, Plasma-cell tumor induction in (NZB × BALB/c)$F_1$ hybrid mice, *J. Natl. Cancer Inst.* **37**:135 (1966).
130. Good, R. A., and B. W. Papermaster, Ontogeny and phylogeny of adaptive immunity, *Adv. Immunol.* **4**:1 (1964).
131. Grabar, P., R. Fauvert, P. Burtin, and L. Hartman, Étude sur les protéines du myélome; l'analyse immuno-électrophorétique des sérums de 30 malades, *Rev. Franc. Etud. Clin. Biol.* **1**:175 (1956).
132. Gray, W. R., W. J. Dreyer, and L. E. Hood, Mechanism of antibody synthesis: size differences between mouse kappa chains, *Science* **155**:465 (1967).
133. Greenberg, L. J., and J. W. Uhr, DNA–RNA hybridization studies of immuno-

globulin-synthesizing tumors in mice, *Cold Spring Harbor Symp. Quant. Biol.* **32**:243 (1967).

134. Grey, H. M., and H. G. Kunkel, H chain subgroups of myeloma proteins and normal 7*S* gamma globulin, *J. Exp. Med.* **120**:253 (1964).

135. Grubb, R., Agglutination of erythrocytes coated with "incomplete" anti-Rh by certain rheumatoid arthritic sera and some other sera. The existence of human serum groups, *Acta Path. Microbiol. Scand.* **39**:195 (1956).

136. Grubb, R., *in* "Nobel Symposium 3, Gammaglobulins," (J. Killander, ed.), p. 301, Almquist and Wiksell, Stockholm (1967).

137. Grubb, R., and A. B. Laurell, Hereditary serological human serum groups, *Acta Path. Microbiol. Scand.* **39**:390 (1956).

138. Grubb, R., and B. Swahn, Destruction of some agglutinins but not of others by two sulfhydryl compounds, *Acta Path. Microbiol. Scand.* **43**:305 (1958).

139. Grüneberg, H., The case for somatic crossing over in the mouse, *Genet. Res.* **7**:58 (1966).

140. Hamers, R., and C. Hamers-Casterman, Molecular localization of A chain allotypic specifities in rabbit IgG (7*S* gamma-globulin), *J. Mol. Biol.* **14**:288 (1965).

141. Hamers, R., C. Hamers-Casterman, and A. S. Kelus, Un gène nouveau intervenant dans la synthèse de la gamma-globuline du lapin, *Arch. Int. Physiol.* **73**:147 (1965).

142. Hamers, R., C. Hamers-Casterman, and S. Lagnaux, A new allotype in the rabbit linked with As1 which may characterize a new class of IgG, *Immunology* **10**:399 (1966).

143. Harboe, M., A new hemagglutinating substance in the Gm system, anti-Gmb, *Acta Path. Microbiol. Scand.* **47**:191 (1959).

144. Harboe, M., Interactions between red cells coated with incomplete anti-D and rheumatoid sera, *Acta Path. Microbiol. Scand.* **50**:383 (1960).

145. Harboe, M., J. Deverill, and H. C. Godal, Antigenic heterogeneity of Waldenström type gamma-M-globulins, *Scand. J. Haemat.* **2**:137 (1965).

146. Harboe, M., J. Lundevall, A new type in the Gm system, *Acta Path. Microbiol. Scand.* **45**:357 (1959).

147. Harboe, M., C. K. Osterland, M. Mannik, and H. G. Kunkel, Genetic characters of human γ-globulins in myeloma proteins, *J. Exp. Med.* **116**:719 (1962).

148. Heller, G., A. S. Jacobson, and M. H. Kolodny, Modification of hemagglutination test for rheumatoid arthritis, *Proc. Soc. Exp. Biol. Med.* **72**:316 (1949).

149. Heremans, H., Les Globulines Seriques du Système Gamma, Masson et Cie, Paris (1960).

150. Heremans, H., J. Clausen, M. Th. Heremans, and R. Rask Nielson, Immuno-electrophoretic characteristics of normal mouse serums as a basis for studying pathological changes in serums of mice carrying transplantable malignant growths, *J. Natl. Cancer Inst.* **22**:45 (1959).

151. Herzenberg, L. A., A chromosome region for gamma-2a- and beta-2A-globulin H-chain isoantigens in the mouse, *Cold Spring Harbor Symp. Quant. Biol.* **29**:455 (1964).

152. Herzenberg, L. A., J. D. Minna, and L. A. Herzenberg, The chromosome region for immunoglobulin heavy chains in the mouse: allelic electrophoretic mobility differences and allotype suppression, *Cold Spring Harbor Symp. Quant. Biol.* **32**:181 (1967).

153. Herzenberg, L. A., and N. L. Warner, Genetic control of mouse immunoglobulins, *in* "Regulation of the Antibody Response" (B. Cinader, ed.), Charles B. Thomas, Springfield, in press.

154. Herzenberg, L. A., N. L. Warner, and L. A. Herzenberg, Immunoglobulin isoantigens

(allotypes) in the mouse. I. Genetics and cross-reactions of the 7S γ-2a-isoantigens controlled by alleles at the Ig-1 locus, *J. Exp. Med.* **121**:415 (1965).

155. Herzenberg, Leonore A., and L. A. Herzenberg, Suppression of a γG-globulin allotype in mice by antiallotype antibodies, *in* "Genetic Variations in Somatic Cells," p. 227, Academia Publishing House, Praha (1965).
156. Herzenberg, Leonore A., L. A. Herzenberg, R. C. Goodlin, and E. C. Rivera, Immunoglobulin synthesis in mice. Suppression by anti-allotype antibody, *J. Exp. Med.* **126**:701 (1967).
157. Hess, M., and R. Butler, Anti-Gm specificities in sera of Rhesus monkeys immunized with human gamma globulin, *Vox Sang.* **7**:93 (1962).
158. Hill, R. L., R. Delaney, R. E. Fellows, Jr., and H. E. Lebovitz, The evolutionary origins of the immunoglobulins, *Proc. Natl. Acad. Sci. U.S.* **56**:1762 (1966).
159. Hill, R. L., H. E. Lebovitz, R. E. Fellows, Jr., and R. Delaney, *in* "Nobel Symposium 3, Gammaglobulins," (J. Killander, ed.), p. 109, Almquist and Wiksell, Stockholm (1966).
160. Hill, W. C., and J. Cebra, Retention of antibody activity by γM-subunits, *Fed. Proc.* **24**:634 (1965).
161. Hilschmann, N., *in* "Nobel Symposium 3, Gammaglobulins," (J. Killander, ed.), p. 33, Almquist and Wiksell, Stockholm (1967).
162. Hilschmann, N., and L. C. Craig, Amino acid sequence studies with Bence-Jones proteins, *Proc. Natl. Acad. Sci. U.S.* **53**:1403 (1965).
163. Hirose, S., and A. G. Osler, Interaction of rheumatoid factors with aggregated subunits of human gamma globulin, *J. Immunol.* **94**:927 (1965).
164. Hood, L. E., W. R. Gray, and W. J. Dreyer, On the evolution of antibody light chains, *J. Mol. Biol.* **22**:179 (1966).
165. Hood, L. E., W. R. Gray, and W. J. Dreyer, On the mechanism of antibody synthesis: a species comparison of L chains, *Proc. Natl. Acad. Sci. U.S.* **55**:826 (1966).
166. Hood, L. E., W. R. Gray, B. G. Sanders, and W. J. Dreyer, Light-chain evolution, *Cold Spring Harbor Symp. Quant. Biol.* **32**:133 (1967).
167. Hong, R., B. Pollara, and R. A. Good, A model for colostral IgA, *Proc. Natl. Acad. Sci. U.S.* **56**:602 (1966).
168. Houston, E. W., S. E. Ritzmann, and W. C. Levin, Chromosomal aberrations common to three types of monoclonal gammopathies, *Blood* **29**:214 (1967).
169. Howell, D. S., J. M. Malcolm, and R. Pike, The FII agglutinating factors in serums of patients with nonrheumatic diseases, *Am. J. Med.* **29**:662 (1960).
170. Humphrey, J., D. M. V. Parrot, and J. East, Studies on globulin and antibody production in mice thymectomized at birth, *Immunol.* **7**:419 (1964).
171. Ingram, V. M., "Hemoglobin and Its Abnormalities," Charles Thomas, Co., Springfield (1961).
172. Inman, J. K., Differences in amino acid composition associated with allotypic specificities of rabbit γG-immunoglobulin Fd fragments, *Fed. Proc.* **26**:479 (1967).
173. Irvin, G. L., J. C. Eustace, J. L. Fahey, Enhancement activity of mouse immunoglobulin classes, *J. Immunol.* **99**:1085 (1967).
174. Ishizaka, K., and T. Ishizaka, Physicochemical properties of reaginic antibody. I. Association of reaginic activity with an immunoglobulin other than gamma-A- or gamma-G-globulin, *J. Allergy* **37**:169 (1966).
175. Ishizaka, K., T. Ishizaka, and M. M. Hornbrook, Physicochemical properties of human reaginic antibody. IV. Presence of a unique immunoglobulin as a carrier of reaginic activity, *J. Immunol.* **97**:75 (1966).
176. Jerne, N. K., A. A. Nordin, and C. Henry, The agar plaque technique for recognizing

antibody-producing cells, *in* "Cell Bound Antibodies" (B. Amos and H. Koprowski, eds.), Wistar Inst. Press (1963).
177. Johansson, S. G. O., and H. Bennich, *in* "Nobel Symposium 3, Gammaglobulins" (J. Killander, ed.), p. 193, Almquist and Wiksell, Stockholm (1967).
178. Kabat, E. A., *in* "Nobel Symposium 3, Gammaglobulins" (J. Killander, ed.), p. 127, Almquist and Wiksell, Stockholm (1967).
179. Kelus, A. S., *in* "Nobel Symposium 3, Gammaglobulins" (J. Killander, ed.), p. 329, Almquist and Wiksell, Stockholm (1967).
179a. Kelus, A. S., in preparation.
180. Kelus, A. S., and P. G. H. Gell, *in* "Proc. 11th Int. Cong. Genet. The Hague" (Sjgeerst, ed.), Vol. 1, p. 194 (1963).
181. Kelus, A. S., and P. G. H. Gell, An allotypic determinant specific to rabbit macroglobulin, *Nature* **206**:313 (1965).
182. Kelus, A. S., and P. G. H. Gell, Immunoglobulin allotypes of experimental animals, *Prog. Allergy* **11**:141 (1967).
183. Kelus, A. S., J. R. Marrick, and C. B. Richard, *in* "Protides of the Biological Fluids," Vol. 9 (H. Peeters, ed.), p. 176, American Elsevier, New York (1961).
184. Kelus, A. S., and J. K. Moor-Jankowsky, Serum protein antigens of hereditary character, *in* "Protides of the Biological Fluids," Vol. 9 (H. Peeters, ed.), p. 193, American Elsevier, New York (1961).
185. Killander, J. (ed.), "Nobel Symposium 3, Gammaglobulins," Almquist and Wiksell, Stockholm (1967).
186. Klemperer, M. D., E. R. Halbrook, and H. H. Fudenberg, Gm(2D) a new hereditary gamma-globulin factor, *Am. J. Hum. Genet.* **18**:433 (1966).
187. Koshland, M. E., Primary structure of immunoglobulins and its relationship to antibody specificity, *J. Cell Physiol.* **67**:(suppl. 1), 33 (1966).
188. Koshland, M. E., Location of specificity and allotypic amino acid residues in antibody Fd fragments, *Cold Spring Harbor Symp. Quant. Biol.* **32**:119 (1967).
189. Koshland, M. E., and S. M. Engelberger, Differences in the amino acid composition of two purified antibodies from the same rabbit, *Proc. Natl. Acad. Sci. U.S.* **50**:61 (1963).
190. Kronvall, G., Gm(f) activity of human gamma-globulin fragments, *Vox Sang.* **10**:303 (1965).
191. Kuff, E. L., M. Potter, K. R. McIntyre, and N. E. Roberts, Studies on microsome fractions from a plasma cell neoplasm producing only Bence-Jones protein, *Fed. Proc.* **21**:154 (1962).
192. Kuff, E. L., M. Potter, K. R. McIntyre, and N. E. Roberts, The *in vitro* synthesis of specific secretory protein by an ascites plasma-cell tumor, *Biochemistry* **3**:1707 (1964).
193. Kunkel, H. G., Myeloma proteins and antibodies, The Harvey Lectures, Ser. 59, p. 219 (1964).
194. Kunkel, H. G., J. C. Allen, H. M. Grey, L. Martensson, and R. Grubb, A relationship between the H-chain groups of 7S γ-globulin and the Gm system, *Nature* **203**:413 (1964).
195. Kunkel, H. G., and R. A. Prendergast, Subgroups of gamma-A immune globulins, *Proc. Soc. Exp. Biol. Med.* **122**:910 (1966).
196. Kunkel, H. G., W. J. Yount, and S. D. Litwin, Genetically determined antigen of the Ne subgroup of gamma globulin: detection by precipitin analysis, *Science* **154**:1041 (1966).
197. Lamm, M. E., and P. A. Small, Jr., Polypeptide chain structure of rabbit immunoglobulins. II. Gamma-M-immunoglobulin, *Biochemistry* **5**:267 (1966).

198. Lawler, S. D., A genetical study of the Gm groups in human serum, *Immunology* 3:90 (1960).
199. Lennox, E. S., and M. Cohn, Immunoglobulins, *Ann. Rev. Biochem.* 36:365 (1967).
200. Lennox, E. S., P. M. Knopf, A. J. Munro, and R. M. E. Parkhouse, A search for biosynthetic subunits of light and heavy chains of immunoglobulins, *Cold Spring Harbor Symp. Quant. Biol.* 32:249 (1967).
201. Leskowitz, S., Immunochemical study of rabbit γ-globulin allotypes, *J. Immunol.* 90:98 (1963).
202. Lichter, E. A., Isoimmunization with Human gamma-G-immunoglobulins, *Proc. Soc. Exp. Biol. Med.* 122:231 (1966).
203. Lichter, E. A., Rabbit gamma-A- and gamma-M-immunoglobulins with allotypic specifities controlled by the *a* locus, *J. Immunol.* 98:139 (1967).
204. Lieberman, R., and S. Dray, Five allelic genes at the Asa locus which control gamma-globulin allotypic specificities in mice, *J. Immunol.* 93:584 (1964).
205. Lieberman, R., and S. Dray, Maternal–fetal mortality in mice with isoantibodies to paternal gamma-globulin allotypes, *Proc. Soc. Exp. Biol. Med.* 116:1069 (1964).
206. Lieberman, R., S. Dray, and M. Potter, Linkage in control of allotypic specificities on two different gamma-G-immunoglobulins, *Science* 148:640 (1965).
207. Lieberman, R., and M. Potter, Close linkage in genes controlling gamma-A and gamma-G heavy-chain structure in BALB/c mice, *J. Mol. Biol.* 18:516 (1966).
208. Lieberman, R., and M. Potter, Polymorphism of heavy-chain genes in immunoglobulins of wild mice, *Science* 154:535 (1966).
209. Litwin, S. D., and H. G. Kunkel, Studies on the major subgroup of human γG-globulin heavy chains using two new genetic factors, *Fed. Proc.* 25:371 (1966).
210. Litwin, S. D., and H. G. Kunkel, A gamma-globulin genetic factor related to Gm(a) but localized to a different portion of the same heavy chains, *Nature* 210:866 (1966).
211. Litwin, S. D., and H. G. Kunkel, Genetic factors of human gamma globulin detected by rabbit antisera, *Transfusion* 6:140 (1966).
212. Lummus, Z. L., Properties of light chains from rabbit immunoglobulins, Ph.D. dissertation, Univ. of Fla., April 1966.
213. Lyon, M. F., Sex chromatin and gene action in the mammalian X chromosome, *Am. J. Hum. Genet.* 14:135 (1962).
214. McCamish, J., A heat-labile skin-sensitizing activity of mouse serum, *Nature* 214:1228 (1967).
215. McIntyre, K. R., R. M. Asofsky, M. Potter, and E. L. Kuff, Macroglobulin-producing plasma-cell tumor in mice: identification of a new light chain, *Science* 150:361 (1965).
216. McIntyre, K. R., and M. Potter, Studies of thirty different Bence-Jones protein producing plasma cell neoplasms in an inbred strain of mouse, *J. Natl. Cancer Inst.* 33:631 (1964).
217. MacKenzie, M. R., and H. F. Deutsch, Studies with rhesus monkeys antisera to human γ-M-globulins (γ-M), *J. Immunol.* 95:87 (1965).
218. Mage, R., and S. Dray, Persistent altered phenotypic expression of allelic gamma-G-immunoglobulin allotypes in heterozygous rabbits exposed to isoantibodies in fetal and neonatal life, *J. Immunol.* 95:525 (1965).
219. Mage, R., R. A. Reisfeld, and S. Dray, An evaluation of the number of b4 allotypic determinants on rabbit gamma-G-immunoglobulin using double-labeled, soluble complexes with univalent antibody, *Immunochemistry* 3:299 (1966).
220. Mannik, M., and H. G. Kunkel, Classification of myeloma globulins, Bence-Jones proteins, and macroglobulins into two groups on the basis of common antigenic determinants, *J. Exp. Med.* 116:859 (1962).

221. Mannik, M., and H. G. Kunkel, Two major types of normal 7S γ-globulin, *J. Exp. Med.* **117**:213 (1963).
222. Mannik, M., and H. Metzgar, Hybrid antibody molecules with allotypically different L-polypeptide chaips, *Science* **148**:383 (1965).
223. Marchalonis, J., and G. M. Edelman, Phylogenetic origins of antibody structure. I. Multichain structure of immunoglobulins in the smooth dogfish *(Mustelus canis)*, *J. Exp. Med.* **122**:601 (1965).
224. Marchalonis, J., and G. M. Edelman, Phylogenetic origins of antibody structure. II. Immunoglobulins in the primary immune response of the bullfrog, *Rana catesbiana*, *J. Exp. Med.* **124**:901 (1966).
225. Marchalonis, J., and G. M. Edelman, Polypeptide chains of immunoglobulins from the smooth dogfish *(Mustelis canis)*, *Science* **154**:1567 (1966).
226. Marrack, J. R., C. B. Richards, and A. Kelus, Antigenic specificity of hydrolysis products of γ-globulins, *in* "Protides of the Biological Fluids," Vol. 9 (H. Peeters, ed.), p. 200, American Elsevier, New York (1961).
227. Martensson, L., Gm characters of M-components, *Acta Med. Scand.* **367**:87 (1961).
228. Martensson, L., On the relationships between the gamma-globulin genes of the Gm system. A study of Gm gene products in sera, myeloma globulins, and specific antibodies with special reference to the gene Gm, *J. Exp. Med.* **120**:1169 (1964).
229. Martensson, L., Genes and immunoglobulins, *Vox Sang.* **11**:521 (1966).
230. Martensson, L., and H. H. Fudenberg, Gm genes and gamma-G-globulin synthesis in the human fetus, *J. Immunol.* **94**:514 (1965).
231. Martensson, L., E. Van Loghem, H. Matsumoto, and J. Neilsen, Gm(s) and Gm(t): genetic determinants of human gamma globulin, *Vox Sang.* **11**:393 (1966).
232. Masseyeff, R., M. Daquo, and J. Gombert, Information Exchange Group No. 5, Memo No. 299.
233. Mellors, R. C., and L. Korngold, The cellular origin of human immunoglobulins (gamma-2, gamma-1M, gamma-1A), *J. Exp. Med.* **118**:387 (1963).
234. Meltzer, M., E. C. Franklin, H. H. Fudenberg, and B. Frangione, Single peptide differences between gamma-globulins of different genetic (Gm) types, *Proc. Natl. Acad. Sci. U.S.* **51**:1007 (1964).
235. Merryman, C., and B. Benacerraf, Studies on the structure of mouse antikodies, *Proc. Soc. Exp. Biol. Med.* **114**:372 (1963).
236. Merwin, R. M., and G. H. Algire, Induction of plasma-cell neoplasms and fibrosarcomas in BALB/c mice carrying diffusion chambers, *Proc. Soc. Exp. Biol. Med.* **101**:437 (1959).
237. Merwin, R. M., and L. W. Redman, Induction of plasma-cell tumors and sarcomas in mice by diffusion chambers placed in the peritoneal cavity, *J. Natl. Cancer Inst.* **31**:997 (1963).
238. Metzger, H., and F. Miller, Characterization of a human macroglobulin. I. The molecular weight of its subunit, *J. Biol. Chem.* **240**:3325 (1965).
239. Migita, S., and F. N. Putnam, Antigenic relationship of Bence-Jones proteins, myeloma globulins, and normal human γ-globulins, *J. Exp. Med.* **117**:81 (1963).
240. Milstein, C., Interchain disulphide bridge in Bence-Jones proteins and in gamma-globulin B chains, *Nature* **205**:1171 (1965).
241. Milstein, C., Variations in amino acid sequence near the disulphide bridges of Bence-Jones proteins, *Nature* **209**:370 (1966).
242. Minna, J. D., G. M. Iverson, and L. A. Herzenberg, Identification of a gene locus for gamma-G-1 immunoglobulin H chains and its linkage to the H-chain chromosome region in the mouse, *Proc. Natl. Acad. Sci. U.S.* **58**:188 (1967).

243. Mishell, R., and J. L. Fahey, Molecular and submolecular localization of two isoantigens of mouse immunoglobulins, *Science* **143**:1440 (1964).
244. Mota, I., The mechanism of anaphylaxis. I. Production and biological properties of "mast-cell-sensitizing" antibody, *Immunology* **7**:681 (1964).
245. Mota, I., Biological characterization of mouse "early" antibodies, *Immunology* **12**:343 (1967).
246. Mota, I., and J. M. Peixoto, A skin-sensitizing and thermolabile antibody in the mouse, *Life Sciences* **5**:1723 (1966).
247. Nanney, D. L., *in* "Biological Organization at the Cellular and Super Cellular Level," p. 91, Academic Press, New York (1963).
248. Natvig, J. B., Gm(g)—A "new" gamma-globulin factor, *Nature* **211**:318 (1966).
249. Natvig, J. B., and H. Kunkel, Detection of genetic antigens utilizing gamma globulins coupled to red blood cells, *Nature* **215**:68 (1967).
250. Niall, H. D., and P. Edman, Two structurally distinct classes of kappa-chains in human immunoglobulins, *Nature* **216**:262 (1967).
251. Nisonoff, A., F. C. Wissler, and L. N. Lipman, Properties of the major component of a peptic digest of rabbit antibody, *Science* **132**:1770 (1960).
252. Nossal, G. J. V., A. Szenberg, G. L. Ada, and C. M. Austin, Single-cell studies on 19*S* antibody production, *J. Exp. Med.* **119**:485 (1964).
253. Nussensweig, V., and B. Benacerraf, Quantitative variations in L-chain types in guinea pig anti-hapten antibodies, *J. Exp. Med.* **124**:805 (1966).
254. Nussensweig, V., and B. Benacerraf, Presence of identical antigenic determinants in the Fd fragments of gamma-1- and gamma-2- guinea pig immunoglobulins, *J. Immunol.* **97**:171 (1966).
255. Nussensweig, V., and B. Benacerraf, *in* "Nobel Symposium 3, Gammaglobulins," (J. Killander, ed.), p. 223, Almquist and Wiksell, Stockholm (1967).
256. Nussensweig, V., M. E. Lamm, and B. Benacerraf, Presence of two types of L polypeptide chains in guinea pig 7*S* immunoglobulins, *J. Exp. Med.* **124**:787 (1966).
257. Nussenzweig, R. S., C. Merryman, and B. Benacerraf, Electrophoretic separation and properties of mouse antihapten antibodies involved in passive cutaneous anaphylaxis and passive hemolysis, *J. Exp. Med.* **120**:315 (1964).
258. Ohno, S., C. Weiler, J. Poole, L. Christian, and C. Stenius, Autosomal polymorphism due to pericentric inversions in the deer mouse *(Peromyscus maniculatus)* and some evidence of somatic segregation, *Chromosoma* **18**:177 (5966).
259. Olins, D. E., and G. M. Edelman, The antigenic structure of the polypeptide chains of human γ-globulin, *J. Exp. Med.* **116**:635 (1962).
260. Onoue, K., Y. Yagi, A. L. Grossberg, and D. Pressman, Number of binding sites of rabbit macroglobulin antibody and its subunits, *Immunochemistry* **2**:401 (1965).
261. Onoue, K., Y. Yagi, and D. Pressman, Multiplicity of antibody proteins in rabbit anti-*p*-azobenzenearsonate sera, *J. Immunol.* **92**:173 (1964).
262. Onoue, K., Y. Yagi, and D. Pressman, Isolation of rabbit IgA antihapten antibody and demonstration of skin-sensitizing activity in homologous skin, *J. Exp. Med.* **123**:173 (1966).
263. Ouchterlony, O., Diffusion-in-gel methods for immunological analysis, *Progr. Allergy* **6**:30 (1962).
264. Oudin, J., Sérologie-Réaction de précipitation spécifique autre des sérums d'animaux de même espèce, *Compt. Rend.* **242**:2489 (1956).
265. Oudin, J., Sérologie-l'allotypie de certaine antigènes protéidiques du sérum, *Compt. Rend.* **242**:2606 (1956).

266. Oudin, J., Allotypy of rabbit serum protein. I. Immunochemical analysis leading to the individualization of seven main allotypes, *J. Exp. Med.* **112**:107 (1960).
267. Oudin, J., Allotypy of rabbit serum protein. II. Relationship between various allotypes 1. Their common antigenic specificities, their distribution in a simple population: genetic implications, *J. Exp. Med.* **112**:125 (1960).
268. Oudin, J., On the unusual behavior of certain antiallotype antibodies, *Compt. Rend.* **254**:2877 (1962).
269. Oudin, J., Genetic regulation of immunoglobulin synthesis, *J. Cell. Physiol.* **67**:(Suppl. 1), 77 (1966).
270. Ovary, Z., Passive cutaneous anaphylaxis in the mouse, *J. Immunol.* **81**:355 (1958).
271. Ovary, Z., Immediate reactions in the skin of experimental animals provoked by antibody-antigen interactions, *Prog. Allergy* **5**:459 (1958).
272. Ovary, Z., Reverse passive cutaneous anaphylaxis in the guinea pig with horse, sheep, or hen antibodies, *Immunology* **3**:19 (1960).
273. Ovary, Z., Immunological methods, *in* "CIONS Symposium," (J. S. Ackroyd, ed.), p. 259, Blackwell Scientific Publications, Oxford (1964).
274. Ovary, Z., The structure of various immunoglobulins and their biologic activities, *Ann. N.Y. Acad. Sci.* **129**:776 (1966).
275. Ovary, Z., W. S. Barth, and J. L. Fahey, The immunoglobulins of mice. 3. Skin-sensitizing activity of mouse immunoglobulins, *J. Immunol.* **94**:410 (1965).
276. Ovary, Z., B. Benacerraf, and K. J. Bloch, Properties of guinea pig $7S$ antibodies. II. Identification of antibodies involved in passive cutaneous and systemic anaphylaxis, *J. Exp. Med.* **117**:951 (1963).
277. Pain, R. H., The molecular weights of the peptide chains of $\gamma$-globulin, *Biochem. J.* **88**:234 (1963).
278. Papermaster, B. W., The clonal differentiation of antibody-producing cells, *Cold Spring Harbor Symp. Quant. Biol.* **32**:447 (1967).
279. Pernis, B., and G. Chiappino, Identification in human lymphoid tissues of cells that produce group 1 or group 2 gamma globulins, *Immunology* **7**:500 (1964).
280. Pernis, B., G. Chiappino, A. S. Kelus, and P. G. H. Gell, Cellular localization of immunoglobulins with different allotypic specificities in rabbit lymphoid tissues, *J. Exp. Med.* **122**:853 (1965).
281. Perham, R., E. Appella, and M. Potter, Light chains of mouse myeloma proteins: partial amino acid sequence, *Science* **154**:391 (1966).
282. Pilgrim, H. I., *in* "Proc. International Conference on the Morphological Precursors of Cancer," University of Perugia, Italy (1961), p. 671.
283. Polmar, S. H., and A. G. Steinberg, Dependence of a Gm(b) antigen on the quarternary structure of human gamma globulin, *Science* **145**:928 (1964).
284. Porter, R. R., The hydrolysis of rabbit $\gamma$-globulin and antibodies with crystalline papain, *Biochem. J.* **73**:119 (1959).
285. Porter, R. R., *in* "Nobel Symposium 3, Gammaglobulins" (J. Killander, ed.), p. 81, Almquist and Wiksell, Stockholm (1967).
286. Potter, M., E. Appella, and S. Geisser, Variations in the heavy polypeptide chain structure of gamma myeloma immunoglobulins from an inbred strain of mice and a hypothesis as to their origin, *J. Mol. Biol.* **14**:361 (1965).
287. Potter, M., and C. R. Boyse, Induction of plasma-cell neoplasms in strain BALB/c mice with mineral oil and mineral oil adjuvants, *Nature* **193**:1086 (1962).
288. Potter, M., W. J. Dreyer, E. L. Kuff, and K. R. McIntyre, Heritable variation in Bence-Jones protein structure in BALB/c mice: Relation to gamma globulin, *Fed. Proc.* **22**:649 (1963).

289. Potter, M., W. J. Dreyer, E. L. Kuff, and K. R. McIntyre, Heritable variation in Bence-Jones protein structure in an inbred strain of mice, *J. Mol. Biol.* **8**:814 (1964).

290. Potter, M., and J. L. Fahey, Studies on eight transplantable plasma-cell neoplasms of mice, *J. Natl. Cancer Inst.* **24**:1153 (1960).

291. Potter, M., J. L. Fahey, and H. I. Pilgrim, Abnormal serum protein and bone destruction in transmissible mouse plasma cell neoplasms, *Proc. Soc. Exp. Biol. Med.* **94**:327 (1957).

292. Potter, M., and E. L. Kuff, Myeloma globulins of plasma-cell neoplasms in inbred mice. I. Immunoelectrophoresis of serum, with rabbit antibodies prepared against microsome fractions of the neoplasms, *J. Natl. Cancer Inst.* **26**:1109 (1965).

293. Potter, M., and E. L. Kuff, Disorders in the differentiation of protein secretion in neoplastic plasma cells, *J. Mol. Biol.* **9**:537 (5964).

294. Potter, M., and R. Lieberman, Genetics of immunoglobulins in the mouse, *Adv. Immunol.* **7**:91 (1967).

295. Potter, M., R. Lieberman, and S. Dray, Isoantibodies specific for myeloma gamma-G and gamma-H immunoglobulins of BALB/c mice, *J. Mol. Biol.* **16**:334 (1966).

296. Potter, M., and R. C. MacCardle, Histology of developing plasma cell neoplasia induced by mineral oil in BALB/c mice, *J. Natl. Cancer Inst.* **33**:497 (1964).

297. Potter, M., and C. L. Robertson, Development of plasma cell neoplasms in BALB/c mice after intraperitoneal injection of paraffin-oil adjuvant, heat-killed staphylococcus mixtures, *J. Natl. Cancer. Inst.* **25**:847 (1960).

298. Poulik, M. D., and J. Shuster, Heterogeneity of H chains of myeloma proteins: susceptibility to papain and trypsin, *Nature* **204**:577 (1964).

299. Pretty, H., H. H. Fudenberg, H. Perkins, and F. Gerbode, Anti-γ-globulin antibodies after open heart surgery, *Blood*, in press.

300. Putnam, F. W., Structural evolution of kappa and lambda light chains, *in* "Nobel Symposium 3, Gammaglobulins," (J. Killander, ed.), p. 45, Almquist and Wiksell, Stockholm (1967).

301. Putnam, F. W., S. Migita, and C. W. Easley, Structural and immunochemical relationships among Bence-Jones proteins, *in* "Protides of the Biological Fluids," Vol. 10 (H. Peeters, ed.), p. 93, American Elsevier, New York (1962).

302. Putnam, F. W., T. Shinoda, K. Titani, and M. Wikler, Immunoglobulin structure: variation in amino acid sequence and length of human lambda light chains, *Science* **157**:1050 (1967).

303. Rask-Neilson, R., and H. Gormsen, On occurrence of plasma-cell leukemia in various strains of mice, *J. Natl. Cancer Inst.* **16**:1137 (1956).

304. Rask-Neilson, R., H. Gormsen, and J. Clausen, A transplantable plasma-cell leukemia in mice associated with the production of β-paraprotein, *J. Natl. Cancer Inst.* **22**:509 (1959).

305. Reisfeld, R. A., S. Dray, and A. Nisonoff, Differences in amino acid composition of rabbit gamma-G-immunoglobulin light polypeptide chains controlled by allelic genes, *Immunochemistry* **2**:155 (1965).

306. Rockey, J. H., and H. G. Kunkel, Unusual sedimentation and sulfhydryl sensitivity of certain isohemagglutinins and skin-sensitizing antibody, *Proc. Soc. Exp. Biol. Med.* **110**:101 (1962).

307. Ropartz, C., J. Lenoir, and L. Rivat, A new inheritable property of human sera: the Inv factor, *Nature* **189**:586 (1961).

308. Ropartz, C., L. Rivat, and P. Y. Rousseau, Le Gm(b) et ses problèmes, *Vox Sang.* **8**:717 (1963).

309. Ropartz, C., L. Rivat, and P. Y. Rousseau, Deux nouveaux facteurs des systèmes héréditaires des gamma globulins le Gm(e) et l'Inv(1), in "Proc. 9th Cong. Int. Soc. Blood Transfusion, Mexico, 1962," pp. 455–58 (1964).
310. Ropartz, C., L. Rivat, P. Y. Rousseau, H. H. Fudenberg, R. Molter, and C. Salmon, Seven new human serum factors presumably supported by the gamma-globulins, *Vox Sang.* **11**:99 (1966).
311. Rose, H. M., C. Ragan, E. Pearce, and M. O. Lipman, Differential agglutination of normal and sensitized sheep erythrocytes by sera of patients with rheumatoid arthritis, *Proc. Soc. Exp. Biol. Med.* **68**:1 (1948).
312. Rothfield, N. F., B. Frangione, and E. C. Franklin, Slowly sedimenting mercaptoethanol-resistant antinuclear factors related antigenically to M immunoglobulins ($\gamma$-1-M-globulin) in patients with systemic lupus erythematosus, *J. Clin. Invest.* **44**:62 (1965).
313. Rowe, D. S., and J. L. Fahey, A new class of human immunoglobulins. I. A unique myeloma protein, *J. Exp. Med.* **121**:171 (1965).
314. Scharff, M. D., A. L. Shapiro, and B. Ginsberg, The synthesis, assembly, and secretion of gamma globulin polypeptide chains by cells of a mouse plasma cell tumor, *Cold Spring Harbor Symp. Quant. Biol.* **32**:235 (1967).
315. Sell, S., Immunoglobulin M allotypes of the rabbit: identification of a second specificity, *Science* **153**:641 (1966).
316. Sell, S., Isolation and characterization of rabbit colostral IgA, *Immunochemistry* **4**:49 (1967).
317. Seth, S. K., A. Nisonoff, and S. Dray, Hybrid molecules of rabbit gamma globulin formed by recombination of half molecules of gamma globulins differing in genotype at two loci, *Immunochemistry* **2**:39 (1965).
318. Shapiro, A., M. Scharff, J. Maizel, and J. W. Uhr, Polyribosomal synthesis and assembly of the H and H chains of gamma globulin, *Proc. Natl. Acad. Sci. U.S.* **56**:216 (1966).
319. Silverstein, A. M., Ontogeny of the immune response, *Science* **144**:1423 (1964).
320. Singer, J., and R. Doolittle, Antibody active sites and immunoglobulin molecules, *Science* **153**:13 (1966).
321. Small, P. A., and M. E. Lamm, Polypeptide chain structure of rabbit immunoglobulins. I. Gamma-G-immunoglobulin, *Biochemistry* **5**:259 (1966).
322. Small, P. A., R. A. Reisfeld, and S. Dray, Peptide differences of rabbit gamma-G-immunoglobulin light chains controlled by allelic genes, *J. Mol. Biol.* **11**:713 (1965).
323. Small, P. A., R. A. Reisfeld, and S. Dray, Peptide maps of rabbit gamma-G-immunoglobulin heavy chains controlled by allelic genes, *J. Mol. Biol.* **16**:328 (1966).
324. Smithies, O., Gamma-globulin variability: a genetic hypothesis, *Nature* **199**:1231 (1963).
325. Smithies, O., G. E. Connell, and G. E. Dixon, Chromosomal rearrangements and the evolution of haptoglobin genes, *Nature* **196**:232 (1962).
326. Speiser, P., Uber Antikörperbildung von Säuglingen und Ein bisher unbekanntes, dem Erythroblastosemechanismus Konträres Phänomen mit anscheinend immunogenetisch obligatem charakter, *Wien Med. Wochen.* **113**:966 (1963).
327. Speiser, P., and D. Mikertz, Beobachtungen über gehäuftes Auftreten von Anti-Gma bei bis zu 2 Jahre alten Kindern nebst Untersuchungen über Antigenverwandtschaft zwischen Gm(a) und Gm(x) mit Pocken-, BCG-, und Poliomyelitisantigen, *Blut* **10**:425 (1964).
328. Steinberg, A. G., Progress in the study of genetically determined human gamma globulin types (the Gm and Inv groups), *Prog. Med. Genet.* **2**:1 (1962).

329. Steinberg, A. G., Studies on the Gm factors: Comparison of the agglutinators in serum from patients with rheumatoid arthritis and in serum from healthy donors, *Arth. Rheum.* **5**:331 (1965).

330. Steinberg, A. G., B. Giles, and R. Stauffer, A Gm-like factor present in Negroes and rare or absent in whites: its relation to $Gm^a$ and $Gm^x$, *Am. J. Hum. Genet.* **12**:44 (1960).

331. Steinberg, A. G., and R. Goldblum, A genetic study of the antigens associated with the Gm(b) factor of human gamma globulin, *Am. J. Hum. Genet.* **17**:133 (1965).

332. Steinberg, A. G., and J. A. Wilson, Hereditary globulin factors and immune tolerance in man, *Science* **140**:303 (1963).

333. Steinberg, A. G., and J. A. Wilson, Studies on hereditary gamma globulin factors: evidence that Gm(b) in whites and Negroes is not the same and the Gm-like is determined by an allele at the Gm locus, *Am. J. Hum. Genet.* **15**:96 (1963).

334. Steinberg, A. G., J. A. Wilson, and S. Lanset, A new human gamma globulin factor determined by an allele at the Inv locus, *Vox Sang.* **1**:151 (1962).

335. Stelos, P., and W. H. Taliaferro, Comparative study of rabbit hemolysins to various antigens. II. Hemolysins to the Forssman antigen of guinea pig kidney, human type A red cells, and sheep red cells, *J. Infect. Dis.* **104**:105 (1959).

336. Stemke, G. W., Allotypic specificities of A- and B-chains of rabbit gamma globulin, *Science* **145**:403 (1964).

337. Stemke, G. W., A study of soluble complexes and uncombined material in antigen–antibody reactions involving allotypic specificities of purified rabbit gamma globulin, *Immunochemistry* **2**:359 (1965).

338. Stemke, G. W., and R. J. Fischer, Rabbit 19*S* antibodies with allotypic specificities of the *a*-locus group, *Science* **150**:1298 (1965).

339. Stiehm, E. R., and H. H. Fudenberg, Antibody to gamma globulin in infants and children exposed to isologous gamma globulin, *Pediatrics* **35**:229 (1965).

340. Stiehm, E. R., and H. H. Fudenberg, Serum levels of immune globulins in health and disease: a survey, *Pediatrics* **37**:715 (1966).

341. Stone, W. H., and M. R. Irwin, Blood groups in animals other than man, *Adv. Immunol.* **3**:315 (1963).

342. Takakura, K., W. B. Mason, and B. P. Hollander, Studies on the pathogenesis of plasma cell tumors. I. Effects of cortisol on development of plasma cell tumors, *Cancer Res.* **26**:596 (1966).

343. Takakura, K., H. Yamada, and B. P. Hollander, Studies on the pathogenesis of plasma cell tumors. II. The role of mast cells and pituitary glycoprotein hormones in the inhibition of plasma cell tumorigenesis, *Cancer Res.* **26**:2464 (1966).

344. Takakura, K., H. Yamada, A. H. Weber, and B. P. Hollander, Studies on the pathogenesis of plasma cell tumors: effects of sex hormones on the development of plasma cell tumors, *Cancer Res.* **27**:932 (1967).

345. Takatsuki, K., and E. F. Osserman, Structural differences between 2 types of "heavy-chain" disease proteins and myeloma globulins of corresponding types, *Science* **145**:499 (1964).

346. Terres, G., and W. Wolins, Enhanced immunological sensitization of mice by the simultaneous injection of antigen and specific antiserum. I. Effect of varying the amount of antigen relative to antiserum, *J. Immunol.* **86**:361 (1961).

347. Terry, W. D., and J. L. Fahey, Subclasses of human gamma-2-globulin based on differences in the heavy polypeptide chains, *Science* **146**:400 (1964).

348. Terry, W. D., J. L. Fahey, and A. G. Steinberg, Gm and Inv factors in subclasses of human IgG, *J. Exp. Med.* **122**:1087 (1965).

349. Thorbecke, G. J., B. Benacerraf, and Z. Ovary, Antigenic relationship between two types of 7S guinea pig gamma globulins, *J. Immunol* **91**:670 (1963).
350. Thorpe, N., N. L. Warner, G. M. Hockwald, and S. H. Ohanian, Immunogublin production by the bursa of young chickens, *Immunology* **15**:123 (1968).
351. Thorpe, N., and H. Deutsch, Studies on papain-produced subunits of human gamma-G-globulins. I. Physicochemical and immunochemical properties of gamma-G-globulin Fc fragments, *Immunochemistry* **3**:317 (1966).
352. Thorpe, N., and H. Deutsch, Studies on papain-produced subunits of human gamma-G-globulins. II. Structures of peptides related to the genetic Gm activity of gamma-G-globulin Fc fragments, *Immunochemistry* **3**:329 (1966).
353. Titani, K., E. Whitley, Jr., L. Avogardo, and F. W. Putnam, Immunoglobulin structure: Partial amino acid sequence of a Bence-Jones protein, *Science* **149**:1090 (1965).
354. Todd, C. W., Allotypy in rabbit 19S protein, *Biochem. Biophys. Res. Commun.* **11**:170 (1963).
355. Todd, C. W., and J. K. Inman, Comparison of the allotypic combining sites on H-chains of rabbit IgG and IgM, *Immunochemistry* **4**:407 (1967).
356. Tomasi, C. B., E. M. Tan, A. Solomon, and R. A. Prendergast, Characteristics of an immune system common to certain external secretions, *J. Exp. Med.* **121**:101 (1965).
357. Uhr, J. W., and J. B. Baumann, Antibody formation, II. The specific anamnestic response, *J. Exp. Med.* **113**:959 (1961).
358. Uhr, J. W., and M. S. Finkelstein, Antibody formation. IV. Formation of rapidly and slowly sedimenting antibodies and immunological memory to bacteriophage $\phi$X 174, *J. Exp. Med.* **117**:457 (1963).
359. Utsumi, S., and F. Karush, The subunits of purified rabbit antibody, *Biochemistry* **3**:1329 (1964).
360. Vaerman, J. P., and J. F. Heremans, Subclasses of human immunoglobulin A based on differences in the alpha polypeptide chains, *Science* **153**:647 (1966).
361. Vaerman, J. P., H. H. Fudenberg, C. Vaerman, and W. Mandy, On the significance of the heterogeneity in molecular size of human serum gamma-A-globulins, *Immunochemistry* **2**:263 (1965).
361a. Vaz, N. M., N. L. Warner, and Z. Ovary, in preparation.
362. Vierucci, A., Gm groups and anti-Gm antibodies in children with Cooley's anaemia, *Vox Sang.* **10**:82 (1965).
363. Voisin, G. A., R. G. Kinsky, and F. K. Jansen, Transplantation immunity: localization in mouse serum of antibodies responsible for haemagglutination, cytotoxicity, and enhancement, *Nature* **210**:138 (1966).
364. Vyas, G. N., H. H. Fudenberg, H. M. Pretty, and E. R. Gold, A new rapid method for genetic typing of human immunoglobulins, *J. Immunol.* **100**:274 (1968).
365. Waaler, E., On occurrence of factor in human serum activating specific agglutination of sheep blood corpuscles, *Acta Path. Microbiol Scand.* **17**:172 (1940).
366. Waller, M., R. D. Hughes, J. E. Townsend, E. C. Franklin, and H. H. Fudenberg, New serum group, Gm(p), *Science* **142**:1321 (1963).
367. Waller, M., and J. Vaughan, Use of anti-Rh sera for demonstrating agglutination activating factors in rheumatoid arthritis, *Proc. Soc. Exp. Biol. Med.* **92**:198 (1956).
367a. Warner, N. L., in preparation.
367b. Warner, N. L., in preparation.
368. Warner, N. L., and L. A. Herzenberg, Immunoglobulin isoantigens (allotypes) in the mouse. 3. Detection of allotypic antigens with heterologous antisera, *J. Immunol.* **97**:525 (1966).

368a. Warner, N. L., and L. A. Herzenberg, in preparation.
369. Warner, N. L., and L. A. Herzenberg, Immunoglobulin isoantigens (allotypes) in the mouse. IV. Allotype specificities common to two distinct immunoglobulin classes, *J. Immunol.* **99**:675 (1967).
370. Warner, N. L., L. A. Herzenberg, and G. Goldstein, Immunoglobulin isoantigens (allotypes) in the mouse. II. Allotypic analysis of three gamma-G2-myeloma proteins from (NZB × BALB/c) F1 hybrids and of normal gamma-G2-globulins *J. Exp. Med.* **123**:707 (1966).
370a. Warner, N. L., and M. R. Mackenzie, in preparation.
370b. Warner, N. L., and M. A. S. Moore, in preparation.
371. Warner, N. L., and R. Wistar, Immunoglobulins in NZB/BL mice. I. Serum immunoglobulin class of erythrocyte autoantibody, *J. Exp. Med.* **127**:169 (1968).
372. Warner, N. L., N. M. Vaz, and Z. Ovary, Immunoglobulin classes in antibody responses in mice. I. Analysis by biological properties, *Immunology* **14**:725 (1968).
373. Wilheim, E., and M. E. Lamm, Absence of allotype b4 in the heavy chains of rabbit γG-immunoglobulin, *Nature* **212**:846 (1966).
374. Willson, C., D. Perrin, M. Cohn, F. Jacob, and J. Monod, Non-inducible mutants of the regulator gene in the "lactose" system of *Escherichia coli*, *J. Mol. Biol.* **8**:582 (1964).
375. Wilson, J. A., and A. G. Steinberg, Antibodies to gamma globulin in the serum of children and adults, *Transfusion* **5**:516 (1965).
376. Wollheim, F. A., and R. Williams, Studies on the macroglobulins of human serum. II. Heterogeneity of antigenic determinants among M-components in Waldenström's macroglobulinemia, *Acta Med. Scand.* **179**(445):115 (1966).
377. World Health Organization, *Nomenclature for Human Immunoglobulins* **30**:447 (1964).
378. Wortis, H. H., R. B. Taylor, and D. W. Dresser, Antibody production studied by means of the LHG assay. I. The splenic response of CBA mice to sheep erythrocytes, *Immunology* **11**:603 (1966).
379. Wunderlich, J., and L. A. Herzenberg, Genetics of a gamma globulin isoantigen (allotype) in the mouse, *Proc. Natl. Acad. Sci. U.S.* **49**:592 (1963).
380. Yount, W. J., M. M. Dorner, H. G. Kunkel, and E. A. Kabat, Studies on human antibodies. VI. Selective variations in subgroup composition and genetic markers, *J. Exp. Med.* **127**:633 (1968).
381. Zvaifler, N. J., and E. L. Becker, Rabbit anaphylactic antibody, *J. Exp. Med.* **123**:935 (1966).
382. Zvaifler, N. J., and E. L. Becker, The demonstration of anaphylactic antibody in the primary response of rabbits, *Int. Arch. Allergy* **31**:465 (1967).

*Chapter 4*

# Human Genetics of Membrane Transport with Emphasis on Amino Acids

Charles R. Scriver
and Peter Hechtman

*The deBelle Laboratory for Biochemical Genetics*
*McGill University–Montreal Children's Hospital Research Institute*
*Montreal, Canada*

## INTRODUCTION

This chapter is concerned with membrane transport and its genetic control in man. A discussion in this context would be unmanageable if one were to consider all the known physical and chemical aspects of cell membranes, their relevant functions, and the inherited disorders thereof. On the other hand, since no one can yet define what the critical physical and chemical features of biological membranes are, nor define precisely how the process of membrane transport is accomplished,[163] it is still necessary to consider transport as a rather black-box phenomenon. We do know of several rare inherited disorders of membrane transport in man and in other species which are viewed with great interest because of the insight they bring concerning the organization and function of membrane transport processes.

The following discussion is limited primarily to the genetics of amino acid transport in man because of our own particular interests, and because most of the basic principles of transport genetics can be covered within this limitation. An excellent general discussion of inherited disorders of membrane function is available elsewhere.[169]

## MEMBRANE TRANSPORT

### General Comments

The idea of the cell as a biological unit differentiated from its environment was first developed based on the observations of Nageli in 1844 (cited by

Scott[193]). Working with plant cells, he demonstrated a semi-permeable diffusion barrier dividing the interior of the cell from the exterior. Although the barrier was invisible to the microscopy of his own time, the simple osmotic experiments performed by Nageli confirmed its physical presence adequately. He also found that a new protoplasmic surface identical to the original disrupted surface grew quickly around extruded cell protoplasm. Nageli gave the name *plasmamembran* to this surface layer. All subsequent work has been an attempt to define more precisely the nature of the surface diffusion barrier. Workers such as Pfeffer[158] and Overton[150] further developed the osmotic concepts applicable to biological cells, but, as Homer Smith has so whimsically stated,[219] "On the whole, a century elapsed during which the terms 'membrane,' 'cell membrane,' and 'plasma membrane' appear in many papers, settling here and there in subordinate clauses, less rarely appearing as the grammatical subject of a sentence, before the ghost acquired bones and flesh and became a matter of proper scientific interest." It was Chambers who gave the plasma membrane its first rigorous definition by means of micropuncture and dissection methods.[21-23]

Across this membrane there occurs the traffic of free molecules which participate in the commerce of cell metabolism and biosynthesis; products and by-products of this metabolism must also leave the cell by crossing the same plasma membrane. This traffic is more elegantly termed "biological transport." The same process, when it occurs between intracellular compartments across internal membranes, is likely to be of equal importance and subject to those laws which also govern transport across the plasma membrane. This regulatory process thus establishes and maintains the remarkable difference in composition between intracellular and extracellular fluids.

Membranes probably played an important role in early chemical evolution,[20] and later in cellular or biological evolution. Living biological cells without membranes are unknown. Transport across membranes is thus a universal function, essential for survival. In multicellular organisms, such as man, this function has been specialized to such a degree in such organs as the intestine and the renal tubule that survival is impossible if these transport tissues are ablated.

The matrix for function of transport in all membranes is an aggregation of lipids and proteins, the precise chemical structure and physical disposition of which is still a subject of considerable debate.[124,147,153,163,228] The actual mechanisms by which molecules are moved across the barrier is also still very much a "black box"[153,163,228]. And yet, despite our ignorance and the frustration derived therefrom, there is fascination in what can be observed and surmised concerning the nature of membrane transport.

## Descriptive Terms

Before proceeding with a description of the transport processes in man which are affected by mutation, it is useful to define the terms which will be used in the discussion. There are a number of mechanisms whereby a molecule such as an amino acid can gain access to the interior of the cell.[24] For example, *chemical modification* of a solute may occur in or on the membrane with or without significant translocation. This appears to play an important role in the uptake of monosaccharides in some systems.[4,126,216] There is believed to be no significant chemical modification of amino acids during the actual uptake process into mammalian cells,[24] although isolated examples of uptake of conjugated amino acid derivatives have been described;[5] but again, these do not account for the greater part of amino acid access. Molecules may enter cells by *passive diffusion*, the velocity of diffusion being a linear function of their partition coefficient between lipid and aqueous phases; yet amino acids, which are hydrophilic and which should thus be held to the external aqueous phase, penetrate into cells across hydrophobic intact biological membranes at rates greater than can be accounted for by diffusion. Amino acids must therefore gain access to the cell by some other process.

*Transfer in bulk phase* occurs when the extracellular fluid containing the solute is engulfed by the cell. The engulfing process is known as *pinocytosis*,[99] and it occurs regularly in some cells of the body; however, it is not a mechanism which can account for the observed rates of uptake of free amino acids in most tissues.

It is clear then that some agency must mediate the uptake of free amino acids, and, in fact, there are several forms of *mediated transport.* If the transport of the ampholyte occurs against a concentration gradient, and energy is expended to achieve the uptake, then the process is said to be *active.* If the mediated transport is not against a gradient, or energy is not expended, then some form of *facilitated diffusion* accounts for the process. Mediated diffusions may involve *exchange*,[92,104] and if the influx of one molecule is opposed by efflux of another molecule of the same species and employing the same transport mechanism, homoexchange or counterflow is said to exist; when the molecules which exchange across the membrane are different the process is one of *heteroexchange.* In the latter case it is possible for the influx to occur against a gradient with little or no requirement for energy.

The assumption inherent in all proposals for mediated transport is that the solute combines with a reactive site[24,147,153,228] on the surface of the membrane, following which translocation across the membrane occurs. How energy is applied to the transport is unknown, and there is no single hypothesis which has yet explained the process of translocation. Several recent reviews have discussed these and related topics in transport.[42,94,109,124,147,153,228]

## Genetic Variation

The inability to define by direct analysis the physical and chemical features of membrane transport systems for free amino acids and other solutes has forced the investigator to utilize information gained by other means, such as the study of mutant transport phenotypes. For example, much of our current understanding of membrane transport has been derived from the study of transport mutants in nonhuman species (Table I). It is apparent from the mutants listed in Table I that microorganisms have yielded most of this information. By contrast, much less is known about mutant transport phenotypes in vertebrates (Table I), and a recent review[135] of the hereditary metabolic phenotypes discovered in nonhuman vertebrates catalogs very few inborn errors of transport. If we want the best opportunity for studying the hereditary variation of membrane transport in vertebrates, it is to man that we must turn, for in this species a respectable number of aberrant transport phenotypes have been identified (Table II). In each condition listed in this table there is clear, or strongly suggestive, evidence that the trait is inherited according to Mendelian laws. There are many mutations at the genetic loci which control the specific transport processes of the cell, and a detailed analysis of the mutant amino acid transport phenotypes in man shows that the genetic control of transport mechanisms is highly refined. In fact, it is evident that the sophistication of genetic control which we have come to accept for the synthesis of hemoglobin or glucose-6-phosphate dehydrogenase, for example, is present also for a function as important to cellular economy as membrane transport.

## CHARACTERISTICS OF THE TRANSPORT PROCESS

The subsequent portions of this chapter are confined primarily to a discussion of amino acid transport in man. This process, like the transport of the other solutes referred to in Table I, involves facilitated movement of a particular class of free molecules across cell membranes. A *carrier*, or some form of mediator, is involved in the transfer process. Recent investigations in man, supported by experiments in nonhuman systems, have contributed information about the characteristics of the membrane components used in the transport of amino acids.

**TABLE I.  Transport Mutations of Nonhuman Species**

| Mutation affecting transport of | Species | Substrates included | Substrates excluded | References |
|---|---|---|---|---|
| I. In bacteria | | | | |
| A. Amino Acids | | | | |
| Proline | *Escherichia coli* | L-Azetidine-2-carboxylate, 3,4-dehydroproline | L-Hydroxyproline, DL-pipecolate | 112, 120, 133, 241, 253 |
| Aromatic amino acids | *Salmonella typhimurium* | L-Phenylalanine, L-tyrosine, L-tryptophan, L-histidine | — | 60 |
| Histidine | *Escherichia coli* | — | Arginine | 215 |
| Glutamic acid | *Escherichia coli* | — | — | 85 |
| Glutamic acid | *Streptococcus faecalis* | L-Aspartate | — | 96 |
| D-Serine | *Escherichia coli* | L-Serine, L-alanine, glycine | Arginine | 189 |
| Arginine | *Escherichia coli* | Canavanine, lysine, ornithine | Serine, alanine, cystine | 189 |
| Glycine | *Escherichia coli* | — | L-Serine, glycyl-glycine | 129 |
| Dipeptides | *Escherichia coli* | Glycyl-glycine, other dipeptides | Glycine | 121 |
| Oligopeptides | *Escherichia coli* | Triornithine, triarginine, trilysine, dilysylcadverine | Amino acids, lysine, tetrapeptides | 156 |

**TABLE I** (*continued*)

| Mutation affecting transport of | Species | Substrates included | Substrates excluded | References |
|---|---|---|---|---|
| **B. Sugars** | | | | |
| L-α-Glycerol phosphate | *Escherichia coli* | — | Glycerol | 36 |
| β-Glucosides | *Escherichia coli* | — | — | 187 |
| β-Galactosides | *Escherichia coli* | — | Other sugars | 33 |
| Carbohydrates | *Staphylococcus aureus,* and *Aerobacter aerogenes* | Monosaccharides, disaccharides, polyols | Amino acids, dicarboxylic acids, glycerol | 53, 234 |
| **C. Drugs** | | | | |
| Amethopterin | *Diplococcus pneumoniae* | — | — | 217 |
| **D. Ions** | | | | |
| Orthophosphate | *Bacillus cereus* | Orthophosphate, pyrophosphate, arsenate | Organic phosphates | 180 |
| Sulfate | *Salmonella typhimurium* | Chromate, vanadate, thiosulphate | — | 154, 155 |
| Potassium | *Escherichia coli* | Sodium efflux | — | 132 |
| **II. In fungi** | | | | |
| **A. Amino Acids** | | | | |
| Histidine | *Neurospora crassa* (linkage group V) | Arginine, lysine | Neutral and acidic amino acids | 258 |
| Neutral amino acids | *Neurospora crassa* (linkage group IV) | Tryptophan, leucine, serine, histidine, (other neutrals) | Arginine, lysine | 128, 227 |
| Cationic amino acids | *Neurospora crassa* (linkage group I) | Tryptophan, arginine, lysine (modifier gene effect) | — | 226 |
| Neutral amino acids | *Neurospora crassa* (linkage group V) | Acidic and neutral amino acids, arginine | Lysine | 103 |
| Selected substrates | *Neurospora crassa* (linkage group I) | Neutral, acidic potassium | Lysine, glucose, acetate (membrane | 113 |

| | | | | |
|---|---|---|---|---|
| Arginine | *Saccharomyces cerevisiae* | Lysine, ornithine, histidine | All other amino acids | 81 |
| Lysine | *Saccharomyces cerevisiae* | | All other amino acids | 80 |
| Methionine | *Saccharomyces cerevisiae* | Ethionine | All other amino acids | 74 |
| B. Sugars | | | | |
| Isomaltose | *Saccharomyces cerevisiae* | | — | 86 |
| C. Purines | | | | |
| Purines (axg) | *Aspergillus nidulans* | Hypoxanthine, guanine, adenine | — | 43 |
| Purines (uap) | *Aspergillus nidulans* | Xanthine, uric acid | — | 43 |
| III. In Metazoa: vertebrate (nonhuman) | | | | |
| A. Amino Acids | | | | |
| Cystine | *Canis familiaris* (dog) | Lysine, ornithine, arginine | All other amino acids | 34a, 238, 251 |
| Cystine[a] | *Mustela vison* (mink) | ? | — | 148 |
| B. Purines | | | | |
| Uric acid | *Canis familiaris* (dog) (dalmatian) | Allantoin | — | 90, 251 |
| C. Vitamins | | | | |
| Riboflavin | *Gallus gallus* (chicken) | | — | 35 |
| D. Ions | | | | |
| Potassium | *Trichosurus vulpecula* (possum) | Sodium efflux | — | 6 |
| Potassium | *Ovis aries* (sheep) | Sodium efflux | — | 122 |
| Potassium | *Capra hircus* (goat) | Sodium efflux | — | 55 |
| E. Drugs | | | | |
| Amethopterin | *Mus musculus* L51784 leukemia cells[b] | | — | 64, 119 |

[a] Cystine identified by chemical methods; excretion pattern of other amino acids not investigated.
[b] Probably a somatic mutation; trait identified in tumor cells.

TABLE II.  Transport Mutations of Man

| Substrates affected | Trait | Tissue[a] | Mode of inheritance | Ref. |
|---|---|---|---|---|
| **I. Amino Acids** | | | | |
| *Specific groups of amino acids* | | | | |
| Cystine, lysine, ornithine, arginine | The "classical" cystinurias | Kidney (intestine) | Autosomal recessive | 10, 123, 168 |
| Lysine, ornithine, arginine | Hyperdibasicaminoaciduria | Kidney (intestine) | Autosomal recessive (or dominant) | 116, 250 |
| Imino acids and glycine | Imino-glycinuria | Kidney (intestine) | Autosomal recessive | 178, 200 |
| Neutral amino acids (except imino acids and glycine) | Hartnup disease | Kidney (intestine) | Autosomal recessive | 7, 106 |
| *Single amino acids* | | | | |
| Cystine | Hypercystinuria | Kidney | Autosomal recessive | 18 |
| Tryptophan | Blue diaper syndrome | Intestine | Autosomal recessive (?)[b] | 49 |
| Methionine | Methionine malabsorption syndrome | Intestine | Autosomal recessive (?)[b] | 100 |
| **II. Monosaccharides** | | | | |
| Glucose | Renal glucosuria | Kidney | Undecided | 125 |
| Glucose and galactose | Glucose-galactose malabsorption | Intestine; kidney? | Autosomal recessive | 188 |
| **III. Electrolytes, water, and others** | | | | |
| Phosphate | Familial hypophosphatemic rickets | Kidney; intestine (?) | X-linked dominant | 19, 252 |
| Calcium (Parathyroid hormone binding to membrane) | Pseudohypoparathyroidism | Kidney, intestine, bone | Autosomal dominant | 9, 137 |

| Substance / transport | Disorder | Tissue[a] | Inheritance[b] | Reference |
|---|---|---|---|---|
| Calcium (vitamin D binding to membrane?) | Vitamin D dependency | Gut; bone? | Autosomal recessive (or dominant?) | 162 |
| Bicarbonate | Renal tubular acidosis | Kidney | Autosomal recessive | 69 |
| Hydrogen ion | Renal tubular acidosis | Kidney | Autosomal dominant | 221 |
| Chloride | Congenital chloridorrhea | Intestine | Autosomal recessive | 213 |
| Sodium | Hereditary spherocytosis | Erythrocyte | Autosomal dominant | 56 |
| Sodium and potassium | ATPase deficiency, hemolytic anemia | Erythrocyte | Autosomal recessive | 105 |
|  | Other mechanisms | Erythrocyte | Autosomal recessive (?) | 89 |
|  |  |  | (Unknown) | 262 |
| Water | Diabetes Insipidis (Vasopressin resistant) | Kidney | X-linked recessive | 149 |
| Vitamin B$_{12}$ | Vitamin B$_{12}$ malabsorption | Intestine | Autosomal recessive | 75, 79 |
| **IV. General, and Others** |  |  |  |  |
| Amino acids | Rowley–Rosenberg–Busby syndrome | Kidney; muscle? | Not known | 181, 185 |
| Amino acids, monosaccharides, electrolytes, water, etc. | Fanconi syndrome | Kidney, intestine | Autosomal recessive for many of its causes | 127 |
|  | Lowe–Terrey–Maclachlan syndrome | Kidney, intestine | X-linked recessive | 1 |
| Glucose-glycine | Glucoglycinuria | Kidney | Autosomal dominant | 114 |
| Gluco-aminoaciduria | Luder–Sheldon syndrome | Kidney | Autosomal dominant | 100a, 134, 214a |

[a] Parentheses indicate tissues which are affected in some forms of the trait and not in others (see discussion on genetic heterogeneity).

[b] Inheritance of trait not yet proven rigorously.

## Relevance of Transport to the Distribution of Amino Acids in Body Fluids

### Plasma–Tissue Distribution Ratios

To detect abnormal distributions of amino acids in body fluids one must first know the normal distribution. Consequently, recognition of the various forms of hyperaminoacidemia or hyperaminoaciduria[50,51,182,198,199] has required careful determination of normal values in the human subject under a variety of prescribed conditions.[182] It is now apparent that membrane transport plays an important role in the establishment and maintenance of these "normal" distributions.

Van Slyke and Meyer[242] were the first to describe the distribution of free amino acids between plasma and tissue water. Their important paper describes a concentration gradient in the dog for amino acids distributed between the tissues and the plasma; amino acids are held inside the cells, in the free state, at concentrations which are higher than in the plasma.

Little was done with this observation until Christensen and colleagues undertook a detailed evaluation of its significance.[25,31] Christensen[25] has proposed that the tissues act as reservoirs for amino acids (Fig. 1), thereby sustaining an extracellular equilibrium which is perturbed very little by normal metabolic and nutritional events. One factor which helps to establish this equilibrium appears to be the cell plasma membrane, as indicated by a number of seemingly unrelated observations:

1. The concentration of individual amino acids in the plasma of human subjects has been measured, and the normal range has been established.[182] Subjects of similar age living in America,[98,202] Africa,[223] and Europe,[17] and who presumably have diets of different protein and amino acid composition, have remarkably similar plasma amino acid profiles.

2. Man ingests his protein at isolated moments of the day, at which time the amino acid intake from the intestine may be ten times greater than the free amino acid pool in extracellular fluids. Yet there is remarkably little diurnal fluctuation in plasma amino acid concentration,[57,58,260] and there is no important change in amino acid excretion in urine.[202,223]

3. Amino acid concentrations in human plasma are lower during periods of growth than in the adult,[182] even though protein intake per kilogram of body weight in the child is higher than in the adult. Christensen and Streicher[31] and Noall and colleagues[146] showed that the distribution ratio (amino acids in tissues): (amino acids in extracellular fluids) is higher in the young animal than in the adult.

4. Introduction of a metabolically inert amino acid at high concentrations *in vivo* impedes tubular conservation of certain amino acids, and

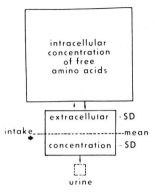

Fig. 1. Distribution of free amino acids (or other analogous metabolites) in body water. Note that largest pool and greatest concentration is found intracellularly.[242] Size of extracellular pool has statistical limits (e.g., normal plasma amino acid values).[182] Uptake across membrane into reservoir of cells serves to regulate size of extracellular pool during times of fluctuating intake. Loss of amino acids, etc., into urine by mammals, including man, is small, because of tubular transport of solute across membranes back into cells.

depletes liver of one third to two thirds of its free intracellular amino acid pool.[29] Competition for transport explains this observation.

Thus, with regard to the concentration of amino acids in plasma and tissues, it appears that the ability of tissues to take up these free solutes and to hold them is an important factor in sustaining the observed equilibrium. To achieve this, the amino acids must pass cell membranes, an event influenced by many factors.

## Plasma–Urine Distribution

The intervention of membrane transport in the final distribution of amino acids in body fluids is evident in the formation of urine. Less than 3–5% of the filtered amino acid load is actually excreted in the bladder urine, indicating that net absorption occurs during tubular transit. In studies employing nonmetabolizable amino acids in man[28] and in the rat[28,30] Christensen's group showed that renal tubular absorption *in vivo* from urine into plasma occurs against a concentration gradient across the tubular epithelial sheet.

Accurate measurement of the endogenous renal clearance rates of individual free amino acids became feasible with the advent of improved elution chromatography on ion-exchange resin columns. Subsequently, a considerable body of data was developed concerning renal clearance of amino acids by the human subject under a variety of normal physiological conditions.[17,182] Endogenous renal clearance rates indicate something about the characteristics of net tubular absorption of amino acids; low values indicate avid reabsorption, and high values, by comparison, point to greater tubular rejection of the filtered solute. The data shown in Fig. 2 show that the short-chain aliphatic neutral amino acids are less well reabsorbed than those with longer carbon side chains at similar concentrations in plasma. These characteristics of amino acid uptake by human kidney *in vivo* parallel those found in the intestine of other mammals.[62,130,201,255] It appears that the lipophilic property of the side chain is a decisive factor in determining the accessibility of an amino acid to bind with its reactive site for transport across the membrane.

Another characteristic of amino acid transport by human kidney is also shown in Fig. 2. The clearance of L-proline rises steeply when its concentration in plasma reaches a certain level, indicating rapid saturation of the binding sites, whereas the same characteristic is not seen at comparable concentrations in plasma of L-phenylalanine. The difference in the renal clearance of these two molecules indicates that the kidney absorbs them in different ways. A number of the features of membrane transport are thus identified from these simple, but indirect, measurements of renal uptake of amino acids.

### Characteristics Which Can Be Determined in vivo and in vitro

### Saturability

Saturation kinetics for the uptake of glucose [$T_m$(glucose)] by kidney *in vivo* were described first in the dog[214] and then in man[220] using the classical technique of intravenous infusion of the solute, measurement of the filtered and excreted amounts, and calculation of the amount of net absorption at various filtered loads. Saturation kinetics in vivo for the absorption of many other substrates, including amino acids were subsequently defined for dog kidney.[160,218] However, it was not until recently that this feature of

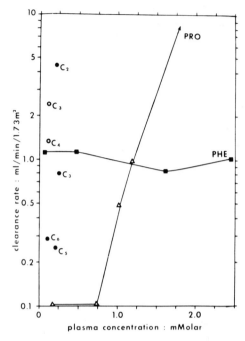

Fig. 2. Renal clearance of amino acids varies with respect to their chemical structure and their concentration in plasma. Closed circles at left numbered $C_2$, $C_3$, etc., indicate neutral aliphatic amino acids with 2, 3, etc. carbon atoms; open circles indicate hydroxy–aliphatic neutral amino acids. Note decreasing clearance (i.e., better net tubular absorption) with increasing side-chain length. Triangles and squares show clearance of L-proline and L-phenylalanine, respectively. Renal transport of the former saturates early in both normal and hyperprolinemic subjects;[200] phenylalanine transport has not been saturated in a phenylketonuric subject, even at 25 times the normal substrate concentration.

amino acid absorption was also demonstrated conclusively for human kidney *in vivo* (Fig. 3); L-proline[203] and hydroxy-L-proline[205] both exhibit a maximal rate of tubular reabsorption ($T_m$).

Saturable membrane transport of amino acids has been investigated intensively *in vitro* (Fig. 3) using the rat kidney cortex slice technique;[171] saturable uptake by human kidney slices has also been studied by this technique.[67,170] Several other tissues of man and other mammals also show

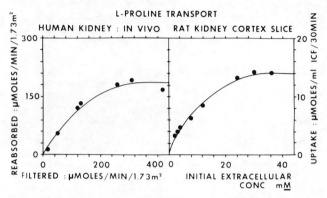

Fig. 3.   Evidence for a mediated mode of entry of polar solutes into cells. Membrane transport of amino acids is saturable and concentrative, as shown by data on uptake of L-proline by human kidney *in vivo* (left), and by rat kidney cortex slices *in vitro* (right). (Data taken from *in vivo* work by Scriver et al.[203] and from *in vitro* studies by Mohyuddin and Scriver.[140])

evidence for a saturable migration of amino acids.* The *in vitro* studies show that solutes such as amino acids also use a nonsaturable diffusional migration, which is probably mediated,[3] in addition to the saturable component, which is of prime importance physiologically.

## Concentrative Uptake

Amino acid transport by human kidney *in vivo* takes place against a concentration gradient; Christensen and Clifford[28] employed the metabolically inert amino acid 1-aminocyclopentanecarboxylic acid to demonstrate this feature of renal absorption in man.

Human tissues have also been studied *in vitro*; leucocytes,[174] kidney cortex,[67,170] intestinal mucosa,[143,237] and cultured skin fibroblasts[161] are each capable of concentrative uptake of amino acids. Moreover, the distribution ratio (free amino acids of red blood cells): (free amino acids of plasma) is usually greater than 1.0, again pointing to concentrative uptake

---

*Several reports of particular interest have appeared since a review of these aspects of transport by Johnstone and Scholefield;[109] they include descriptions of uptake into human white cells[174] and red cells,[13,257] human intestine,[143,237] human skin fibroblasts,[161] rat muscle,[15,54] rat renal papilla,[131] rat glomeruli,[136] rat bone,[63] and other organs of the rat,[144] isolated rabbit kidney tubules,[93,107,142] mouse pancreas,[12] and brain.[14]

even in these cells.[13,257] An expenditure of metabolic energy is required by tissues which can sustain concentrative uptake.

## Specificity of the Transport Process

At one time it was customary to think that amino acids were transported by relatively nonspecific mechanisms which bound all amino acids. However, the selective nature of most hereditary hyperaminoacidurias (see Table II, for example) indicates that a number of selective membrane transport systems serve the transport of amino acids into cells.

### Preference for the L-Stereo Isomer.
Studies in the living human subject indicate the clear preference of renal transport systems for the L-enantiomorphs of amino acids.[16] Piel and Harper[159] and Efron et al.[52] documented a high renal clearance rate for D-methionine in contrast to the normal low renal clearance of the L-methionine.[17,202,223] Although mammalian tissues do transport the D-isomers of amino acids by mediated processes,[151] the affinity of reactive sites for the D-enantiomorph is many times less than for the natural isomer.

### Chemical Specificity.
Many types of investigation indicate that some chemical specificity is required of an amino acid for its binding by a reactive membrane site.[24] Chemical modification of selected test solutes reveals that free carboxyl and amino groups are necessary for mediated uptake of amino acids, while the $\alpha$-hydrogen is not. Covalent linkage of the carboxyl or amino groups in peptide bonds relegates peptides to transport sites which are segregated from those used by the constituent free amino acids. A clear segregation of peptide and amino acid transports has been shown for human kidney in vivo[195] and rodent intestine in vitro,[145] as well as in other biological systems (Table I).

Higher distribution ratios between the cell water and the extracellular space, and greater affinity for uptake can be discerned when the amino group is alpha- rather than beta- or omega- to the carboxyl group. In man a simple demonstration of this is seen in the high renal clearance of $\beta$-alanine compared to the low clearance of $\alpha$-L-alanine.[207]

Selective interactions in vivo between amino acids have been identified during uptake by rat kidney[76,254] (Fig. 4), by mouse kidney,[73] and by dog kidney.[243–245,247] Comparable selective interactions during renal absorption are also found in man. Robson and Rose[166] showed that when cationic ("dibasic") amino acids such as lysine, ornithine, or arginine are infused intravenously into human subjects net tubular absorption of the other dibasic amino acids is depressed; the absorption of cystine was also depressed.

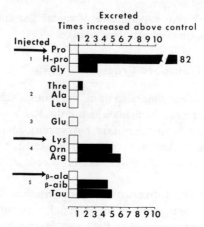

Fig. 4. Evidence for ability of transport sites to recognize chemical and molecular specificity. Example of specific interactions between groups of amino acids during tubular absorption *in vivo* in rat; these interactions represent a process of competitive inhibition, as shown by further experiments *in vitro*.[254] The "injected" amino acid is delivered into the peritoneum or the cardiac ventricle; urine collection is performed in the subsequent hour(s). The concentration of amino acids in urine is then compared with that of the control (preinjection) urine sample. Note that interactions are essentially confined to the chemical group to which the injected amino acid belongs. Numbers on left refer to transport groups: (1) iminoglycine; (2) other neutrals; (3) anionic; (4) cationic (dibasic); (5) β-amino. A series of different membrane sites must exist to accomodate this range of specificity.

The imino acids proline and hydroxyproline, and the neutral α-amino acid glycine, manifest selective interaction during tubular transport in man.[203,205] Selective interaction has also been identified for the β-amino acids during uptake by human kidney *in vivo*.[207] Each of these patterns of interaction has also been documented *in vitro* in kidney and in other tissues.[26,254] Under *in vitro* conditions it can be shown that competitive inhibition for binding occurs between the individual members of the substrate groups. Such evidence suggests that a group of chemically related amino acids can share a common reactive site, although it does not exclude the possibility that a single amino acid may have access to more than one transport system.[26,27,254]

The above-mentioned studies indicate the presence of several recognition sites on the membrane, each with a preference for a certain chemical group of amino acids. At present five "common" systems have been described in human kidney (Fig. 5) which facilitate the migration of cationic amino acids, anionic amino acids, neutral aliphatic and ring-structured amino acids, neutral imino (secondary) acids and glycine, and the $\beta$-amino compounds, respectively. These shared, or "common," systems operate at substrate concentrations which exceed the usual physiological range. They have been described so far primarily in kidney and intestine, where their capacity to mediate uptake at high solute concentration may confer a nutritional advantage.[224] Few studies have been carried out to determines whether high-capacity, shared-transport systems also occur on cell membranes of other tissues. The work of Blasberg and Lajtha[14] does suggest that such transport systems are present in the brain of mouse.

**Multiplicity of Systems Available to Individual Substrates.** There is another pattern of specificity for the cellular uptake of amino acids (Fig. 5). In this case the specificity is expressed in relation to the concentration of the solute. Moreover, qualitative characteristics such as $Na^+$ dependence and selective effects of inhibitors also identify a multiplicity of carriers serving migration of individual amino acids. It is increasingly

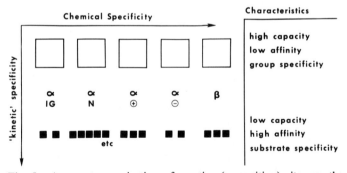

Fig. 5. Apparent organization of reactive (recognition) sites on the plasma membrane for amino acid uptake by mammalian kidney and intestine. Sites have at least two types of specificity; one for the chemical nature of solute, another with respect to the concentration of substrate. Specificity is broad, capacity is great, and affinity for substrate is low when the substrates are at "high" concentration (i.e., above the usual plasma concentration range); sites for uptake at low substrate concentration have the opposite characteristics.

apparent that different modes of access are used by amino acids when the substrate presents itself at different concentrations. Two studies in man show this particularly well. Rosenberg and colleagues[170] found evidence *in vitro* for more than one mode of lysine uptake by human kidney cortex slices. When the reciprocal of the rate of uptake was plotted against the reciprocal of the substrate concentration (Lineweaver and Burk plot) a biphasic regression was obtained. The mode of lysine transport utilized at the low or physiological concentrations of the substrate was characterized by its high affinity and low capacity; the other mediation was used at relatively high concentrations of substrate, and it was characterized by its low affinity, but high capacity. In another study by Scriver and Wilson[200,208] it was found that human kidney absorbed imino acids and glycine by two modes *in vivo*, each with different kinetic characteristics which resembled those described for lysine in terms of capacity and affinity.

These studies, indicating heterogeneity of amino acid transport in man, were preceded by a series of interesting reports by Christensen,[26,27] who described amino acid uptake by mouse ascites tumor cells and other tissues; these studies clearly drew attention to the multiple mediations available to a single amino acid.[26,27] Other groups have described uptake of individual amino acids by heterogeneous modes in rat kidney[140,206,212] and in bone cells.[63] The phenomenon is thus evident in several species and tissues. It has also been documented in microorganisms.[117] Therefore, it would appear that heterogeneity of uptake is an important feature of membrane transport. Whether it is characteristic of all tissues in metazoans, such as man, is still unknown.

## Other Characteristics

Several characteristics of membrane transport of amino acids have been delineated in mammalian tissues *in vitro* which do not lend themselves to the equivalent documentation *in vivo* in man. A thermal coefficient has been described for uptake into rat kidney cortex slices,[171,191,254] as well as in many other tissues. Since the $Q10$ for uptake of several amino acids is in the vicinity of 2.0, this can be taken as further evidence that transport of amino acids is both mediated and energy-dependent, and that it does not occur by passive diffusion. However, aerobic metabolism is not essential to achieve concentrative transport; leucocytes[174] and renal papilla[131] can both accumulate amino acids under anaerobic conditions.

A number of studies reveal that the uptake of many amino acids, particularly of neutral amino acids with short side chains,[152] is dependent on $Na^+$; this feature has been well documented, for example, in kidney,[66,206,235] gut,[172] bone,[63] and leucocytes.[174] The $Na^+$ dependence is usually linked to concentrative uptake, whereas uptake of one amino acid during exchange with another amino acid inside the cell may not require the presence of sodium ion.[108] Information of this nature illuminates, but still does not clarify, how energy derived from cellular metabolism is used to achieve concentrative transport. The dependence of concentrative transport upon metabolic energy is evident from experiments in which the exposure of cells to inhibitors of metabolic energy production abolishes concentrative transport.

It is possible that energy is applied primarily to pump $Na^+$ from the cell's interior to the extracellular space, in order to establish an electrochemical asymmetry at the membrane; when this takes place amino acid uptake can occur. If a molecule of amino acid can substitute for $Na^+$, so that the former moves perforce "downhill" out of the cell, then a second amino acid could move "uphill" into the cell in terms of its own concentration gradient during an exchange reaction, even in the absence of $Na^+$, and without energy expenditure at the time of the exchange.[152]

There is also some evidence that $Na^+$ participates in amino acid transport as a ternary complex with the amino acid [–A–] and the membrane carrier [–C–] in the form [–ACNa–].[101,206] How this influences the solute's traversal across the cell membrane is still undefined.

The availability of ATP for the process of membrane transport has been demonstrated in various ways. It has been suggested that a membrane ATPase may itself be the carrier for cations,[94] but the relevance of these observations to amino acid transport is unknown. For instance, the amino acid "permeases" of microorganisms, which have many features in common with the equivalent transport systems in mammalian tissues have no $Na^+$ dependence, and yet they exhibit energy dependence.

Concentrative uptake requires that the membrane carrier should first receive its solute on the outer surface of the membrane. The carrier must then undergo a modification at the inner surface of the membrane, which reduces its affinity for the substrate, releasing it into the interior of the cell. Thus, it is possible that the mechanism of release, the return of the carrier to the original position, and its reconstitution to a state receptive for binding of the next molecule of substrate at the outer surface are each processes dependent on metabolic energy. If these are the basic requirements for reversible substrate binding, it is not surprising that the number of models which have been proposed to accomodate the available data with hypotheses are almost as numerous as the investigators in the field!

## Influence of Hormones and Vitamins on Transport Processes

The participation of hormones, such as antidiuretic, parathyroid, and steroid hormones, and vitamins, such as vitamin D, in the transport of electrolytes and water across membranes is well known. Mutations which modify the specific membrane sites at which these hormones act will alter membrane transport of the appropriate substrate.

The influence of hormones and vitamins on nonelectrolyte transport is more nebulous, and at present hormone- or vitamin-dependent mutant transport phenotypes for amino acids are unknown in man, to our knowledge. Insulin does influence amino acid uptake in muscle,[54] but it has no effect on this process in kidney, intestine, or brain. Its effect is twofold: by increasing the affinity of the carrier mechanism for amino acids, and by initiating synthesis of membrane transport proteins. Recent work by Elsas and Rosenberg[54a] has shown that there is apparent turnover in membrane transport proteins being observed over a 3-hr period in mammalian kidney. Hormones may therefore act to modulate the rate of turnover of membrane proteins which participate in transport reactions. In this case a change in the rate of the reaction would be observed without any alteration in the affinity of the membrane for the substrate. Alternatively, the hormone may combine with the transport site, or near it, at which time a conformational change in the site occurs which modulates the migration of substrate. In this case one anticipates a change in the $Km$ of the transport reaction. It is well known that hormonal effects on transport are frequently limited to certain classes of substrate and in certain tissues.[24] Such specificity implies that genetic regulation in the expression of the hormone-binding site in a given cell may be one source of hormonal and tissue specificity in transport reactions. We anticipate that there will be new and considerable activity in this area of transport research, and that inherited disorders of hormone-dependent amino acid transport will come to be recognized.

Parathyroid hormone impairs renal transport of amino acids *in vivo* in man[41,68] and rat.[82] The postulated role of vitamin D in membrane transport of amino acids[110] is only indirect and can be accounted for in terms of its complex relationship to calcium metabolism and parathyroid activity.[82]

Observations which at first intimated that vitamin $B_6$ and biotin participate in membrane transport have, after more intensive study, required a more conservative interpretation. For example, the work of Holden's group[95,97] on pyridoxine- and biotin-dependent transport phenotypes in *Lactobatillus* showed that it was the capacity of the organism to withstand osmotic pressure after solute transport, and not migration of solutes, which was affected through interference in cell wall synthesis. Membrane transport was only impaired secondarily because of the osmotic fragility of the cells. Since these observations were made the interest in the role of vitamin $B_6$ in membrane transport of amino acids has waned.[24] Neither pyridoxal or pyridoxal phosphate functions as a carrier, nor do carbonyl reagents, which inhibit vitamin $B_6$-dependent reactions, inhibit transport of amino acids.

Again, it is probable that the obvious changes in amino acid distribution observed in the vitamin $B_6$-deficient rat[165] were the result of cellular changes secondary to $B_6$-dependent metabolic events, and were not due to any direct participation of the vitamin in membrane transport.

## Influence of Metabolism on Transport

Metabolic energy is required to achieve concentrative uptake, except under certain conditions of exchange diffusion. Moreover, substrates which have been transported into the cell may participate in the processes of energy metabolism. Therefore, it is conceivable that the metabolic fate of a particular solute might affect the characteristic of its own transport. Some consideration has been given to this problem,[139] but experiments in this vein are still not very numerous.

Is cellular transport of solute impeded when its normal catabolism is blocked? For instance, in phenylketonuria the principal degradative pathway of phenylalanine is completely blocked at the first step of catabolism. As a result, the concentration of phenylalanine in body fluids rises manyfold above the normal level. Yet, phenylalanine transport in kidney, measured in terms of net tubular absorption, is not impeded,[17b,230] and the normal efficiency of its renal clearance is unaltered (see Fig. 2). In this, as in other examples of "the blocked catabolic mutant," the aberrant metabolic event tends to "isolate" the normal transport event; uptake can then be studied to the same advantage as when metabolically inert compounds, such as $\alpha$-aminoisobutyric acid (AIB)[121] and 1-aminocyclopentanecarboxylic acid (ACPC),[2] are used to study transport. Useful studies of membrane transport have indeed been performed in microorganisms using blocked catabolic mutants for this specific purpose.[91] The many human hereditary amino-acidopathies[50,51,182,199] which are, in essence, "blocked catabolic mutants" could be equally well used for a better understanding of membrane transport phenomena in man.

Does the normal intracellular catabolism of the substrate affect the kinetics of its own uptake? This is an important question if experiments are performed under steady-state conditions, where the distribution ratio of amino acid in the intracellular space relative to the extracellular space achieves a constant value. If the isotopically labeled substrate is catabolized, the identity of the radiochemical isotope inside the cell at equilibrium may be different from the radiochemical introduced into the system at the beginning of the experiment, depending on the rate of metabolic conversion of the accumulated substrate. Yet, the measurement of net accumulation depends only on measurement of isotope distribution; true uptake may not actually be measured if the metabolic fate of the isotope is ignored.

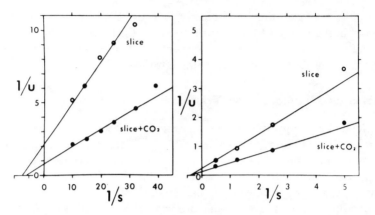

Fig. 6. Effect of substrate catabolism after uptake on the kinetics of substrate uptake. Studies by Mohyuddin and Scriver[140] are depicted in which oxidation and retention of L-proline were measured after uptake by rat kidney cortex slices. When catabolism is accounted for the apparent rate constant ($V_{max}$), but not the binding constant ($Km$), of the substrate is affected. This applies whether migration is studied at low concentration of substrate (left), or at high concentration (right). Transport at these different concentration ranges occurs on a specific and a common site, respectively.

The effect of catabolism on the kinetics of L-proline uptake into rat kidney cortex slices has been studied.[140] Mohyuddin and Scriver found that up to 60% of L-proline underwent conversion to other metabolites and to $CO_2$ during a 40-min incubation of rat kidney cortex slices. Nonetheless, there was no difference in the $Km$ value for uptake of L-proline by the slices, whether or not the intracellular conversion of the label was taken into account. On the other hand, the observed rate of uptake and $V_{max}$ was considerably altered by the metabolic conversion (Fig. 6).

An *in vivo* study of this type of problem revealed no alteration in the absorption of L-proline by kidney in human subjects with familial hyperprolinemia,[203] which is another form of blocked catabolic mutant.

Thus, estimates of the specificity and binding affinity of transport systems are apparently not influenced by cellular metabolism of the substrate, whereas estimates of the rate or capacity for its transport might be greatly compromised by such events.

### Summary and Interpretation of the Characteristics of Membrane Transport Systems

Transport of amino acids and other polar solutes across intact biological membranes is a mediated and saturable process which usually is concentrative and requires metabolic energy. Sodium ion is also required for active transport of many neutral amino acids.

It is apparent that two types of specificity are offered by amino acid transport systems. One form recognizes chemical differences between the molecules which bind to the reactive site or transport carrier; the other form of specificity offers, to a single substrate, the option to be transported at more than one reactive site, the option being determined by the concentration of the substrate and the affinity constants of the different transport systems.

Migration of substrate across the membrane is mediated by macromolecular mechanisms within which the features of specificity reside. Only proteins are capable of exhibiting the degree of specificity which is required for transport. Preliminary studied suggest that membrane "transport" proteins have a molecular weight of about 30,000.[153] How the transport protein* carries the solute across the lipoprotein membrane is still an enigma.[153]

Two approaches among several illuminate the origin and nature of membrane reactive sites or carriers. One is the study of ontogeny of transport processes; the other is the study of genetic mutants which ablate a single transport system. Both approaches can refine our appreciation of the exquisite organization of membrane transport functions. The ultimate analysis will, of course, require isolation and characterization of the individual membrane components which comprise each part of the specific transport mechanisms.

## ONTOGENY OF MEMBRANE TRANSPORT SYSTEMS

Distinctive developmental patterns of various transport processes would be indicative of discrete genetic control of the specific activity of these functions. The study of transport ontogeny provides another way to characterize their individuality.

A number of investigations have shown that intestinal transport systems "mature," in terms of their concentrative capacity, prior to birth. This pattern of change in the specific activity of transport functions thus appears to be preparative for extrauterine life rather than adaptive to that environment. Wilson and Lin[256] showed that the rabbit intestine exhibits concentrative uptake of glucose, galactose, L-tyrosine, and L-histidine on the third day of life. Histidine is transported actively prior to birth, and concentrative uptake occurs under aerobic and anaerobic conditions; the latter property disappears, however, during the first week of life. Deren and

---

* Or carrier, permease, translocase, or "here-to-there'ase,"[169] as it has been called by others.

associates[47] pursued an extensive study of perinatal maturation of membrane transport systems in rabbit intestine. They observed that concentrative uptake of α-methyl glucoside appeared at the 22nd day of fetal life, and that the ability to concentrate this solute increased abruptly from the 24th to the 30th day. Since the uptake of α-methyl glucoside was inhibited by glucose and phlorizin, it was assumed that the relevant specific transport site had developed during this period. However, these workers did not study phlorizin inhibition of α-methyl glucoside transport prior to the 22nd day to determine whether the site was also present prior to this date. Thus, we do not know whether it was merely the ability to concentrate the solute, or the ability to bind and concentrate substrate, which developed after the 22nd day of fetal life. This point was particularly evaluated in an investigation of the uptake of L-lysine and betaine by gut during fetal development.[47] Figure 7 shows a specific pattern to the appearance of concentrative uptake of the two solutes. Lysine uptake becomes strongly concentrative on the 24th day; yet it is only on the 28th day that betaine

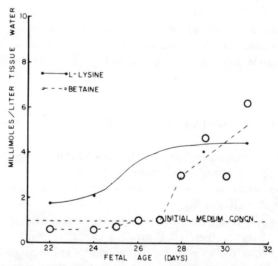

Fig. 7.  Change in specific activity of transport systems in rabbit intestine during ontogeny. Deren *et al.*[47] measured concentrative uptake of amino acids by intestinal rings obtained at different stages of fetal development. Lysine transport develops a concentrative component before, and independent of, betaine transport. The two solutes are known to be transported by different mechanisms. Independent genetic control of the two systems is implied by this observation.

transport also develops this property. Lysine and betaine are transported by separate membrane sites in mammalian intestine.[83,84] Moreover, there is no evidence that different sources of metabolic energy are used to achieve uptake from the two types of membrane sites. Thus, this observation suggests that the two transport systems develop independently. These qualitative differences in the specific activity of the two transport systems also dismiss the proposal that concentrative uptake merely parallels the increase in surface area of the transport membrane as villi and microvilli mature.[47] A noteworthy observation in this regard has been reported by States and Segal,[227a] who investigated the ontogeny of L-cystine transport in rat intestine. They observed that fetal transport withstands anaerobic conditions and $Na^+$ deprivation, and that augmented rates of uptake, which coincided with the period of the maximum postnatal growth rate, were achieved with an augmented $V_{max}$ for cystine uptake, but with no alteration in the $Km$ of transport.

The renal tubule, whose functional and structural characteristics, with regard to membrane transport, closely resemble those of the intestine, also exhibits distinctive patterns of perinatal development. Webber[246] has studied urinary excretion of amino acids in relation to plasma amino acid levels in the rat pup. Certain amino acids, such as proline and glycine, are cleared into urine at higher rates in the two-week-old pup when compared to the older animal. Subsequent investigation of this phenomenon in vitro[248] using the kidney cortex slice technique showed that initial rates of uptake of most amino acids are slower in the immature kidney, but that the uptake ratio in the immature kidney of the accumulated solute at equilibrium could differ strikingly from the mature kidney. No clear explanation for these observations is apparent at the moment, although Webber and Cairns[248] have suggested that dissimilarity of efflux characteristics might account for the differences in concentrative capacity; subsequent work by Webber[246a] has shown that efflux of substrate from fetal kidney slices is diminished.

The pattern of aminoaciduria in early infancy is quite different from that of the adult;[17,194] tubular absorption of amino acids is about 10–15 % less efficient in the infant. However, imino acids and glycine, in particular, are less efficiently absorbed by the human infant, and only in the second six months of life does the kidney absorb these solutes completely as in the mature subject. The postnatal maturation of iminoglycine absorption may reflect the appearance of the high-capacity, low-affinity type of membrane site (see Fig. 5) which is shared by this specific group of solutes. Since transport of imino acids and glycine in particular is compromised, a genetic basis for the change in the specific activity of this membrane transport function is implicated. The likelihood that the well established morphological changes in glomerular-tubular relationships at this age[61] could account for this phenomenon is small.

Spencer[224] has suggested that transport ontogeny may recapitulate its own phylogeny. If an elaborate deployment of transport systems emerges only late in fetal development during mammalian ontogeny, perhaps more-primitive organisms may exhibit membrane transport functions lacking sophisticated specificity and concentrative properties. Certainly, micro-organisms have membrane transport systems which are sophisticated by any of the criteria mentioned earlier; but whether protozoa such as amoeba and paramecium have complex membrane transport functions has yet to be investigated. Representative studies of membrane transport in non-mammalian metazoan tissue, such as flounder intestine[184] and star fish digestive glands,[59] indicate that mediated and concentrative uptake of solutes occurs in the digestive tracts of these creatures, but little has been done to characterize further the cellular transport mechanisms at these levels of evolution.

## HUMAN GENETICS OF MEMBRANE TRANSPORT (AMINO ACIDS)

The identification of mutant transport phenotypes has been an important aid to the description of membrane transport systems. The recognition of genetic control for specific transport functions is only one obvious by-product of such observations. As with the biochemical studies cited earlier, the human inborn errors of amino acid transport show that groups of structurally related amino acids share common transport sites, and that within these groups there are marked differences of affinity and capacity for transport of the individual solutes by the common system. Mutant phenotypes have also revealed that a single amino acid may be transported at more than one site. The individual loci which control transport sites may express a variety of mutant alleles. Thus, many "transport" mutations are found in man, some of which share a common phenotype, while others produce widely divergent specific phenotypes.

### Evidence for Several Genetic Loci Controlling Membrane Transport of Amino Acids

Proteins in the membrane would appear to be the only macromolecules with sufficient specificity to discriminate among several substrates and provide the properties of recognition sites for transport. Mutations which delete functions used by specific substrates thus offer further evidence that membranes comprise, in part, a mosaic of specific transport proteins.

The observed effects of mutation suggest that many loci control amino acid transport. Mutations in man cause impairment of amino acid transport in three ways: there are those which affect a specific amino acid; others will affect only a selective group of amino acids; and there are those which affect transport of amino acids in general, as well as the transport of other solutes.

## Loci Controlling Reactive Sites Used by Different Amino Acids

There are seven hereditary transport traits which reflect the occurrence of several gene loci for reactive membrane sites (Table II). These are the classical cystinurias, the iminoglycinurias, Hartnup disease, and the hyperdibasicaminoacidurias, in each of which a group of amino acids is involved, plus three conditions in which the transport of only a single amino acid is impaired: hypercystinuria, the "blue diaper" syndrome, and methionine malabsorption. We do not intend to review the clinical aspects of these traits; key references in Table II indicate where more-extensive descriptions are available.

The mutations which affect transport of the cationic (dibasic) amino acids lysine, ornithine, and arginine, and the neutral amino acid cystine, illustrate the concept of a mosaic of membrane reactive sites particularly well.

In 1951 Dent and Rose[46] proposed that (classical) cystinuria was an inborn error of amino acid transport; they suggested this, having shown that it was net tubular absorption, and not endogenous metabolism, which was abnormal in the trait. The prior discovery of an excessive excretion of lysine and arginine[261] and of ornithine[229] in the urine of patients with cystinuria helped them to reach this conclusion. Dent and Harris[45] subsequently found Mendelian inheritance for the trait and a distinct segregation of this form of "cystinuria" from other causes of cystinuria. Dent and Rose[46] noted that lysine, arginine, ornithine, and cystine were structurally similar, since each had two amino groups, or a guanidino and an amino group, separated by four to six carbon or sulfur atoms; this encouraged them to propose a common transport system for the four substrates. A simple explanation for the complex aminoaciduria in this Mendelian trait was therefore found. A number of *in vivo* studies in man,[166] rat,[254] and dog,[186,247] testing for competitive interaction between dibasic amino acids, did nothing to dissuade investigators that the "dibasic" amino acids and their chemically neutral bed-fellow, cystine, shared a common transport systems.

Matters rested easily until Rosenberg *et al.*[176] presented the disturbing, but unavoidable, evidence that L-cystine is not transported at the site which mediates uptake of the dibasic amino acids in rat kidney cortex slices; this finding was confirmed later by others.[212,254] To make matters even more difficult to understand, a segregated mode of cystine transport was also found in *human* kidney,[67] and it was shown that L-cystine uptake *in vitro* was *not* impaired in human cystinuric kidney. Furthermore, although *net* tubular *absorption* of L-cystine *in vivo* is clearly depressed,[38,72] there is also evidence for net tubular *secretion* of cystine.[38,72] Clearance data also suggest that there are separate mechanisms for the excretion of cystine and the dibasic amino acids.[38] Furthermore, other evidence derived from a study of renal extraction of amino acids from blood[70,71,179] suggests that urinary cystine is derived from the renal plasma, and not just from glomerular filtrate. These observations led to additional investigations proving that cystinuria cannot be interpreted as a disorder of L-cysteine transport either *in vivo*[65,179] or *in vitro*.[210] L-Cystine and L-cysteine are, in fact, transported by separate systems in kidney.[211]

In the absence of any demonstrable interactions between the two sulfur amino acids and the cationic amino acids during influx into kidney cells it is therefore difficult to accept the original Dent–Rose hypothesis as an explanation for the hyperdibasicaminoaciduria and cystinuria of the classical cystinuric trait. One must therefore find another interpretation. Schwartzman *et al.*[190,192] found a specific interaction between intracellular dibasic amino acids and L-cysteine during *efflux* from kidney cells. They suggested that the cystinuric trait in kidney might reflect some defect in the control of efflux, a conclusion of some interest in view of the evidence for "net tubular secretion" of dibasic amino acids and cystine *in vivo* in classical cystinuria.[38,72] An excess of cysteine efflux could account for this controversial observation; it might also explain the excretion of the mixed disulfide[70] and the exaggerated renal arterial/venous extraction ratio for cysteine, but not for cystine, in cystinuria.[10,70,71,179]

The problem of cystinuria is complicated further because cystine and dibasic amino acids do share a common uptake mechanism in mammalian intestine,[83,236,237] contrary to the situation in kidney. The intestinal system is not shared by L-cysteine.[173] Uptake of dibasic amino acids and of cystine (but not of cysteine) is impaired in some forms of classical cystinuria.[143,173,179,237] Rosenberg and colleagues[175] found that intestinal transport of cystine and dibasic amino acids is seriously impaired only in some homozygous cystinuria patients (type I), while in others there is only modestly impaired intestinal transport (type II); homozygous patients without any impairment of intestinal transport were considered to be a third genotypic variant (type III). All three types of homozygotes apparently have an equivalent loss of tubular transport.

These challenging and seemingly contradictory observations offer two important insights. First, there is evidence for genotypic heterogeneity in the trait; this is discussed in more detail on p. 253. Secondly, there is support for the concept of reactive site mosaicism, as shown by the segregation of uptake mechanisms for cationic amino acids, cystine, and cysteine. The latter conclusion gains further support from other mutant phenotypes which reveal segregation of cystine and dibasic amino acid transport.[18,116,250]

Brodehl and colleagues[18] found two siblings with isolated hypercystinuria unaccompanied by increased urinary excretion of the dibasic compounds. The renal clearance of cystine was increased, and its net tubular absorption was only about 75 % of the normal value.

A second hereditary trait has been described in which renal tubular absorption of the cationic amino acids is specifically impaired, while cystine reabsorption is normal.[116,250]* (See also p. 250.) Thus, the hypercystinuric and hyperdibasicaminoaciduric traits are complementary to classical cystinuria and each other, and may be viewed as experiments of nature distinct from cystinuria; they indicate a clear segregation of uptake systems for cystine and the cationic amino acids.

On the basis of existing evidence, the following proposal can be made concerning the deployment of membrane systems for transport of this particular group of substrated in kidney, and perhaps in other tissues as well.

Influx Systems.  Several sites exist on the outer surface of the membrane; one for cystine uptake, another for cysteine, and one or more for uptake of dibasic amino acids, at least one of which is common to lysine, arginine, and ornithine.

Efflux Systems.  At least one system is common to the dibasic compounds and L-cystine; other modes of efflux may also exist. The lower specificity of an efflux system compared to the specificity of the equivalent influx system(s) is in keeping with the findings of Oxender and Christensen.[152]

We have given considerable attention to a description of mutant transport phenotypes affecting cationic amino acids and cystine because this particular constellation of traits illustrates well how difficult it may be to relate findings *in vitro* to the clinical data. Hereditary traits can be helpful in the interpretation of such data.

## Loci Controlling Different Reactive Sites Used by the Same Amino Acid

The homozygote retains much of the normal transport capacity in most inborn errors of amino acid transport. Previous discussions of these traits

---

* A mutant strain of *E. coli*[189] is also of interest in this context; this "permease" mutant is defective in its ability to take up lysine, arginine, and ornithine, but not cystine.

TABLE III.   Apparent Failure of Some Mutant Amino Acid Transport Traits
in Man to Observe Expected Gene Dosage Effect[a]

| Trait | Substrate | Percent of tubular transport function lost[b] | |
|---|---|---|---|
| | | Heterozygote | Homozygote |
| Hereditary renal | Proline | 0 | 20 |
| iminoglycinuria | Hydroxyproline | 0 | 35 |
| | Glycine | 10 | 30 |
| Hartnup | Serine | 0 | 70 |
| | Leucine | 0 | 12 |
| | Neutral group | 0 | 35 |

| Trait | Substrate | Types | | |
|---|---|---|---|---|
| | | Type I | II & III | All types[c] |
| Classical | Cystine | 0 | 6 | 80 |
| cystinuria | Lysine | 0 | 13 | 65 |
| | Ornithine | 0 | 1 | 70 |
| | Arginine | 0 | 1 | 44 |

[a] Recalculated from previous data.[198]
[b] Calculated approximately, and at endogenous plasma amino acid concentration.
[c] Data of Crawhall et al.[38] show net tubular secretion in some patients: range of values for per cent loss of transport were: cystine, 91–223; lysine, 30–125; ornithine, 14–71; arginine, 5–141.

have addressed themselves primarily to the qualitative aspects of the relevant *hyperaminoaciduria*; rather less attention has been paid to the equivalent quantitative aspects of the abnormal transport.

Table III shows how little of the endogenous tubular absorption is actually lost by homozygotes in classical cystinuria and in the Hartnup and imino glycinuric traits. There are several possibilities for the persistence of a significant quantity of the relevant transport function under these conditions (Fig. 8):

1. The mutation might decrease the affinity of the site for its substrate (curve 2, Fig. 8). In this case the total capacity for uptake, $T_m$ or $V_{max}$,* may not be decreased, but the ability of the site to bind substrate would be less efficient. Thus, at given concentrations of substrate, less is taken up by the tubular cell, and more is excreted in urine. This is reflected as a lowered

*The former is the relevant physiological parameter,[160,218] the latter is the equivalent Michaelis–Menten parameter.

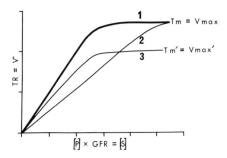

Fig. 8. Theoretical plots of transport data.
(1) Normal saturation kinetics. When tubular
reabsorption (TR) is measured *in vivo* at
various filtered loads (plasma conc. [P] × GFR)
a maximum rate of tubular absorption ($T_m$) is
defined; the physiological terms are equivalent
to the respective Michaelis–Menten terms ($v$, $S$,
and $V_{max}$). (2) Absorption (transport) when
the site is modified and binding at the reactive
site is impaired. (3) Absorption when affinity
of site is unchanged, but rate of transfer is
inhibited; effect is analogous to noncompetitive
inhibition. A mutation which slightly alters
conformation of the reactive site would result
in curve 2. Mutation causing impaired *transfer*
of solute after normal binding would produce
curve 3.

plasma threshold for urinary excretion *in vivo*, or as unusual "splay" in
the $T_m$. The equivalent transport $Km$ will be elevated in this situation.

2. The mutation might affect the number of transport sites of one species
available to the substrate (curve 3, Fig. 8). In this case the binding of substrate
is unaltered, but the total capacity ($T_m$ or $V_{max}$) is decreased.

3. A third possibility* assumes that more than one species of sites,

* Woolf and colleagues[259] developed an argument similar to that shown in Fig. 8, which
served to interpret a heterozygous transport trait. They discussed the genetic basis of
hereditary renal glucosuria which is considered by many to be a Mendelian dominant.
Two forms of glucose $T_m$ called types *A* and *B* by Reubi,[164] and respectively analagous
to curves 3 and 2 in Fig. 8, are found in renal glucosuria. Woolf *et al.* suggested that
the two forms of titration curve can be accounted for by mutant alleles which affect
either the quantity of available glucose-binding sites (type *A* glucosuria), or the structure
of those sites, so that about half are normal, and half are altered in their affinity for
glucose binding (type *B* glucosuria).

each with different transport kinetics, is used by the substrate. At any given concentration the kinetics of uptake of a single substrate by the sites is distributed among them according to the equation

$$\text{Total uptake} = \frac{V_{\max_1}[S]}{Km_1 + S} + \frac{V_{\max_2}[S]}{Km_2 + S} + \cdots + \frac{V_{\max_n}[S]}{K_{m_n} + S}$$

where $V_{\max_1}$ and $Km_1$ refer to the kinetic constants for the first species of sites, etc., and $[S]$ is the substrate concentration.

Genetic deletion of one system will alter the kinetics of substrate uptake, which was heretofore spread over several systems.

Investigations have been performed in subjects with the iminoglycinuric trait[178,200,208] which show that the third proposal is probably the correct interpretation for the transport phenotype of this trait. At low concentrations of substrate, tubular absorption of filtered proline by heterozygotes is complete [Fig. 9(a)]; Fig. 9(a) shows that mutant subjects have an impaired L-proline $T_m$ and a gene dosage effect is apparent. Moreover, the heterozygote transports proline efficiently at the lower concentrations, indicating efficient binding. The mutant homozygote still transports some proline at all concentrations; this process saturates at low concentrations, in contrast to the system found in normal subjects. These observations exclude possibility 1 as the mode of gene expression. Possibility 2 is also excluded because the persistent transport in homozygotes, and some of the residual function in heterozygotes, has qualitative characteristics which are different from those expected, were the appearance of the trait to depend only on the presence of a greatly reduced number (or capacity) of normal sites. Possibility 3 suggests that a transport system, which is used predominantly at substrate concentrations extending beyond the usual physiological range, and which is shared by the imino acids and glycine, has been deleted in the trait. Another type of transport is thus exposed; this residual type operates with high affinity and low total capacity at physiological concentrations of substrate [Fig. 9(b)], however, a small amount of each substrate is also carried on a high-capacity, low-affinity system shared by all three substrates. The mutant transport gene in hereditary renal iminoglycinuria ablates only the "common" system in homozygotes. The residual capacity for iminoglycine transport on the other systems is small, but quite efficient under normal endogenous conditions, so that homozygotes appear to retain considerable function (see Table III). Figure 9 also shows a gene dosage effect in heterozygous and homozygous proline $T_m$ data.

The foregoing interpretation of the iminoglycinuric trait was possible inasmuch as the qualitative and quantitative characteristics of iminoglycine

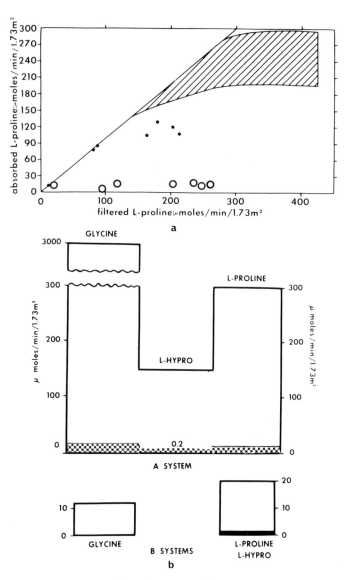

Fig. 9. A demonstration of two types of membrane transport for a single substrate (see Fig. 5). (a) The renal $T_m$ for proline for normal subjects (hatched), a heterozygote with hereditary renal iminoglycinuria (closed circles), and a homozygote with the same trait (open circles).[200] The presence of two types of proline transport is implied; (b) a translation in graphic terms of this concept. The proposed specificity and capacity of the various transport systems for imino acids and glycine identified in human kidney *in vivo* are depicted.

transport by human kidney had been determined *in vivo*.[200,203,205] Comparable data on the transport of other amino acids by human kidney has not yet been published; hence, it would still be difficult to identify, in like manner, the basis of the phenotype in the other inborn errors of amino acid transport. Nonetheless, a similar interpretation would explain the persistence of efficient transport at physiological concentrations of substrate in the mutant homozygous phenotypes of cystinuria and Hartnup disease, for example.

If there are specific sites for the migration of individual amino acids, in addition to the shared sites, one can anticipate mutant transport phenotypes involving only one amino acid. Hypercystinuria[18] seems to be one of these traits. Perhaps methionine malabsorption[83] and tryptophan malabsorption[82] are also phenotypes wherein intestinal transport, but not renal transport, of single amino acids is affected by mutation.

## Loci Apparently Controlling the Transfer of Substrates across Membranes

There are mutations which are different from those described above and which produce traits known as the Fanconi syndrome,[127] "Busby" syndrome,[181,185] and Lowe–Terrey–MacLachlan syndrome.[1] In these conditions there is a *generalized* impairment of amino acid transport; moreover, the transport of other solutes, including glucose, bicarbonate, potassium, and phosphate, may also be impaired. It is difficult to conceive how a single mutation could affect many different specific reactive sites simultaneously. Therefore, it is more likely that such mutations affect some other component of the transport mechanism which is linked to the different reactive sites. If *binding* of solute at a reactive site comprises one of the basic components of the transport process, another component must provide the mechanism for *transfer* of substrate across the membrane; this is followed by release of the solute on the opposite side of the membrane and return of the component to its initial state on the initial surface for a new cycle. When active transport occurs energy is expended to maintain a concentration gradient. Thus, an impaired supply of energy, or an alteration in the component achieving transfer, would affect the influx component of a concentrative mechanism, causing a depression of intracellular uptake, or of net tubular absorption.

It is believed that events occur in the Fanconi syndrome which impinge upon the supply of metabolic energy used for transport. A number of causes for a disturbance of this nature can be identified. For example, heavy-metal poisoning[78] and maleic acid[88] both produce generalized hyperaminoaciduria *in vivo* as part of the syndrome. Rosenberg and Segal[183] showed that maleic acid is a noncompetitive inhibitor of amino acid uptake by kidney cortex slices *in vitro*, an observation which implicates the process of transfer, rather than the binding of substrate, in this mode of transport inhibition.

The site of inhibition, be it acquired or inherited, is thus confined primarily to the second phase of transport after the binding of substrate has taken place. This assumption is supported by the data of Robson and Rose.[166] They observed a brisk competitive inhibition of arginine transport superimposed by the presence of lysine in a patient with the Fanconi syndrome; this suggests that the site at which this interaction occurred was still normally receptive; thus, the prior inhibition of transport in this patient with the syndrome was at some other stage of the mechanism.

Surprisingly, there has been little work done to document more precisely the altered functional characteristics acquired by patients with generalized disorders of transport, such as the Fanconi syndrome. In one patient with abnormal tubular transport affecting phosphate, glucose, and glycine[204] it was shown: (1) that the glucose $T_m$ was depressed without "splay" (see curve 3, Fig. 8) in a manner analogous to Reubi's type $A$ glucosuria; (2) that the glycine reactive site was unaltered in its response to competitive inhibition by L-proline; and (3) that the proline $T_m$ was depressed without splay, but insufficiently to produce prolinuria at the normal endogenous plasma concentration.* These observations indicate that the affinity of each of the transport sites for its respective solutes was unaltered, and that the inhibition of solute transfer involved the transfer mechanism. Many more studies of this nature in patients with various forms of the Fanconi syndrome would be interesting, and are necessary.

The striking morphological changes found in the proximal tubule of patients with various forms of the Fanconi syndrome[44] develop progressively after birth,† and are assumed to be secondary manifestations of the prolonged inhibition of cell function.[102] One consequence of the reduction of tubular volume and surface area which accompanies these changes will be a reduction in the number of transport sites on the luminal surface of the nephron available to the substrate. Structural changes of this nature will reduce the capacity of transport processes and cause a reduction in observed $T_m$ (curve 3, Fig. 8).

Another feature of the Fanconi syndrome and similar traits, which has received little attention, concerns intestinal transport of substrates in such conditions. One might ask: If there is a generalized inhibition of transport in the renal tubule, is the same disturbance demonstrable in the intestine? Our own preliminary investigations† reveal that intestinal absorption of two amino acids used as test solutes (L-proline and L-lysine hydrochloride)

---

*C. R. Scriver, unpublished observation.
† H. Goldman and C. R. Scriver, unpublished observations.

is impaired in patients with the Fanconi syndrome. Bartsocas[8] has identified a defect in intestinal absorption of amino acids in Lowe's syndrome. Presumably, the inhibitory phenomenon again affects the translocation of solute, rather than its binding to available sites.

At the present time it is assumed that hereditary traits, such as cystinosis,[209] the recessively inherited adult form of the Fanconi syndrome,[45,127] and the dominantly inherited forms,[100a,134,214a] "tyrosinosis,"[197] and other inherited causes of the syndrome,[50,199] produce inhibition of membrane transport as secondary phenomena through some form of inhibition of the energy supply for transport.*

Although one can speculate about the general nature of the transport defect in the generalized traits, such as the Fanconi syndrome, there is no information concerning the exact site of the primary phenotype in these diseases. Inheritance patterns indicate Mendelian inheritance for each of the traits, and there is sufficient evidence to believe that many different genetic loci are represented. Whether the inhibition of energy supply is always acquired as a sequel to a primary accumulation of a toxic metabolite, as appears to occur in the classical example of galactosemia,[40] or whether some traits involve mutations directly affecting energy production in transport cells, has yet to be determined.

## Genetic Heterogeneity Within Loci

### Phenotypic Variation

Phenotypic variation occurs in a number of mutant transport traits. It will be shown that such variation may reflect the presence of several mutant alleles at the relevant gene locus. Therefore, is is necessary to define the clinical trait precisely in order to interpret it properly. The phenotypic variants of classical cystinuria, renal iminoglycinuria, and hyperdibasicaminoaciduria will be discussed to illustrate this point.

**Classical Cystinuria.**  One form of mammalian cystinuria exhibits an interesting phenotypic artefact. Canine cystinuria, like its human counterpart, is a disorder of renal tubular conservation of cystine and the cationic amino acids.[34a,238-240] However, in this species cystinuria is found predominantly in male dogs,[238,239] an observation which has caused some workers to suggest $X$-linked inheritance for the canine trait, in contrast to autosomal

---

*The *Neurospora* mutant, in which a generalized membrane transport defect is found (the work of Kappy and Metzenberg[113] cited here in Table I), might be an analogous model system which warrants more study from this viewpoint.

linkage of the human trait. It is more likely, however, that sex influences only the *detection* of the trait in dogs, and not its inheritance. Detection of canine cystinuria is virtually dependent on stone formation; calculi are detected predominantly in the male dog because of the antomy of the os penis and the urethral exit from the bladder.

Human cystinuria can be attributed to more than one mutant autosomal allele. When the presence of abnormal amino acid excretion was used as the index for case finding by Harris *et al.*[87] they observed two modes of inheritance for the classical cystinuric trait. They called one form "completely recessive," because heterozygous carriers showed no evidence of the trait; the second form was called "incompletely recessive," because heterozygotes excreted a modest excess of the relevant amino acids. Similar observations were made with different analytical methods during the later investigations of Crawhall *et al.*[37] With the advent of yet more sensitive methods of amino acid analysis Rosenberg and colleagues[175] reinvestigated the problem and concluded that the classical cystinuric trait actually comprised three different genotypes (Table IV). They observed the following:

1. All homozygotes have a similar degree of hyperaminoaciduria *in vivo* and a similar degree of inhibition of amino acid uptake by kidney cortex slices. Thus, on the basis of the "kidney" phenotype, there is no heterogeneity of the phenotype in homozygous cystinuria.

2. Homozygotes have three "intestinal" phenotypes. Some patients (type I) have greatly impaired absorption of L-cystine (but not of L-cysteine) from the intestine into plasma *in vivo*; moreover, concentrative uptake by intestinal mucosa *in vitro* of cystine, lysine, and arginine is ablated. Another group of patients (type II) have impaired cystine absorption *in vivo* and

TABLE IV.   Phenotypes for Three Genetically Distinct Forms of
Classical Human Cystinuria[a]

| Proposed genotype | Urinary phenotype | | Intestinal phenotype; homozygotes |
|:---:|:---:|:---:|:---:|
| | Homozygotes | Heterozygotes | |
| I | $++++^{b}$ | 0 | $++++^{d}$ |
| II | $++++$ | $++^{c}$ | $+++$ |
| III | $++++$ | $+$ | $+$ |

[a] From Rosenberg *et al.*[175]
[b] Degree of specific hyperaminoaciduria involving cystine, lysine, ornithine, and arginine.
[c] Degree of specific hyperaminoaciduria.
[d] Degree of impairment in the mediated uptake of amino acids *in vivo* and *in vitro*.

severely inhibited uptake of amino acids *in vitro*. The third phenotype (type III) exhibits only modest impairment of concentrative amino acid uptake *in vivo* and *in vitro*.

3. There are three types of heterozygotes (Fig. 10). Those with homozygous offspring of type I intestinal phenotype have normal aminoaciduria (completely recessive); those whose homozygous relatives are of type II or type III phenotype have a slightly excessive specific aminoaciduria (incomplete recessive); type II heterozygotes have a hyperaminoaciduria which is statistically greater than the type III trait.

These data indicate the presence of at least three mutant alleles for the cystinuric phenotype. Further studies (see below) have discerned whether the heterogeneity is caused by mutant alleles at different autosomal loci, or at the same gene locus.

**Renal Iminoglycinuria.** Two mechanisms have been identified whereby excessive urinary excretion of L-proline, hydroxy-L-proline, and glycine may occur. The first produces the trait by a "combined" mechanism.[184,198] Competitive inhibition of uptake of the other two substrates which share the common iminoglycine transport system will produce specific iminoglycinuria in the presence of sufficiently high concentrations of either imino acid. Thus, hyperprolinemia[203] and hydroxyprolinemia[205] can each be accompanied by an iminoglycinuric phenotype. The affinity of glycine for the common system is too low to allow it to act as a competitive inhibitor of imino acid uptake *in vivo* or *in vitro*.[254] Iminoglycinuria caused by this *combined* mechanism, where saturation and competitive inhibition at a shared site occur simultaneously, can therefore be discriminated from iminoglycinuria caused by autosomal recessive mutations which directly affect the common transport system.

Renal iminoglycinuria[178,200] can be distinguished from the "combined" form of iminoglycinuria by the pure renal mechanism underlying its appearance.* A bias in ascertainment at one time also suggested that the trait was accompanied by mental retardation and central nervous system dysfunction.[77,111,141,232] Several pedigrees have now been sufficiently studied[178,200,249] to show that the trait is the result of a harmless autosomal recessive mutation, affecting membrane transport of this trio of substrates.

---

*The normal newborn infant has iminoglycinuria[194] which persists up to six months after birth. Neonatal iminoglycinuria can be attributed to reduced efficiency of tubular absorption of the imino acids and glycine.[17] The apparent ontogenetic significance of this phenomenon was discussed in the previous section.

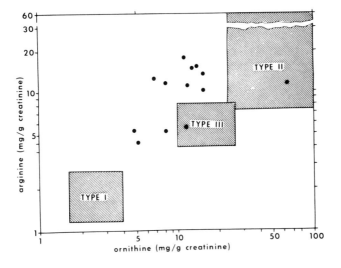

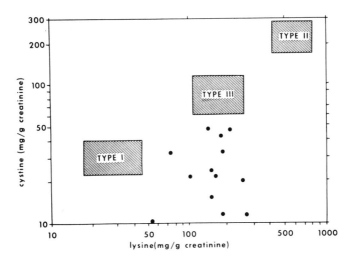

Fig. 10.   The hatched areas in the two graphs indicate amino acid excretion in cystinuric heterozygotes.[168,177] The differences in excretion rates are statistically significant, and they reveal three distinct phenotypes resulting from three different human cystinuric genotypes.[175] Thus, cystinuria is a heterogeneous trait. The closed circles show amino acid excretion in a dominant human trait in which transport of cationic acids alone is abnormal.[250] A second gene must therefore control cationic amino acid transport in a manner which is segregated from cystine transport.

The following features indicate the presence of phenotypic and genetic heterogeneity within the trait:

1. All homozygotes have a decreased capacity for tubular absorption of proline, hydroxyproline, and glycine, without elevation of the plasma concentrations of these substrates [Fig. 9(a)]. However, when the plasma concentration of imino acids is low, hyperiminoaciduria may not occur,[200] because an alternate system for transport of imino acids [Fig. 9(b)] achieves complete absorption of these substrates.

2. Some homozygotes have normal uptake of L-proline into plasma from the intestine after administration of L-proline by mouth;[178,200] others have an impaired rate of absorption[77,141] (Fig. 11).

3. If the plasma concentration of glycine exceeds about 0.10 m$M$, most obligate heterozygotes for this trait exhibit hyperglycinuria. However, one obligate heterozygote has been found free of hyperglycinuria despite an adequate concentration of glycine in plasma.[200] Heterozygotes without hyperglycinuria have also been identified in other pedigrees.[232] (Unfortunately, the glycine content of plasma was not reported in the latter patients.)

The presence of more than one mutant genotype is required to explain the two homozygous phenotypes (gut and kidney defect, or kidney defect alone), and the two heterozygous phenotypes (with or without hyper-glycinuria) which occur in the mutant iminoglycine transport trait. The additional phenotypic variation (e.g., presence or absence of iminoaciduria in homozygotes) at first suggestive of variable penetrance of the trait, is readily explained in terms of the established characteristics of membrane transport for the imino acids and glycine.

**Hyperdibasicaminoaciduria.** Two forms of an interesting specific hyperaminoaciduria have been described recently; one type appears in Finland[116,157] as a recessive trait, while the second form appears as a dominant trait in French Canadians.[250] The trait affects renal transport of the cationic amino acids only (Fig. 10); cystine transport is normal. This condition again emphasizes the apparent segregation of membrane transport systems used for uptake of cystine and for cationic amino acids.

The dominantly inherited French-Canadian type of hyperdibasicamino-aciduria might well be the heterozygous form of the condition found in Finland, since the latter, which affects sibs and has occurred in a consanguinous lineage, appears to be an autosomal recessive trait.[116] However, certain facts argue against this assumption. The Finnish trait is

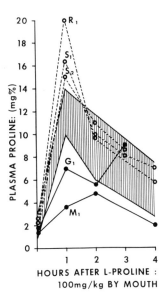

Fig. 11. Evidence for genetic
heterogeneity in the iminoglycinuric trait. The graph
shows the response in plasma
proline concentration after an
L-proline load by mouth. Two
responses have been recorded
for mutant homozygotes. Some
patients[178,200] have a normal
response (hatched area representing the normal response);
others have an impaired response,[77,141] indicating an intestinal transport defect. Both
types of homozygote have the
same renal phenotype.

symptomatic, with gastrointestinal intolerance of protein, vomiting, diarrhea,
failure to thrive, hepatomegally, and cirrhosis; the blood urea concentration
is depressed, and hyperammonemia occurs readily after nitrogen loading.
The dominant French-Canadian trait, by contrast, is asymptomatic. The
difference in clinical expression of the traits might reflect only a dosage
effect for a pair of mutant alleles. However, there are important discrepancies
between the heterozygous phenotypes of the French-Canadian and Finnish
traits; hyperdibasicaminoaciduria occurs in the former, but not in the latter.
Moreover, intestinal absorption of lysine is modestly impaired in French-

Canadian heterozygotes,[250] whereas there is no intestinal transport defect, either *in vivo* or *in vitro*, even in the homozygotes of the Finnish trait.[115] These differences suggest genotypic heterogeneity at the locus responsible for transport of cationic amino acids. Whether the two mutant alleles actually occur at the same locus could be determined by studying mutant homozygotes born to heterozygotes of equivalent and of dissimilar phenotypes. However, the opportunity to demonstrate allelism or nonallelism has not yet arisen with respect to the hyperdibasicaminoaciduric trait. (As will be shown below, cystinuria and renal iminoglycinuria have once again proven themselves most useful for the investigation of this particular type of question.)

**Hartnup Disease.** This condition is yet another example of phenotypic heterogeneity. The typical patient with Hartnup disease exhibits a specific hyperaminoaciduria involving certain neutral $\alpha$-amino acids;[7,106] the trait is the result of a transport defect[39] which also affects intestinal transport of certain neutral amino acids.[138,196] All of the clinical and biochemical features of the disease[106] can be attributed to the membrane transport defect. However, unusual cases of Hartnup disease have been described[51,225] in which the typical clinical and "urinary" phenotypes were present, but in which there was no apparent evidence for an intestinal transport defect. These patients are therefore probable examples of a second "Hartnup" genotype. They constitute further evidence for the prevalence of the phenomenon of genetic heterogeneity. Seakins and Ersser[208a] described an unusual patient in whom the intestinal trait was partially evident only under loading conditions, and in whom lysine transport was impaired, while histidine transport was not; it is possible that this patient has yet another variant of the Hartnup phenotype.

**Cystinosis.** Phenotypic heterogeneity is again well illustrated by this complicated trait. The origin of cystine storage in this trait is still unclear, and its relation to the impairment of transport is also unknown. Yet, cystine storage in itself is probably not as serious as was once suspected; this interpretation is encouraged by the recent discovery of a benign adult form of cystinosis[188a] in which there is no deterioration of renal transport functions, and no impairment of growth and development, despite the fact that homozygotes retain cystine in tissues 30–50 times above the normal level. This type of cystinosis is not found in pedigrees in which the classical and fatal childhood type occurs. Two different genotypes must therefore account for "cystinosis." The possibility that a third mutant allele also causes "cystinosis" is suggested by the discovery of another pedigree in which two sibs have cystine storage in tissues and the Fanconi syndrome. Both sibs are alive and outwardly well in their second decade, with normal stature and no evidence of renal failure.*

## Allelism

Does the genetic heterogeneity of the transport traits, such as cystinuria, renal iminoglycinuria, etc., occur at a single locus, or at different loci which control different components of the relevant transport mechanism? If it occurs at different loci, then "double heterozygotes," that is, subjects receiving one mutant, but dissimilar allele, from each parent, would synthesise about half of the gene product controlled by each of the alleles; such hetero-allelic individuals should be no more severely affected than a simple heterozygote for either allele. On the other hand, if the alleles are at the same locus, then the "double heterozygote" (or heteroallelic "homozygote") cannot synthesize any normal gene product controlled by that locus. Consequently, homozygous and doubly heterozygous phenotypes should be similar if the different mutant alleles are at the same locus.

**Cystinuria.** It has been assumed in this discussion that classical cystinuria is an autosomal recessive trait resulting from defective synthesis of a membrane macromolecule controlling the uptake of the cationic amino acids and cystine. At least three different homozygous genotypes are associated with the same phenotype (Tables III and IV).

Rosenberg and colleagues[167,177] have investigated several critical pedigrees exhibiting intrafamilial heterogeneity of the classical cystinuric genotypes [Fig. 12(left)]. The simple heterozygotes in these pedigrees were classified as type I, II, or III mutant genotype; it was then found that cystinuric offspring of matings where genotypes I–II, I–III, or II–III were paired were indistinguishable from each other with respect to their renal transport defect; moreover, each of the "double heterozygotes" resembled classical homozygotes of presumed genotypes I–I, II–II, and III–III.

Intestinal transport was also studied in the mixed heterozygotes; all double heterozygotes showed greatly impaired intestinal transport of lysine and arginine *in vitro*. On the other hand, a mixture of types I and III genotypes caused only modest impairment of intestinal uptake of cystine *in vivo*, in accordance with the prediction made by Rosenberg's group (see Table IV).

Such observations constitute the first direct evidence for allelism in a heterogeneous trait such as classical cystinuria.

**Iminoglycinuria.** A situation comparable to that described for classical cystinuria has also been found in the iminoglycinuric trait. It has

* H. Goldman, J. Dossetor, and C. Scriver, unpublished data.

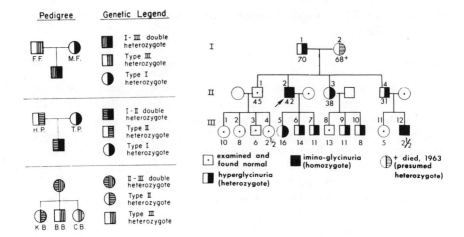

Fig. 12. Evidence that the genotypic heterogeneity in cystinuria and iminoglycinuria (see other evidence of this in Figs. 10 and 11) is, in each case, dependent on allelism at the relevant gene locus. Pedigrees with intrafamilial genotypic heterogeneity are shown on the left for cystinuria[168] and on the right for iminoglycinuria.[200] In cystinuria, matings of different genotypes produced the same homozygous renal phenotype, which was no different from the classical homozygous cystinuric phenotype.

been stated[232] that some obligate iminoglycinuric heterozygotes do not manifest the hyperglycinuria* which is believed to be the hallmark of the heterozygote in other pedigrees.[178,200]

This phenotypic heterogeneity probably indicates genetic heterogeneity and allelism, as shown in one important pedigree[200] [Fig. 12(right)]. In this family one grandson [subject III.12, Fig. 12(right)] had renal iminoglycinuria on every occasion between the age of $2\frac{1}{2}$ and $3\frac{1}{2}$ years when urine amino acids were examined. Since he is too old to have the normal iminoglycinuria of infancy, he is assumed to be homozygous for the trait. This boy's father [II.4, Fig. 12(right)] has hyperglycinuria, as expected of an obligate heterozygote. However, his mother [II.5, Fig. 12(right)], who has been examined on three occasions, has no hyperglycinuria and has a normal renal clearance of glycine; hence, her heterozygous phenotype is at variance with that of her husband. Her son must therefore be a doubly mutant heterozygote, yet one whose phenotype resembles that of the homozygotes in the same pedigree. Therefore, it can be postulated that two mutant alleles affect transport of the imino acids and glycine, and that they occur at the same gene locus.

*The dominantly inherited hyperglycinuric trait observed in an Ashkenazic Jewish pedigree[48] has been reinterpreted[200] as a display of the heterozygous phenotype for familial iminoglycinuria; the latter mutation has been described at least three times in Ashkenazic Jews.[178,200,249]

*Summary*

Several genetic loci control membrane reactive sites at which amino acids bind prior to their transfer across the membrane. Unmistakable traits, such as classical cystinuria and hyperdibasicaminoaciduria, point to a refined genetic control of membrane sites which, in this instance, can unequivocally discriminate between cystine and the structurally similar, but chemically different, cationic (dibasic) amino acids. Additional evidence also suggests that transport sites on the external surface of the membrane are probably under different genetic control from those on the internal surface. There is further evidence that more than one gene controls the uptake of a single amino acid, because its uptake may occur at several membrane sites. Such an assumption helps to explain, for example, the occurrence of classical cystinuria and isolated hypercystinuria in man. The recognition of intrafamilial heterogeneity in the phenotypic expression of some mutant traits has also provided a useful opportunity to document allelism within some of the individual gene loci.

There are other genes which appear to control the transfer of substrate across the membrane once it has been bound at the recognition sites controlled by the aforementioned genes. Whereas some species of protein must constitute the basis for specificity of the recognition sites, it is not at all clear what type of mechanism or membrane structure constitutes the transfer phase of transport. One can only presume from the genetic evidence that the transfer mechanism at least involves a different portion of the recognition site complex, or that it is a different structure which is related physically and biochemically in some way to the binding site.

## GENETIC CONTROL OF TRANSPORT SYSTEMS IN VARIOUS TISSUES

The activities of several genes which control amino acid transport in man resemble those of transport genes found in other organisms. For example, the Hartnup mutation of man[7,106] (Table II) mimics a transport mutation affecting neutral amino acids in *Neurospora*[128,227] (Table I); cystinuria in the dog[238] resembles human cystinuria. And yet, despite this sophisticated awareness allowing investigators to make such comparisons, relatively little is known about the expression of transport genes in different organs and tissues of man. It is known, for example, that transport systems which appear in mammalian intestine tend to be found also in kidney; both organs are epithelialized structures with obvious morphological and functional similarities. But it has yet to be proven adequately whether membrane transport systems which are present in epithelial cells are duplicated, for example, in leucocytes, skin, and liver. The work of Christensen's group suggests that some transport systems which occur in rodent epithelial tissues also function in mouse ascites tumor cells; Christensen has also described in detail some trans-species and trans-tissue (nonhuman) characteristics of membrane transport.[27]

Amino acid uptake by human peripheral leucocytes has been studied by Rosenberg and Downing.[174] These cells concentrate amino acids by mediated membrane systems whose characteristics resemble those used for uptake of amino acids at low concentrations by kidney. Leucocytes accumulate cationic amino acids by a common system which excludes cystine. The $Km$ for lysine uptake is about one-twentieth of that for its uptake by kidney and gut.

It is no surprise, then, that investigators[11,174] should have examined the leucocytes of cystinuric patients; however, it is interesting that no impairment in accumulation of cystine, or of cationic amino acids, was found in cystinuric leucocytes. Two interpretations of this finding are possible. First, the data may indicate that the mutant allele is not expressed in leucocytes, because even normal cells do not have the transport system which is controlled by this gene, and hence, presumably, even the normal allele is not expressed. This conclusion is strongly suggested by the difference in leucocyte and kidney $Km$ lysine values in normal subjects. Alternatively, it is possible that the investigations of cystinuric leucocytes were performed at substrate concentrations which did not actually test for the presence or absence of the transport system modified by the mutant cystinuria allele; this seems to be an unlikely explanation because the concentrations of amino acids used for the study of amino acid transport by leucocytes were equivalent to those used to study gut mucosa and kidney transport *in vitro*. Absence of cationic transport was detected in the latter tissues obtained from cystinuric subjects. Absence of the "cystinuria" transport system, even in normal leucocytes, is thus the more likely reason for nonexpression of the trait in "cystinuric" leucocytes.

Leucocyte transport of amino acids has also been studied in one patient with the renal iminoglycinuric trait.[233] No transport defect was found. Nor was there abnormal incorporation of L-proline into skin fibroblast collagen during a 2-hr incubation period. Tada and colleagues[233] concluded that proline transport in leucocytes and skin was under a different mode of genetic control from that in kidney. However, the concentration of L-proline substrate employed in their experiment does bear on the interpretation of their results. According to their report,[233] incubation was performed with L-proline 0.006 m$M$. It is known that over 95 % of the uptake at this concentration will occur on the low-$Km$ system in rat kidney slices;[140] this is not the system which is affected by the mutant allele in renal iminoglycinuria.[200,208]

Thus, it appears that Tada and co-workers did not actually test for absence of the transport system in leucocytes; their observations should be repeated, using the substrate at much higher concentrations.

Tryptophan transport in peripheral leucocytes has also been examined in Hartnup patients by Tada's group.[233a] Again, the mutant transport trait was not expressed in Hartnup leucocytes, and again the studies were performed at low (0.04 m$M$) substrate concentrations. Thus, whether the investigators failed to observe the mutant trait because it was indeed not expressed, or because it was not actually tested for at the appropriate substrate concentration, still requires elucidation.

It is likely that a number of laboratories will soon begin to report on amino acid transport in cultured human tissue explants. The most available tissue to obtain for culture is the skin fibroblast, but other tissues could also be used for this purpose. With one modest exception,[161] virtually nothing has been done to study the kinetics or the organization of amino acid transport systems in cultured human tissues. The deployment of transport systems in normal cultured tissues will first require investigation before mutant phenotypes can be evaluated in perspective.

Until recently investigation of transport in mammalian kidney was focused largely upon tubular epithelial uptake of substrates *in vivo*, or upon uptake into cortical slices where the majority of cells are of tubular origin. However, studies of amino acid transport have now been made on isolated mammalian renal tubules.[93,107,142] In such preparations the uptake of amino acids obeys Michaelis–Menten kinetics; however, equilibrium is achieved more rapidly than in the slice, and the concentration ratio at equilibrium is usually greater. Others are studying amino acid uptake into isolated glomeruli;[136] in these structures uptake is again mediated, but it is much slower than in the slice or tubule preparations, and the concentration ratio obtained is much less. Whether the diversity of membrane sites used for transport by kidney tubules will also be found in glomeruli remains to be determined. Since the functional and structural characteristics in the two portions of the nephron are sufficiently different, it would not be surprising if different functional characteristics of plasma membranes of these two cell types were found. In this sense, comparisons of glomerular and tubular transport characteristics might serve as a model for the future development of such studies in other tissues.

## TREATMENT AND COUNSELING

Mutations which affect a function as important to the cell as that of membrane transport could have a deleterious effect upon cellular growth and the development of the organism; this is frequently observed with micro-organisms. Preliminary data indicate that cystinuric and Hartnup patients are shorter than average in mean height;[239] if it is true, this observation implies that a hereditary impairment of intestinal and renal transport can compromise the nutrition of the subject. However, most hereditary transport defects of man are strikingly benign in their effect, in contrast to what might be expected. Cystinuria is a serious disorder only when urinary calculi form. Since this is a direct function of cystine solubility, dilution and solubilization of cystine[123] can oversome cystine precipitation; when this is achieved there is no indication that the continued urinary and fecal losses of cystine and cationic amino acids constitute a real hazard to the health and vitality of the patient. Hartnup disease is largely asymptomatic; the trait comes to clinical attention primarily under marginal nutrition conditions which apparently compromise tryptophan-dependent niacin synthesis. The renal iminoglycinuria trait is almost certainly benign.[249]

Thus, a lowered ability of cells to accumulate certain groups of amino acids usually has little direct impact on the viability of the human organism as far as we know. Note, however, that in each case mentioned above the mutant allele controls a high-capacity, shared-transport system. Kepes[117] has speculated that this type of transport serves the organism best in a nutritionally abundant environment; it is the low-capacity systems with high affinity which are perhaps of most importance to sustain protein synthesis, cell replication, and hypertrophy in a starved environment. Would transport mutations which affect only the low-capacity systems for amino acid uptake be harmful to man? Would mutations affecting transport of solutes which normally have access to only one system be harmful to man? As yet we have insufficient experience to know the answers to these questions. It is interesting, however, that two traits affecting intestinal transport of single essential amino acids (methionine and tryptophan, see Table II) are apparently associated with serious clinical manifestations. However, this correlation is tenuous, since so few patients with the latter type of trait have been described.

A number of hereditary transport defects are responsible for what might be termed second-order clinical manifestations. For example, traits which cause the Fanconi syndrome[127] produce demineralization of bone, and rickets or osteomalacia, because of phosphate depletion. In these same traits, dehydration with acidemia results from poor renal conservation of water and bicarbonate. Glucose-galactose malabsorption[188] and congenital chloridorrhea[56] each produce diarrhea through the osmotic effect of the solutes which are poorly absorbed from the intestinal lumen.

Treatment of transport disorders therefore depends on an assessment of the clinical significance of the trait. If symptoms are derived from osmotic effects, it may be possible to eliminate the offending solute from the diet, with benefit to the patient. Where an endogenous deficit occurs as the result of a transport defect, supplementation of the diet with the substrate may offset the defect, presumably because the nonsaturable modes of uptake[3] can be utilized. Alternatively, the end product of the metabolic pathway can be supplied if its deficiency is the determinant of symptoms.

Families bearing mutant transport alleles can usually be counseled clearly on the significance of the trait. A condition like iminoglycinuria is benign; cystinuria is also benign under certain environmental conditions; the cystinotic form of the Fanconi syndrome in childhood almost always has a grave prognosis; the adult form of cystinosis is benign in comparison. With few exceptions, the mutant transport traits are recessively inherited, and the usual predictions can be made concerning their recurrence in siblings and the risk for offspring of affected probands. The frequency of the traits in the population at large is usually unknown. Cystinuria is the best studied, and recent estimates suggest that the homozygotes for all of the pooled genotypes are found about once in 10,000 live births. This means that carriers of cystinuria occur once in 50 live births, but since type II and type III genotypes constitute a minority, it is unlikely that more than half of the heterozygotes can actually be identified in the population by simple methods, such as chromatography of urine amino acids.

Whether a transport trait in a female proband has any influence on fetal development *in utero* has not been studied. However, the placenta is a transport organ which delivers many solutes to the fetus at a fetal–maternal distribution ratio in favor of the fetus.[118] To our knowledge, there has been little investigation into the rate of abortion and still-birth and into fetal growth and development in pedigrees exhibiting mutant maternal transport mutants.


## CONCLUSION

The transport of polar organic solutes across the plasma membrane of cells is achieved by a mediated process which exhibits Michaelis–Menten kinetics. Two components to the migration can be identified. The first involves binding of the substrates to specific and finite areas of the membrane; the degree of specificity which is found in these reactive, or recognition, sites is of such high order that only a species of proteins in the membrane with the requisite genetic control could meet the requirements of such sites. The second component involves transfer of the bound solute across the width of the membrane, and often against a concentration gradient. Transfer of the substrate may involve migration of the carrier or conformational changes in the membrane matrix to allow some form of diffusion of the substrate. Influx of solute appears to be segregated functionally from its efflux.

There are sufficient studies to indicate that plasma membranes are a mosaic of reactive sites. Whether the mosaic is duplicated in all cells in all tissues of the human body is still poorly understood. During mammalian ontogeny various transport systems develop specific activity in gut and kidney at independent rates, suggesting that specific genetic loci control transport processes. This is clearly confirmed through the study of mutant transport traits throughout evolution and in man.

A careful study of amino acid transport in normal human subjects and in those with inborn errors of transport shows that many genetic loci control the many reactive sites required to bind the *different* amino acids. Certain other loci control a series of recognition sites which bind the *same* species of amino acid at different concentrations. The presence of reactive sites which operate with different kinetic characteristics under various environmental conditions would appear to be a very old legacy, and one which serves the cell well under conditions of starvation and of abundance. There are yet other loci which control the transfer of solute after binding has occurred. Predictions which could be made concerning the effect of mutation on the kinetics of binding, or of transfer, are met by the altered characteristics in several mutant transport phenotypes.

Investigation of certain mutant transport traits which exhibit phenotypic heterogeneity has shown that genetic heterogeneity is responsible for most of the former variation. Investigation of appropriate pedigrees exhibiting intrafamilial heterogeneity has revealed that the genotypic heterogeneity must be allelic to account for the observed phenotypes. Thus, within the spectrum of analysis covered in this review there is evidence for genetic diversity of the transport functions, and close correlation between genotype, phenotype, and allelism within the individual gene loci. The similarities between the basic features of "transport genetics" and the genetics of other catalytic functions, such as hemoglobin and glucose-6-phosphate dehydrogenase, are obvious.

What remains of the transport problem? The nature of the reactive site, and how it is associated with the membrane matrix is unknown. The current interest in isolatable transport proteins[153] may eventually allow one to correlate changes in primary sequence of such a membrane protein with the phenotypic effect of a mutant trait. Microorganisms offer the best opportunity for such studies today; culture explants of human tissues may prove of equal value tomorrow.

Fortunately for man, his inborn errors of transport are rare, and more frequently benign than grave; when they are symptomatic it is usually possible to circumvent them by appropriate environmental manipulations. Genetic counseling is thus simplified. The Mendelian nature of the traits, and the ease with which most primary transport traits can be identified, again makes case-finding and pedigree analysis quite simple.

One can anticipate a continued growth in the rate at which inborn errors of membrane transport will be recognized in man. Hopefully, the same will happen in nonhuman vertebrate species, in order to close the gap between our understanding of these phenomena in microorganisms and in ourselves. From each of these experiments of nature in micrococcus, mouse, or man there is a chance to learn more about the plasma membranes of cells.

## ACKNOWLEDGMENTS

The assistance of Mrs. Ileana Archdall and Mrs. Eveline Zifkin with the preparation of this manuscript is greatly appreciated. Dr. Scriver is an Associate of the Medical Research Council of Canada. Preparation of the manuscript was aided in part by a Medical Research Council grant, No. MT-1085.

## BIBLIOGRAPHY

1. Abbassi, V., C. U. Lowe, and P. L. Calcagno, Oculo-cerebro-renal syndrome. A review, *Amer. J. Dis. Child.* **115**:145 (1968).
2. Akedo, H., and H. N. Christensen, Transfer of amino acids across the intestine: A new model amino acid, *J. Biol. Chem.* **237**:113 (1962).
3. Akedo, H., and H. N. Christensen, Nature of insulin action on amino acid uptake by the isolated diaphragm, *J. Biol. Chem.* **237**:118 (1962).
4. Anderson, B., W. Kundig, R. Simoni, and S. Roseman, Further studies of carbohydrate permeases, *Fed. Proc.* **27**:643 (1968).
5. Arias, I. M., M. Furman, D. F. Tapley, and J. E. Ross, Glucuronide formation and transport of various compounds by Gunn rat intestine *in vitro*, *Nature* **197**:1109 (1963).
6. Barker, J. M., Variations in the erythrocyte potassium and sodium in the possum, *Trichosurus vulpecula*, *Nature* **181**:492 (1958).
7. Baron, D. N., C. E. Dent, H. Harris, E. W. Hart, and J. B. Jepson, Hereditary pellagra-like skin rash with temporary cerebellar ataxia, constant renal aminoaciduria and other bizarre biochemical features, *Lancet* **ii**:421 (1956).
8. Bartsocas, C. S., M. L. Levy, J. D. Crawford, and S. Thier, A defect in intestinal amino acid transport in Lowe's syndrome, *Amer. J. Dis. Child.* **117**:93 (1969).
9. Bartter, F. C., Pseudohypoparathyroidism and pseudo-pseudohypoparathyroidism, *in*: The Metabolic Basis of Inherited Disease, 2nd ed., J. B. Stanbury, J. B. Wyngaarden, and D. S Fredrickson, eds. New York, McGraw-Hill Book Co., New York (1966), p. 1024.
10. Bartter, F. C., M. Lotz, S. Thier, L. E. Rosenberg, and J. T. Potts, Jr., Cystinuria. Combined clinical staff conference at the National Institutes of Health, *Ann. Intern. Med.* **62**:796 (1965).

11. Becker, F. F., and H. Green, Incorporation of cystine and lysine by normal and cystinuric leucocytes, *Proc. Soc. Expt. Biol. Med. (N.Y.)* **99**:694 (1958).

12. Bégin, N., and P. G. Scholefield, The uptake of amino acids by mouse pancreas *in vitro*. I. General characteristics, *Biochim. Biophys. Acta* **90**:82 (1964).

13. Björnesjö, K. B., B. Jarnulf, and E. Lausing, Uptake of labeled amino acids into human erythrocytes in disease, *Clin. Chim. Acta* **20**:23 (1968).

14. Blasberg, R., and A. Lajtha, Substrate specificity of steady-state amino acid transport in mouse brain slices, *Arch. Biochem. Biophys.* **112**:361 (1965).

15. Bombara, G., and E. Bergamini, α-Aminoisobutyric acid uptake *in vitro* by the rat extensor digitorum longus muscle after denervation and tenotomy, *Biochim. Biophys. Acta* **150**:226 (1968).

16. Bonetti, E., and C. E. Dent, The determination of optical configuration of naturally occurring amino acids using specific enzymes and paper chromatography, *Biochem. J.* **57**:77 (1954).

17. Brodehl, J., and K. Gellissen, Endogenous renal transport of free amino acids in infancy and childhood, *Pediatrics* **42**:395 (1968).

17a. Brodehl, J., K. Gellissen, and W. Hagge, Die tubuläre Rückresorption der freien Aminosäuren im Säuglings- und Kindesalter, *Mschr. Kinderheilk.* **116**:305 (1968).

18. Brodehl, J., K. Gellissen, and S. Kowalewski, Isolierter defekt der tubulären cystin-Rückresorption in einer Familie mit idiopathischem Hypoparathyroidismus, *Klin. Wochenschrift* **45**:38 (1967).

19. Burnett, C. H., C. E. Dent, C. Harper, and B. J. Warland, Vitamin D resistant rickets: Analysis of twenty-four pedigrees with hereditary and sporadic cases, *Amer. J. Med.* **36**:222 (1964).

20. Calvin, M., Communication: From molecules to Mars, *A.I.B.S. Bull.* **12**:29 (1962).

21. Chambers, R., A micro injection study on the permeability of the starfish egg, *J. Gen. Physiol.* **5**:189 (1923).

22. Chambers, R., The nature of the living cell as revealed by microdissection, *Harvey Lect.* **22**:41 (1926–1927).

23. Chambers, R., and E. L. Chambers, Explorations into the Nature of the Living Cell, Harvard University Press, Cambridge (1961).

24. Christensen, H. N., Reactive sites and biological transport, *Adv. Protein Chem.* **15**:239 (1960).

25. Christensen, H. N., Free amino acids and peptides in tissues, *in*: Mammalian Protein Metabolism, Vol. I, H. N. Munro and J. B. Allison, eds., Academic Press, New York, (1964) p. 105.

26. Christensen, H. N., Methods for distinguishing amino acid transport systems of a given cell or tissue, *Fed. Proc.* **25**:850 (1966).

27. Christensen, H. N., Some transport lessons taught by the organic solute, *Perspect. Biol. & Med.* **10**:471 (1967).

28. Christensen, H. N., and J. A. Clifford, Excretion of 1-aminocyclopentanecarboxylic acid in man and the rat, *Biochim. Biophys. Acta* **62**:160 (1962).

29. Christensen, H. N., and A. M. Cullen, Effects of nonmetabolizable analogs on the distribution of amino acids in the rat, *Biochim. Biophys. Acta* **150**:237 (1968).

30. Christensen, H. N., and J. C. Jones, Amino acid transport models: Renal resorption and resistance to metabolic attack, *J. Biol. Chem.* **237**:1203 (1962).

31. Christensen, H. N., and J. A. Streicher, Association between rapid growth and elevated cell concentrations of amino acids. I. In fetal tissues, *J. Biol. Chem.* **175**:95 (1948).

32. Christensen, H. N., J. A. Streicher, and R. L. Elbinger, Effects of feeding individual

amino acids upon the distribution of other amino acids between cells and extracellular fluid, *J. Biol. Chem.* **172**:515 (1948).

33. Cohen, G. N., and J. Monod, Bacterial permeases, *Bacteriol. Rev.* **21**:169 (1957).
34. Colliss, J. E., A. J. Levi, and M. D. Milne, Stature and nutrition in cystinuria and Hartnup disease, *Brit. Med. J.* **i**:590 (1963).
34a. Cornelius, C. E., J. A. Bishop, and M. H. Schaffer, A quantitative study of aminoaciduria in dachshunds with a history of cystine urolithiasis, *The Cornell Veterinarian* **57**:177 (1967).
35. Cowan, J. W., R. V. Boucher, and E. G. Buss, Riboflavin utilization by a mutant strain of single comb white leghorn chickens. 2. Absorption of radioactive riboflavin from the digestive tract, *Poultry Sci.* **43**:172 (1964).
36. Cozzarelli, N. R., W. G. Freedberg, and E. C. C. Lin, Genetic control of the L-α-glycerol phosphate system in *Escherichia coli, J. Molec. Biol.* **31**:371 (1968).
37. Crawhall, J. C., E. P. Saunders, and C. J. Thompson, Heterozygotes for cystinuria, *Ann. Hum. Genet.* **29**:257 (1966).
38. Crawhall, J. C., E. F. Scowen, C. J. Thompson, and R. W. E. Watts, The renal clearance of amino acids in cystinuria, *J. Clin. Invest.* **46**:1162 (1967).
39. Cusworth, D. C., and C. E. Dent, Renal clearances of amino acids in normal adults and in patients with aminoaciduria, *Biochem. J.* **74**:550 (1960).
40. Cusworth. D. C., C. E. Dent, and F. V. Flynn, The aminoaciduria in galactosemia, *Arch. Dis. Childh.* **30**:150 (1955).
41. Cusworth, D. C., C. E. Dent, and C. R. Scriver, unpublished data.
42. Czaky, T. Z., Transport through biological membranes, *Ann. Rev. Physiol.* **27**:415 (1965).
43. Darlington, A. J., and C. Sacazzocchio, Use of analogues and the substrate sensitivity of mutants in analysis of purine uptake and breakdown in *Aspergillus nidulans, J. Bacteriol.* **93**:937 (1967).
44. Darmady, E. M., and F. Straneck, Microdissection of the nephron in disease, *Brit. Med. Bull.* **13**:21 (1957).
45. Dent, C. E., and H. Harris, The genetics of cystinuria, *Ann. Eugen.* **16**:60 (1951).
46. Dent, C. E., and G. A. Rose, Aminoacid metabolism in cystinuria, *Quart. J. Med.* **20**:205 (1951).
47. Deren, J. J., E. W. Strauss, and T. H. Wilson, The development of structure and transport systems of the fetal rabbit intestine, *Develop. Biol.* **12**:467 (1965).
48. DeVries, A., S. Kochwa, J. Lazebnik, M. Frank, and M. Djaldetti, Glycinuria, a hereditary disorder associated with nephrolithiasis, *Amer. J. Med.* **23**:408 (1957).
49. Drummond, K. N., A. F. Michael, R. A. Ulstrom, and R. A. Good, Blue diaper syndrome: Familial hypercalcemia with nephrocalcinosis and indicanuria, *Amer. J. Med.* **37**:928 (1964).
50. Efron, M. L., Aminoaciduria, *New Eng. J. Med.* **272**:1058 (1965).
51. Efron, M. L., and M. G. Ampola, The aminoacidurias, *Ped. Clin. N.A.* **14**:881 (1967).
52. Efron, M. L., T. C. McPherson, V. E. Shih, C. F. Welsh, and R. A. MacCready, D-methioninuria due to DL-methionine ingestion, *Amer. J. Dis. Child.* **117**:104 (1969).
53. Egan, J. B., and M. L. Morse, Carbohydrate transport in *Staphylococcus aureus*. II. Characterization of the defect of a pleiotrophic transport mutant, *Biochim. Biophys. Acta* **109**:172 (1965).
54. Elsas, L. J., I. Albrecht, and L. E. Rosenberg, Insulin stimulation of amino acid uptake in rat diaphragm: Relationship to protein synthesis, *J. Biol. Chem.* **243**:1846 (1968).
54a. Elsas, L. J., and L. E. Rosenberg, Inhibition of amino acid transport in rat-kidney cortex by puromycin, *Proc. Natl. Acad. Sci. U.S.* **57**:371 (1967).

55. Evans, J. V., and A. T. Phillipson, Electrolyte concentrations in the erythrocytes of the goat and ox, *J. Physiol.* **139**:87 (1957).
56. Evanson, J. M., and S. W. Stanbury, Congenital chloridorrhea or so-called congenital alkalosis with diarrhea, *Gut* **6**:29 (1965).
57. Feigin, R. D., A. S. Klainer, and W. R. Beisel, Circadian periodicity of blood amino acids in adult men, *Nature* **215**:512 (1967).
58. Feigin, R. D., A. S. Klainer, and W. R. Beisel, Factors affecting circadian periodicity of blood amino acids in Man, *Metabolism* **17**:764 (1968).
59. Ferguson, J. C., Transport of amino acids by starfish digestive glands, *Comp. Biochem. Physiol.* **24**:921 (1968).
60. Ferroluzzi-Ames, G., Uptake of amino acids by *Salmonella typhimurium*, *Arch. Biochem. Biophys.* **104**:1 (1964).
61. Fetterman, G. H., N. A. Shuplock, F. J. Philipp, and H. S. Gregg, The growth and maturation of human glomeruli and proximal convolutions from term to adulthood: Studies by microdissection, *Pediatrics* **35**:601 (1965).
62. Finch, L. R., and F. J. R. Hird, The uptake of amino acids by isolated segments of rat intestine. II. A survey of affinity for uptake from rates of uptake and competition for uptake, *Biochim. Biophys. Acta* **43**:278 (1960).
63. Finerman, G. A. M., and L. E. Rosenberg, Amino acid transport in bone: Evidence for separate transport systems for neutral amino and imino acids, *J. Biol. Chem.* **241**:1487 (1966).
64. Fischer, G. A., Defective transport of amethopterin (methotrexate) as a mechanism of resistance to antimetabolite in L5178Y leukemic cells, *Biochem. Pharmacol.* **11**:1233 (1965).
65. Foley, T. H., and D. R. London, Cysteine metabolism in cystinuria, *Clin. Sci.* **29**:549 (1965).
66. Fox, M., S. Thier, and L. Rosenberg, Ionic requirements for amino acid transport in the rat kidney cortex slices: Influence of the extracellular ions, *Biochim. Biophys. Acta* **79**:167 (1964).
67. Fox, M., S. Thier, L. E. Rosenberg, W. Kiser, and S. Segal, Evidence against a single renal transport defect in cystinuria, *New Eng. J. Med.* **270**:556 (1964).
68. Fraser, D., S. W. Kooh, and C. R. Scriver, Hyperparathyroidism as the cause of hyperaminoaciduria and phosphaturia in human vitamin D deficiency, *Ped. Res.* **1**:425 (1967).
69. Fraser, D., and R. B. Salter, The diagnosis and management of the various types of rickets, *Ped. Clin. N.A.* **1958**(May):417.
70. Frimpter, G. W., Cystinuria: Metabolism of the disulfide of cysteine and homocysteine, *J. Clin. Invest.* **42**:1956 (1963).
71. Frimpter, G. W., Cystinuria: Intravenous administration of [35S] cystine and [35S] cysteine, *Clin. Sci.* **31**:207 (1966).
72. Frimpter, G. E., M. Horwith, E. Furth, R. E. Fellows, and D. O. Thompson, Inulin and endogenous amino acid renal clearances in cystinuria: Evidence for tubular secretion, *J. Clin. Invest.* **41**:281 (1962).
73. Gilbert, J. B., Y. Ku, L. L. Rogers, and R. L. Williams, The increase in urinary taurine after intraperitoneal administration of amino acids to the mouse, *J. Biol. Chem.* **235**:1055 (1960).
74. Gits, J. J., and M. Grenson, Multiplicity of the amino acid permeases in *Saccharomyces cerevisiae*. III. Evidence for a specific methionine-transporting system, *Biochim. Biophys. Acta* **135**:507 (1967).
75. Goldberg, L. S., and H. H. Fudenberg, Familial selective malabsorption of vitamin

$B_{12}$ : Reevaluation of an *in vivo* intrinsic factor inhibitor, *New Eng. J. Med.* **279**:405 (1968).

76. Goldman, H., and C. R. Scriver, A transport system in mammalian kidney with preference for β-amino compounds, *Ped. Res.* **1**:212 (1967).

77. Goodman, S. I., C. A. McIntyre, and D. O'Brien, Impaired intestinal transport of proline in a patient with familial iminoaciduria, *J. Ped.* **71**:246 (1967).

78. Goyer, R. A., The renal tubule in lead poisoning. I. Mitochondrial swelling and aminoaciduria, *Lab. Invest.* **19**:71 (1968).

79. Grasbeck, R., R. Gordin, I. Kantero, and B. Kuhlback, Selective vitamin $B_{12}$ malabsorption and proteinuria in young people: syndrome, *Acta Med. Scand.* **167**:289 (1960).

80. Grenson, M., Multiplicity of the amino acid permeases in *Saccharomyces cerevisiae*. II. Evidence for a specific lysine-transporting system, *Biochim. Biophys. Acta* **127**:339 (1966).

81. Grenson, M., M. Mouset, J. M. Wiame, and J. Bechet, Multiplicity of the amino acid permeases in *Saccharomyces cerevisiae*, I. Evidence for a specific arginine-transporting system, *Biochim. Biophys. Acta* **127**:325 (1966).

82. Grose, J., and C. R. Scriver, Parathyroid dependent phosphaturia and aminoaciduria in the vitamin D-deficient rat, *Amer. J. Physiol.* **214**:370 (1968).

83. Hagihira, H., E. C. C. Lin, A. H. Samiy, and T. H. Wilson, Active transport of lysine, ornithine, arginine and cystine by the intestine, *Biochem. Biophys. Res. Commun.* **4**:478 (1961).

84. Hagihira, H., T. H. Wilson, and E. C. C. Lin, Intestinal transport of certain N-substituted amino acids, *Amer. J. Physiol.* **203**:637 (1962).

85. Halpern, Y. S., and M. Lupo, Glutamate transport in wild-type and mutant strains of *Escherichia coli*, *J. Bacteriol.* **90**:1288 (1965).

86. Halvorsen, H. O., H. Okada, and J. Gorman, The role of an alpha-methyl glucoside permease in the induced synthesis of isomaltase in yeast, *in*: The Cellular Functions of Membrane Transport, J. R. Hoffman, ed., Prentice-Hall, Englewood Cliffs, N.J. (1964), p. 171.

87. Harris, H., U. Mittwoch, E. B. Robson, and F. L. Warren, Pattern of amino acid excretion in cystinuria, *Ann. Hum. Genet.* **19**:195 (1955).

88. Harrison, H. E., and H. C. Harrison, Experimental production of renal glycosuria, phosphaturia and aminoaciduria by injection of maleic acid, *Science* **120**:606 (1954).

89. Harvald, B., K. H. Hanel, R. Squires, and T. Trap-Jensen, Adenosine-triphosphatase deficiency in patients with nonspherocytic haemolytic anemia, *Lancet* **ii**:18 (1964).

90. Harvey, A. M., and H. N. Christensen, Uric acid transport: Apparent absence in erythrocytes of the Dalmatian dog, *Science* **145**:826 (1964).

91. Hechtman, P., and C. R. Scriver, β-Alanine transport in a catabolically defective mutant of *Pseudomonas fluorescens*, *Proc. Canad. Fed. Biol. Soc.* **11**:94 (1968).

92. Heinz, E., and P. O. Walsh, Exchange diffusion, transport and intracellular level of amino acids in Ehrlich carcinoma cells, *J. Biol. Chem.* **233**:1488 (1958).

93. Hillman, R. E., I. Albrecht, and L. E. Rosenberg, Transport of amino acids by isolated rabbit renal tubules, *Biochim. Biophys. Acta* **150**:528 (1968).

94. Hokin, L. E., and M. R. Hokin, Biological transport, *Ann. Rev. Biochem.* **32**:553 (1963).

95. Holden, J. T., Transport and accumulation of amino acids by microorganisms, *in*: Amino Acid Pools, Elsevier, New York (1962), p. 566.

96. Holden, J. T., and N. M. Utech, Defective glutamate uptake in a mutant of *S. faecalis*, *Fed. Proc.* **24**:1231 (1965).

97. Holden, J. T., and N. M. Utech, Effect of biotin, pantothenic acid and nicotinic acid deficiencies on amino acid transport in *Lactobacillus plantarium*, *Biochim. Biophys. Acta* **135**:517 (1967).

98. Holt, L. E., Jr., S. E. Snyderman, P. M. Norton, E. Roitman, and J. Finch, The plasma aminogram in kwashiorkor, *Lancet* **ii**:1343 (1963).

99. Holter, H., Problems of pinocytosis, with special regard to amoebae, *Ann. N.Y. Acad. Sci.* **78**:524 (1959).

100. Hooft, C., D. Carton, J. Snoeck, J. Timmermans, I. Antener, C. Van den Hende, and W. Oyaert, Further investigations in the methionine malabsorption syndrome, *Helv. Paed. Acta* **23**:334 (1968).

100a. Hunt, D. D., G. Stearns, J. B. McKinley, E. Froning, P. Hicks, and M. Bontiglio, Long-term study of family with Fanconi syndrome without cystinosis (DeToni–Debre–Fanconi syndrome), *Amer. J. Med.* **40**:492 (1966).

101. Inui, Y., and H. N. Christensen, Discrimination of single transport systems: The Na$^+$ sensitive transport of neutral amino acids in the Ehrlich cell, *J. Gen. Physiol.* **50**:203 (1966).

102. Jackson, J. D., F. G. Smith, N. N. Litman, C. L. Yuile, and H. Latta, The Fanconi syndrome with cystinosis. Electron microscopy of renal biopsy specimens from five patients, *Amer. J. Med.* **33**:893 (1962).

103. Jacobson, E. S., and R. L. Metzenberg, A new gene which affects uptake of neutral and acidic amino acids in *Neurospora crassa*, *Biochim. Biophys. Acta* **156**:140 (1968).

104. Jacquez, J. A., The kinetics of carrier-mediated active transport of amino acids, *Proc. Natl. Acad. Sci. U.S.* **47**:153 (1961).

105. Jandle, J. H., Hereditary spherocytosis, *in*: The Metabolic Basis of Inherited Disease, 2nd ed., J. B. Stanbury, J. B. Wyngaarden, and D. S. Fredrickson, eds., McGraw-Hill, New York (1966), p. 1035.

106. Jepson, J. B., Hartnup disease, *in*: The Metabolic Basis of Inherited Disease, 2nd ed., J. B. Stanbury, J. B. Wyngaarden, and D. S. Fredrickson, eds., McGraw-Hill, New York (1966), p. 1283.

107. Johnston, C. C., P. Bartlett, and C. J. Podsiadly, Transport of α-aminoisobutyric acid by separated rabbit renal tubules, *Biochim. Biophys. Acta* **163**:418 (1968).

108. Johnstone, R. M., and P. G. Scholefield, The need for ions during transport and exchange diffusion of amino acids into Ehrlich ascites carcinoma cells, *Biochim. Biophys. Acta* **94**:130 (1965).

109. Johnstone, R. M., and P. G. Scholefield, Amino acid transport in tumor cells, *Adv. Cancer Res.* **9**:143 (1965).

110. Jonxis, J. H. P., Phosphate metabolism in rickets and tetany, *Helv. Paed. Acta* **14**:49 (1959).

111. Joseph, R., M. Ribierre, J.-C. Job, and M. Girault, Maladie familiale assosciante des convulsions à début très precoce, une hyperalbuminorachie et une hyperamino-acidurie, *Arch. Franc. Pediat.* **15**:374 (1958).

112. Kaback, H. R., and E. R. Stadtman, Proline uptake by an isolated cytoplasmic membrane preparation of *Escherichia coli*, *Proc. Natl. Acad. Sci. U.S.* **55**:920 (1966).

113. Kappy, M. S., and R. L. Metzenberg, Multiple alterations in metabolite uptake in a mutant of *Neurospora crassa*, *J. Bacteriol.* **94**:1629 (1967).

114. Käser, H., P. Cottier, and I. Antener, Glucoglycinuria, a new familial syndrome, *J. Ped.* **61**:386 (1962).

115. Kekomäki, M., Intestinal absorption of L-arginine and L-lysine in familial protein intolerance, *Ann. Ped. Fenn.* **14**:18 (1968).

116. Kekomäki, M., J. K. Visakorpi, J. Perheentupa, and L. Saxén, Familial protein

intolerance with deficient transport of basic amino acids, *Acta Paed. Scand.* **56**:617 (1967).

117. Kepes, A., The place of permeases in cellular organization, *in*: The Cellular Functions of Membrane Transport, J. F. Hoffman, ed., Prentice-Hall, Englewood Cliffs, N.J. (1964), p. 155.

118. Kerr, G. R., and H. A. Waisman, Transplacental ratios of serum-free amino acids during pregnancy in the Rhesus monkey, *in*: Amino Acid Metabolism and Genetic Variation, W. L. Nyhan, ed., McGraw-Hill, New York (1967), p. 429.

119. Kessel, D., T. C. Hall, and D. Roberts, Uptake as a determinant of methotrexate response in mouse leukemias, *Science* **150**:752 (1965).

120. Kessel, D., and M. Lubin, Transport of proline in *Escherichia coli, Biochim. Biophys. Acta* **57**:32 (1962).

121. Kessel, D., and M. Lubin, On the distinction between peptidase activity and peptide transport, *Biochim. Biophys. Acta* **71**:656 (1963).

122. Khattab, A. G. H., J. H. Watson, and R. F. E. Axford, Genetic control of blood potassium concentration in Welsh mountain sheep, *J. Agric. Sci.* **63**:81 (1964).

123. Knox, W. E., Cystinuria, *in*: The Metabolic Basis of Inherited Disease, 2nd ed., J. B. Stanbury, J. B. Wyngaarden, and D. S. Fredrickson, eds., McGraw-Hill, New York (1966), p. 1262.

124. Korn, E. D., Structure of biological membranes, *Science* **153**:1491 (1966).

125. Krane, S. M., Renal glycosuria, *in*: The Metabolic Basis of Inherited Disease, 2nd ed., J. B. Stanbury, J. B. Wyngaarden, and D. S. Fredrickson, eds., McGraw-Hill, New York (1966), p. 1221.

126. Kundig, W., F. D. Kundig, B. Anderson, and S. Roseman, Restoration of active transport of glycosides in *Escherichia coli* by a component of a phosphotransferase system, *J. Biol. Chem.* **241**:3243 (1966).

127. Leaf, A., The syndrome of osteomalacia, renal glucosuria, aminoaciduria, and increased phosphorus clearance (The Fanconi Syndrome), *in*: The Metabolic Basis of Inherited Disease, 2nd ed., J. B. Stanbury, J. B. Wyngaarden, and D. S. Fredrickson, eds., McGraw-Hill, New York (1966), p. 1205.

128. Lester, G., Genetic control of amino acid permeability in *Neurospora crassa, J. Bacteriol.* **91**:677 (1966).

129. Levine, E. M., and S. Simmonds, Metabolite uptake by serine-glycine auxotrophs of *Escherichia coli, J. Biol. Chem.* **235**:2902 (1960).

130. Lin, E. C. C., H. Hagihira, and T. H. Wilson, Specificity of the transport system for neutral amino acids in the hamster intestine, *Amer. J. Physiol.* **202**:919 (1962).

131. Lowenstein, L. M., I. Smith, and S. Segal, Amino acid transport in the rat renal papilla, *Biochim. Biophys. Acta* **150**:73 (1968).

132. Lubin, M., and H. L. Ennis, On the role of intracellular potassium in protein synthesis, *Biochim. Biophys. Acta* **80**:614 (1964).

133. Lubin, M., D. A. Kessel, A. Budreau, and J. D. Gross, The isolation of bacterial mutants defective in amino acid transport, *Biochim. Biophys. Acta* **42**:535 (1960).

134. Luder, J., and W. Sheldon, A familial tubular absorption defect of glucose and amino acids, *Arch. Dis. Childh.* **30**:160 (1955).

135. Lush, I. E., The biochemical genetics of vertebrates except man, *in*: Frontiers of Biology, Vol. 3, A. Neuberger, and E. L. Tatum, eds., North-Holland Pub. Co., Amsterdam (1967).

136. Mackenzie, S., and C. R. Scriver, L-Proline transport in isolated rat glomeruli, *Biochem. Biophys. Acta* (in press).

137. Mann, J. B., S. Alterman, and A. G. Hills, Albright's hereditary osteodystrophy

comprising pseudohypoparathyroidism and pseudopseudohypoparathyroidism, *Ann. Int. Med.* **56**:315 (1962).

138. Milne, M. D., M. A. Crawford, C. B. Girão, and L. W. Loughridge, The metabolic disorder in Hartnup disease, *Quart. J. Med.* **29**:407 (1960).
139. Mitchell, P., Metabolism, transport, and morphogenesis: Which drives which? *J. Gen. Microbiol.* **29**:25 (1962).
140. Mohyuddin, F., and C. R. Scriver, Similarity of L-proline transport systems in kidney of the rat *in vitro*, and of man *in vivo*, *Biochem. Biophys. Res. Commun.* **32**:852 (1968).
141. Morikawa, T., K. Tada, T. Ando, T. Yoshida, Y. Yokoyama, and T. Arakawa, Prolinuria: Defect in intestinal absorption of imino acids and glycine, *Tohoku J. Exp. Med.* **90**:105 (1966).
142. Murthy, L., and E. C. Foulkes, Movement of solutes across luminal cell membranes in kidney tubules of the rabbit, *Nature* **213**:180 (1967).
143. McCarthy, C. F., J. L. Borland, Jr., H. J. Lynch, Jr., E. E. Owen, and M. P. Tyor, Defective uptake of basic amino acids and L-cystine by intestinal mucosa of patients with cystinuria, *J. Clin. Invest.* **43**:1518 (1964).
144. Neame, K. D., Uptake of L-histidine, L-proline, L-tyrosine and L-ornithine by brain, intestinal mucosa, testis, kidney, spleen, liver, heart muscle, skeletal muscle and erythrocytes of the rat *in vitro*, *J. Physiol.* **162**:1 (1962).
145. Newey, H., and D. H. Smyth, Cellular mechanisms in intestinal transfer of amino acids, *J. Physiol.* **164**:527 (1962).
146. Noall, M. W., T. R. Riggs, L. M. Walker, and H. N. Christensen, Endocrine control of amino acid transfer. Distribution of an unmetabolized amino acid, *Science* **126**:1002 (1957).
147. Northcote, D. H., (ed.), Structure and function of membranes, *Brit. Med. Bull.* **24**:99 (1968).
148. Oldfield, J. E., P. H. Allen, and J. Adair, Identification of cystine calculi in mink, *Proc. Soc. Expt. Biol. Med.* **91**:560 (1956).
149. Orloff, J., and M. B. Burg, Vasopressin-resistant diabetes insipidus, *in*: The Metabolic Basis of Inherited Disease, 2nd ed., J. B. Stanbury, J. B. Wyngaarden, and D. S. Fredrickson, eds., McGraw-Hill, New York (1966), p. 1247.
150. Overton, E., Ueber die allgemeinen osmotichen Eigenschaften der Zelle, ihre vermutlichen Ursachen und ihre Bedeutung für die Physiologie, *Vierteljahresschr. Naturforsch., Ges. Zurich* **44**:88 (1899).
151. Oxender, D. L., Stereospecificity of amino acid transport for Ehrlich tumor cells, *J. Biol. Chem.* **240**:2976 (1965).
152. Oxender, D. L., and H. N. Christensen, Distinct mediating systems for the transport of neutral amino acids by the Ehrlich cell, *J. Biol. Chem.* **238**:3686 (1963).
153. Pardee, A. B., Membrane transport proteins, *Science* **162**:632 (1968).
154. Pardee, A. B., and L. S. Prestidge, Cell-free activity of a sulfate-binding site involved in active transport, *Proc. Natl. Acad. Sci. U.S.* **55**:189 (1966).
155. Pardee, A. B., L. S. Prestidge, M. B. Whipple, and J. Dreyfuss, A binding site for sulfate and its relation to sulfate transport into *Salmonella typhimurium*, *J. Biol. Chem.* **241**:3962 (1966).
156. Payne, J. W., and C. Gilvarg, The role of the terminal carboxyl group in peptide transport in *Escherichia coli*, *J. Biol. Chem.* **243**:335 (1968).
157. Perheentupa, J., and J. K. Visakorpi, Protein intolerance with deficient transport of basic amino acids: Another inborn error of metabolism, *Lancet* **ii**:813 (1965).
158. Pfeffer, W., Osmotische Untersuchungen. Studien zur Zellmechanik, Engelmann, Leipzig (1877).

159. Piel, C. F., and H. A. Harper, Excretion of D- and L-methionine in children with generalized aminoaciduria, *J. Ped.* **59**:861 (1961).
160. Pitts, R. F., Physiology of the Kidney and Body Fluids, Year Book Med. Pub., Chicago (1963).
161. Platter, H., and G. M. Martin, Tryptophane transport in cultures of human fibroblasts, *Proc. Soc. Expt. Biol. Med.* **123**:140 (1966).
162. Prader, V. A., R. Illig, and E. Heierli, Eine besondere Form der primären vitamin-D resistenten Rachitis mit Hypocalcämie und autosomaldominantem Erbgang: die hereditäre Pseudo-Mangelrachitis, *Helv. Paed. Acta* **16**:452 (1961).
163. Quastel, J. H., Membrane structure and function, *Science* **158**:146 (1967).
164. Reubi, F. C., Glucose titration in renal glycosuria, *in*: Ciba Foundation Symposium on the Kidney, Little-Brown, Boston (1954).
165. Riggs, T. R., and L. M. Walker, Diminished uptake of $^{14}C$ $\alpha$-amino-isobutyric acid by tissues of vitamin $B_6$ deficient rats, *J. Biol. Chem.* **233**:132 (1958).
166. Robson, E. B., and G. A. Rose, The effect of intravenous lysine on the renal clearances of cystine, arginine, and ornithine in normal subjects, in patients with cystinuria, and Fanconi syndrome, and in their relatives, *Clin. Sci.* **16**:75 (1957).
167. Rosenberg, L. E., Cystinuria: Genetic heterogeneity and allelism, *Science* **154**:1341 (1966).
168. Rosenberg, L. E., Genetic heterogeneity in cystinuria, *in*: Amino Acid Metabolism and Genetic Variation, W. L. Nyhan, ed., McGraw-Hill, New York (1967), p. 341.
169. Rosenberg, L. E., Inherited disorders of membrane function, *in*: Biological Membranes, R. Dowben, ed., Little-Brown, Boston (1969).
170. Rosenberg, L. E., I. Albrecht, and S. Segal, Lysine transport in human kidney: Evidence for two systems, *Science* **155**:1426 (1967).
171. Rosenberg, L. E., A. Blair, and S. Segal, Transport of amino acids by slices of rat-kidney cortex, *Biochim. Biophys. Acta* **54**:479 (1961).
172. Rosenberg, I. H., A. L. Coleman, and L. E. Rosenberg, The role of sodium ion in the transport of amino acids by the intestine, *Biochim. Biophys. Acta* **102**:161 (1965).
173. Rosenberg, L. E., J. C. Crawhall, and S. Segal, Intestinal transport of cystine and cysteine in man: Evidence for separate mechanisms, *J. Clin. Invest.* **46**:30 (1967).
174. Rosenberg, L. E., and S. Downing, Transport of neutral and dibasic amino acids by human leukocytes: Absence of defect in cystinuria, *J. Clin. Invest.* **44**:1382 (1965).
175. Rosenberg, L. E., S. Downing, J. L. Durant, and S. Segal, Cystinuria: Biochemical evidence for three genetically distinct diseases, *J. Clin. Invest.* **45**:365 (1966).
176. Rosenberg, L. E., S. J. Downing, and S. Segal, Competitive inhibition of dibasic amino acid transport in rat kidney, *J. Biol. Chem.* **237**:2265 (1962).
177. Rosenberg, L. E., J. L. Durant, and I. Albrecht, Genetic heterogeneity in cystinuria: Evidence for allelism, *Trans. Assoc. Amer. Phys.* **79**:284 (1966).
178. Rosenberg, L. E., J. L. Durant, and L. J. Elsas, II, Familial iminoglycinuria. An inborn error of renal tubular transport, *New Eng. J. Med.* **278**:1407 (1968).
179. Rosenberg, L. E., J. L. Durant, and J. M. Holland, Intestinal absorption and renal extraction of cystine and cysteine in cystinuria, *New Eng. J. Med.* **273**:1239 (1965).
180. Rosenberg, H., and J. M. La Nauze, The isolation of a mutant of *Bacillus cereus* deficient in phosphate uptake, *Biochim. Biophys. Acta* **156**:381 (1968).
181. Rosenberg, L. E., P. S. Mueller, and D. M. Watkin, A new syndrome: Familial growth retardation, renal aminoaciduria, and corpulmonale. II. Investigation of renal function, amino acid metabolism, and genetic transmission, *Amer. J. Med.* **31**:205 (1961).

182. Rosenberg, L. E., and C. R. Scriver, Amino acid metabolism, *in*: Duncan's Textbook on Diseases of Metabolism, 6th ed., P. Bondy, ed., Saunders, Philadelphia (1969).
183. Rosenberg, L. E., and S. Segal, Maleic acid-induced inhibition of amino acid transport in rat kidney, *Biochem. J.* **92**:345 (1964).
184. Rout, W. R., D. S. T. Lin, and K. C. Huang, Intestinal transport of amino acids and glucose in flounder fish, *Proc. Soc. Expt. Biol. Med.* **118**:933 (1965).
185. Rowley, P. T., P. S. Mueller, D. M. Watkin, and L. E. Rosenberg, Familial growth retardation, renal aminoaciduria, and corpulmonale. I. Description of a new syndrome with case reports, *Amer. J. Med.* **31**:187 (1961).
186. Ruszkowski, M., C. Arasimowicz, J. Knapowski, J. Steffen, and K. Weiss, Renal absorption of amino acids, *Amer. J. Physiol.* **203**:891 (1962).
187. Schaefler, S., and W. K. Maas, Inducible system for the utilization of $\beta$-glucosides in *E. coli*. II. Description of mutant types and genetic analysis, *J. Bacteriol.* **93**:264 (1967).
188. Schneider, A. J., W. B. Kinter, and C. E. Stirling, Glucose-galactose malabsorption. Report of a case with autoradiographic studies of a mucosal biopsy, *New Eng. J. Med.* **274**:305 (1966).
188a. Schneider, J. A., V. Wong, K. Bradley, and J. E. Seegmiller, Biochemical comparisons of the adult and childhood forms of cystinosis, *New Eng. J. Med.* **279**:1253 (1968).
189. Schwartz, J. H., W. K. Maas, and E. J. Simon, An impaired concentrating mechanism for amino acids in mutants of *Escherichia coli* resistant to L-canavanine and D-serine, *Biochim. Biophys. Acta* **32**:582 (1959).
190. Schwartzman, L., A. Blair, and S. Segal, A common renal transport system for lysine, ornithine, arginine, and cysteine, *Biochem. Biophys. Res. Commun.* **23**:220 (1966).
191. Schwartzman, L., A. Blair, and S. Segal, Effect of transport inhibitors on dibasic amino acid exchange diffusion in rat kidney cortex, *Biochim. Biophys. Acta* **135**:136 (1967).
192. Schwartzman, L., A. Blair, and S. Segal, Exchange diffusion of dibasic amino acids in rat-kidney cortex slices, *Biochim. Biophys. Acta* **135**:120 (1967).
193. Scott, D. H., Carl Wilheim von Nägeli, *Nature* **44**:580 (1891).
194. Scriver, C. R., Hereditary aminoaciduria, *in*: Progress in Medical Genetics, Vol. 2, A. Bearn and A. G. Steinberg, eds., Grune and Stratton, New York (1962), p. 83.
195. Scriver, C. R., Glycyl-proline in urine of humans with bone disease, *Canad. J. Physiol. Pharmac.* **42**:357 (1964).
196. Scriver, C. R., Hartnup disease: A genetic modification of intestinal and renal transport of certain neutral alpha-amino acids, *New Eng. J. Med.* **273**:530 (1965).
197. Scriver, C. R., The phenotypic manifestations of hereditary tyrosinemia and tyrosyluria: A hypothesis, *in*: Conference on Hereditary Tyrosinemia, M. Partington, C. R. Scriver, and A. Sass-Kortsak, eds., *Canad. Med. Assoc. J.* **97**:1073 (1967).
198. Scriver, C. R., Amino acid transport in mammalian kidney, *in*: Amino Acid Metabolism and Genetic Variation, W. L. Nyhan, ed., McGraw-Hill, New York (1967), p. 327.
199. Scriver, C. R., Hyperaminoaciduria, *in*: Cecil-Loeb Textbook of Medicine, 12th ed., P. B. Beeson and W. McDermott, eds., Saunders, Philadelphia (1967), p. 1219.
200. Scriver, C. R., Renal tubular transport of proline, hydroxyproline, and glycine. III. Genetic basis for more than one mode of transport in human kidney, *J. Clin. Invest.* **47**:823 (1968).
201. Scriver, C. R., Amino acid transport: Factors influencing uptake in kidney and intestine, *in*: Symposium on Intestinal Absorption and Malabsorption, S. Karger, Basel (1968).

202. Scriver, C. R., and E. Davies, Endogenous renal clearance rates of free amino acids in prepubertal children, *Pediatrics* **36**:592 (1965).
203. Scriver, C. R., M. L. Efron, and I. A. Schafer, Renal tubular transport of proline, hydroxyproline, and glycine in health and in familial hyperprolinemia, *J. Clin. Invest.* **43**:374 (1964).
204. Scriver, C. R., R. B. Goldbloom, and C. C. Roy, Hypophosphatemic rickets with renal hyperglycinuria, renal glucosuria, and glycylprolinuria. A syndrome with evidence for renal tubular secretion of phosphorus, *Pediatrics* **34**:357 (1964).
205. Scriver, C. R., and H. Goldman, Renal tubular transport of proline, hydroxyproline, and glycine. II. Hydroxy-L-proline as substrate and as inhibitor *in vivo*, *J. Clin. Invest.* **45**:1357 (1966).
206. Scriver, C. R., and F. Mohyuddin, Amino acid transport in kidney: Heterogeneity of AIB uptake, *J. Biol. Chem.* **243**:3207 (1968).
207. Scriver, C. R., S. Pueschel, and E. Davies, Hyper-$\beta$-alaninemia associated with $\beta$-aminoaciduria and $\gamma$-aminobutyricaciduria, somnolence and seizures, *New Eng. J. Med.* **274**:636 (1966).
208. Scriver, C. R., and O. H. Wilson, Amino acid transport in human kidney: Evidence for genetic control of two types, *Science* **155**:1428 (1967).
208a. Seakins, J. W. T., and R. S. Ersser, Effects of amino acid loads on a healthy infant with the biochemical features of Hartnup disease, *Arch. Dis. Childh.* **42**:682 (1967).
209. Seegmiller, J. E., T. Friedmann, H. E. Harrison, V. Wong, and J. A. Schneider, Cystinosis. Combined clinical staff conference, at the National Institutes of Health, *Ann. Int. Med.* **68**:883 (1968).
210. Segal, S., and J. C. Crawhall, Transport of cysteine by human kidney cortex *in vitro*, *Biochem. Med.* **1**:141 (1967).
211. Segal, S., and J. C. Crawhall, Characteristics of cystine and cysteine transport in rat-kidney cortex slices, *Proc. Natl. Acad. Sci.* **59**:231 (1968).
212. Segal, S., L. Schwartzman, A. Blair, and D. Bertoli, Dibasic amino acid transport in rat-kidney cortex slices, *Biochim. Biophys. Acta* **135**:127 (1967).
213. Seldin, D. W., and J. D. Wilson, Renal tubular acidosis, *in*: The Metabolic Basis of Inherited Disease, 2nd ed., J. B. Stanbury, J. B. Wyngaarden, and D. S. Fredrickson, eds., McGraw-Hill, New York (1966), p. 1230.
214. Shannon, J. A., and S. Fisher, The renal tubular reabsorption of glucose in the normal dog, *Amer. J. Physiol.* **122**:765 (1938).
214a. Sheldon, W., J. Luder, and B. Webb, A familial tubular absorption defect of glucose and amino acids, *Arch. Dis. Childh.* **36**:90 (1961).
215. Shifrin, S., B. N. Ames, and G. Ferroluzzi-Ames, Effect of the $\alpha$-hydrazino analog of histidine on histidine transport and arginine biosynthesis, *J. Biol. Chem.* **241**:3424 (1966).
216. Simoni, R. D., M. Levinthal, F. D. Kundig, W. Kundig, B. Anderson, P. E. Hartman, and S. Roseman, Genetic evidence for the role of a bacterial phosphotransferase system in sugar transport, *Proc. Natl. Acad. Sci. (U.S.)* **58**:1963 (1967).
217. Sirotnak, F. M., M. G. Sargent, and D. J. Hutchison, Genetically alterable transport of amethopterin in *Diplococcus pneumoniae*. II. Impairment of system associated with various mutant genotype, *J. Bacteriol.* **93**:315 (1967).
218. Smith, H. W., The Kidney: Structure and Function in Health and Disease, Oxford Univ. Press, New York (1958), p. 81.
219. Smith, H. W., The plasma membrane, with notes on the history of botany, *Circulation* **26**:987 (1962).
220. Smith, H. W., W. Goldring, H. Chasis, H. A. Ranges, and S. E. Bradley, The applica-

tion of saturation methods to the study of glomerular and tubular function in the human kidney, *J. Mount Sinai Hosp.* **10**:59 (1943).

221. Soriano, J. R., H. Boichis, H. Stark, and C. M. Edelmann, Jr., Proximal renal tubular acidosis. A defect in bicarbonate reabsorption with normal urinary acidification, *Ped. Res.* **1**:81 (1967).

222. Sorsoli, W. A., K. D. Spence, and L. W. Parks, Amino acid accumulation in ethionine-resistant *Saccharomyces cerevisiae*, *J. Bacteriol.* **88**:20 (1964).

223. Soupart, P., Free amino acids of blood and urine in the human, *in*: Amino Acid Pools, J. T. Holden, ed., Elsevier, New York (1962), p. 220.

224. Spencer, R. P., Evolutionary and genetic history of intestinal amino acid transport, *Amer. J. Clin. Nutr.* **21**:188 (1968).

225. Srikantia, S. G., P. S. Venkatachalam, and V. Reddy, Clinical and biochemical features of a case of Hartnup disease, *Brit. Med. J.* **i**:282–285 (1964).

226. Stadler, D. R., Genetic control of uptake of amino acids in *Neurospora*, *Science* **150**:385 (1965).

227. Stadler, D. R., Genetic control of the uptake of amino acids in *Neurospora*, *Genetics* **54**:677 (1966).

227a. States, B., and S. Segal, Developmental aspects of cystine transport in rat intestinal segments, *Biochim. Biophys. Acta* **163**:154 (1968).

228. Stein, W. D., The Movement of Molecules across Cell Membranes, Academic Press, New York (1967), p. 369.

229. Stein, W. H., Excretion of amino acids in cystinuria, *Proc. Soc. Expt. Biol. Med.* **78**:705 (1951).

230. Sugita, M., K. Sugita, T. Furukawa, and H. Abe, Studies on the transport mechanism of amino acids in the renal tubules. Part I. Studies on the mechanism of amino-aciduria from the analytical standpoint of titration curve, *Japanese Circ. J.* **31**:405 (1967).

231. Surdin, Y., W. Sly, J. Sire, A. M. Bordes, and H. deRobichon–Suzlmajester, Pro-priétés et contrôle génétique du système d'accumulation des acides amines chez *Saccharomyces cerevisiae*, *Biochim. Biophys. Acta* **107**:546 (1965).

232. Tada, K., T. Morikawa, T. Ando, T. Yoshida, and A. Miragawa, Prolinuria: A new renal tubular defect in transport of proline and glycine, *Tohoku J. Expt. Med.* **87**:133 (1965).

233. Tada, K., T. Morikawa, and T. Arakawa, Prolinuria: Transport of proline by leukocytes, *Tohoku J. Expt. Med.* **90**:189 (1966).

233a. Tada, K., T. Morikawa, and T. Arakawa, Tryptophan load and uptake of tryptophan by leukocytes in Hartnup disease, *Tohoku J. Exp. Med.* **90**:337 (1966).

234. Tanaka, S., and E. C. C. Lin, Two classes of pleiotrophic mutants of *Aerobacter aerogenes* lacking components of a phosphoenolpyruvate-dependent phospho-transferase system, *Proc. Natl. Acad. Sci. U.S.* **57**:913 (1967).

235. Thier, S. O., A. Blair, M. Fox, and S. Segal, The effect of extracellular sodium concentration on the kinetics of $\alpha$-aminoisobutyric acid transport in the rat-kidney cortex slice, *Biochim. Biophys. Acta* **135**:300 (1967).

236. Thier, S., M. Fox, and S. Segal, Cystinuria: *In vitro* demonstration of an intestinal transport defect, *Science* **143**:482 (1964).

237. Thier, S. O., S. Segal, M. Fox, A. Blair, and L. E. Rosenberg, Cystinuria: Defective intestinal transport of dibasic amino acids and cystine, *J. Clin. Invest.* **44**:442 (1965).

238. Treacher, R. J., The aminoaciduria of canine cystine-stone disease, *Res. Vet. Sci.* **4**:556 (1963).

239. Treacher, R. J., The aetiology of canine cystinuria, *Biochem. J.* **90**:494 (1964).

240. Treacher, R. J., Quantitative studies on the excretion of the basic amino acids in canine cystinuria, *Brit. Vet. J.* **120**:178 (1964).

241. Tristam, H., and S. Neale, The activity and specificity of proline permease in wild type and analog resistant strains of *Escherichia coli*, *J. Gen. Microbiol.* **50**:121 (1968).

242. Van Slyke, D. D., and G. M. Meyer, The absorption of amino acids from the blood by the tissues, *J. Biol. Chem.* **16**:197 (1913).

243. Webber, W. A., Interactions of neutral and acidic amino acids in renal tubular transport, *Amer. J. Physiol.* **202**:577 (1962).

244. Webber, W. A., Characteristics of acidic amino acid transport in mammalian kidney, *Canad. J. Biochem. Physiol.* **41**:131 (1963).

245. Webber, W. A., Renal tubular reabsorption of α-aminoisobutyric acid, *Canad. J. Physiol. Pharmacol.* **44**:507 (1966).

246. Webber, W. A., Amino acid excretion patterns in developing rats, *Canad. J. Physiol. Pharmacol.* **45**:867 (1967).

246a. Webber, W. A., A comparison of the efflux rates of AIB from kidney cortex slices of mature and newborn rats, *Canad. J. Physiol. Pharmacol.* **46**:765 (1968).

247. Webber, W. A., J. L. Brown, R. F. Pitts, and J. L. Klein, Interactions of amino acids in renal tubular transport, *Amer. J. Physiol.* **200**:380 (1961).

248. Webber, W. A., and J. A. Cairns, A comparison of the amino acid concentrating ability of the kidney cortex of newborn and mature rats, *Canad. J. Physiol. Pharmacol.* **46**:165 (1968).

249. Whelan, D. T., and C. R. Scriver, Cystathioninuria and renal iminoglycinuria in a pedigree. A perspective on counseling, *New Eng. J. Med.* **278**:924 (1968).

250. Whelan, D. T., and C. R. Scriver, Hyperdibasicaminoaciduria: An inherited disorder of amino acid transport, *Ped. Res.* **2**:523 (1968).

251. White, E. G., R. J. Treacher, and P. Porter, Urinary calculi in the dog. I. Incidence and chemical composition, *J. Comp. Path. Ther.* **71**:201 (1961).

252. Williams, T. F., R. W. Winters, and C. H. Burnett, Familial (hereditary) vitamin D-resistant rickets with hypophosphatemia, *in*: The Metabolic Basis of Inherited Disease, 2nd ed., J. B. Stanbury, J. B. Wyngaarden, and D. S. Fredrickson, eds., McGraw-Hill, New York (1966), p. 1179.

253. Wilson, O. H., Amino acid transport in proline auxotrophs of *E. coli*, PhD Thesis, McGill University, 1966.

254. Wilson, O. H., and C. R. Scriver, Specificity of transport of neutral and basic amino acids in rat kidney, *Amer. J. Physiol.* **213**:185 (1967).

255. Wilson, T. H., Intestinal Absorption, Philadelphia, Saunders (1962), Chapt. 5, pp. 110.

256. Wilson, T. H., and E. C. C. Lin, Active transport by intestines of fetal and newborn rabbits, *Amer. J. Physiol.* **199**:1030 (1960).

257. Winter, C. G., and H. N. Christensen, Migration of amino acids across the membrane of the human erythrocyte, *J. Biol. Chem.* **239**:872 (1964).

258. Woodward, C. K., C. P. Read, and V. W. Woodward, *Neurospora* mutants defective in their transport of amino acids, *Genetics* **56**:598 (1967).

259. Woolf, L. I., B. L. Goodwin, and C. E. Phelps, $T_m$-Limited renal tubular reabsorption and the genetics of renal glucosuria, *J. Theoret. Biol.* **11**:10 (1966).

260. Wurtman, R. J., C. M. Rose, C. Chou, and F. F. Larin, Daily rhythms in the concentrations of various amino acids in human plasma, *New Eng. J. Med.* **279**:171 (1968).

261. Yeh, H. L., W. Frankl, M. S. Dunn, P. Parker, B. Hughes, and P. Gyorgy, The urinary excretion of amino acids by a cystinuric subject, *Amer. J. Med. Sci.* **214**:507 (1947).
262. Zarkowsky, H. S., F. A. Oski, R. Sha'afi, S. B. Shohet, and D. G. Nathan, Congenital hemolytic anemia with high-sodium, low-potassium red cells. I. Studies of membrane permeability, *New Eng. J. Med.* **278**:573 (1968).

*Chapter 5*

# Genetics of Disorders of Intestinal Digestion and Absorption

Jean Frézal
and Jean Rey

*Unité de Recherches de Génétique Médicale*
*Hôpital des Enfants Malades*
*Paris 15, France*

## INTRODUCTION

In this review we shall deal with the problems of intestinal absorption, taken in a broad sense, and its disorders. These problems will be considered according to the location of the primary disturbance, i.e., the pancreas or the gut, and to the nutrients which are affected, leading either to generalized or to specific malabsorptions.

The miscellaneous diseases which are emphasized here could also have been grouped from a pathogenetic point of view under different headings: (1) The first group would provide good examples of inborn errors of metabolims in Garrod's sense, such as isolated lipase or trypsinogen deficiency, sucrose and isomaltose intolerance, and, at least in part, lactose intolerance. In such cases the disturbances are due to missing enzymatic activities. (2) In the next group, which is probably rather close to the first one, would be included the two varieties of failure of chylomicron formation which are due to defects of synthesis or to abnormal structures of the B-proteins (the apoprotein which binds lipids to form $\beta$-lipoproteins). (3) The third group would be concerned with abnormalities of mediated transport across the intestinal cell membrane. In many respects this process is reminiscent of an enzyme-catalyzed reaction, and it is no surprise if such processes appear to be under genetic control, as is suggested by the examples already known. Still to be discovered are the precise underlying defect in these cases and the phase of the process which is affected—the binding with the membrane or the carrier transfer through the lipoprotein layers. In any case, one can be sure that consideration of these diseases will give further insight into the problem, particularly into the chemical specificities involved. (4) Cystic fibrosis of the pancreas would constitute by itself our fourth group. It is an hereditary disease, the pathogenesis of which is still obscure. (5) In the preceding groups the genetic mechanism and the mode of inheritance are, as a rule, clearly defined. In a final group we would include celiac disease and milk protein intolerance, in which genetic factors have been suspected, although their intervention has not been conclusively proved. Furthermore, their pathogenesis remains controversial; enzymatic and immunologic disturbances have been evoked. From this point of view, it has seemed relevant to discuss the problems of malabsorption and immunologic deficiencies.

Although this tentative classification might have appeared a more logical scheme, for the sake of convenience we shall consider successively the pancreatic enzyme deficiencies, the malabsorption syndromes, the failures of chylomicron formation, the disturbances in sugar hydrolysis and transfer, the disorders of amino acid transport and, finally, miscellaneous diseases.

## PANCREATIC ENZYME DEFICIENCIES

### Cystic Fibrosis of the Pancreas

Cystic fibrosis of the pancreas (CF) was described by Fanconi et al.[94] in 1936 and recognized as a distinct entity by Andersen[5] in 1938. The eponym "mucoviscidosis" was coined after the suggestion made by Farber[95] that excessive viscosity of mucous secretions was responsible for the manifestations of the disease. However, this hypothesis was no longer tenable after di Sant'Agnese et al.[280] demonstrated that the electrolyte content of sweat and saliva was abnormal, a finding which clearly suggested that CF is indeed a generalized disease of exocrine glands.

### Natural History

In 10–20 % of cases CF is manifested at birth by meconium ileus, which is lethal in a high proportion of cases.[87,140] In most cases the affected children are referred to physicians for failure to thrive, chronic diarrhea, and respiratory disturbances, the severity of which is variable from patient to patient.[200,281,299] Many other symptoms may complicate the clinical picture and sometimes be the presenting complaint; e.g., sinusitis, nasal polyps, rectal prolapse.[21,302] Cirrhosis of the liver is not uncommon, and CF represents one of the main causes of hepatic cirrhosis in childhood.[62,188,282] The evolution and prognosis are dependent in the first place on bronchopulmonary involvement, and, in severe cases, the patients still succumb in the first years of life. Therapeutic advances, notably antibiotics and physical therapy, as well as fat-restricted diet and replacement of pancreatic enzymes, have led to general improvement of the prognosis and extended the expectancy of life.[85]

TABLE I. Age at Diagnosis in 85 Cases of Cystic Fibrosis
Diagnosed in 1963, and in 65 Cases over the Age of 17 Years[a]

| Age at diagnosis, years | Patients seen in 1963, % | Patients over 17 years, % |
|---|---|---|
| Less than 1 | 50 | 12 |
| 1–3 | 24 | 15 |
| 4–9 | 20 | 25 |
| 10–20 | 5 | 43 |
| Over 21 | 1 | 5 |

[a] After Shwachman et al.[304]

However, one wonders if the upward shift of the age distribution is not—at the present time—essentially due to a better knowledge of the several aspects of the disease and of a better recognition of its minor forms. For instance, Shwachman et al.[304] reported 74 patients over the age of 17 years, with a mean age slightly over 20 $\frac{1}{2}$ years for the entire group; the condition of patients is said to be good in about 40 %, and, seven are married. It is pertinent to notice that the diagnosis was made in the first year of life in only eight of these patients, and that approximately half the patients were diagnosed at over 10 years of age (Table I).

## Pancreatic Insufficiency

Pancreatic insufficiency is the consequence of an anatomical lesion of the exocrine gland. It is inconstant in the first years of life, but follows a progressive course.[281,300] Pancreatic insufficiency can be displayed by enzymatic assays of the duodenal juice obtained after intubation. As a rule, they demonstrate a gross reduction of all activities, i.e., lipase, amylase, and proteolytic enzymes. Enzymatic activities have also been measured in slices of pancreatic tissue, with essentially the same results.

Lipase deficiency results, by a disturbance of fat digestion, in massive steatorrhoea, which amounts to 40–80 % of ingested fats. Fat excretion remains roughly proportional to intake, as in most cases of malabsorption syndromes, so that the amount of absorbed lipids is increased as the diet has a higher fat content (personal data). For the most part, the fecal lipids consist of free fatty acids. The pattern of excreted fatty acids is closely similar to that of the ingested fats. These findings prove that a secondary and additional defect of intestinal absorption does not contribute to steatorrhea, but that the triglycerides are hydrolyzed—likely by bacterial action—too far in their way through the small intestine for absorption to take place.[96,253] Steatorrhea disappears when "natural" long-chain triglycerides are replaced by medium-chain triglycerides (MCT)[174] which are hydrolyzed preferentially by residual pancreatic lipase and which can, in its absence, enter the intestinal cells, where they undergo hydrolysis under the action of a lysosomal lipase, an enzyme which has a high affinity for MCT.[244] From a practical point of view, the usefulness of such a replacement remains very questionable; besides the problems raised by the cost of MCT, they are often accepted only reluctantly by patients, due to their bad taste; they can induce ketosis when administered in high doses; finally, the same results can be achieved more conveniently by the prescription of a low-fat diet.

As a consequence of proteolytic enzyme deficiency, fecal nitrogen is increased and can account for more than 50% of the ingested nitrogen. However, the rate of absorbed nitrogen remains sufficient in most cases to assure satisfactory nitrogen retention. In breast-fed infants with a low protein supply, or in infants fed with a soya preparation with a low nitrogen absorption coefficient (about 20% in CF), the amount of absorbed nitrogen becomes the limiting factor which can lead to hypoproteinemia.[98] In these cases pancreatic enzyme replacement therapy has the best indication, as this lowers the fecal nitrogen and makes the nitrogen balance positive.[99] The low-fat diet gives quite similar results, although, in current circumstances, the increase in nitrogen absorption is balanced by urinary losses, so that nitrogen retention, which depends in the first place on the respiratory state, remains unchanged (personal data).

Starch hydrolysis is grossly impaired. However, no fermentation occurs, since the polysaccharide molecules are not "digested" by intestinal bacteria. Tolerance curves with glucose, xylose, sucrose, and lactose are normal.

## Electrolyte Concentrations and Abnormalities in Biological Fluids

The sweat abnormality consists of marked increases in sodium and chloride concentrations, which are present in almost all cases. The rate of sweating and the response to most stimuli are normal. This abnormality is found from birth and persists throughout life. It is unrelated to the severity and clinical aspects of the disease. Therefore, electrolyte (chloride) determination provides the most consistent clue for the diagnosis.[91,281,301]

Several techniques are available for sweat collection. The most convenient method in use consists of collecting it on a gauze pad or filter paper covered with a plastic square and sealed at the edges, placed on a small area of back or forearm skin, after intradermic injection of a parasympatheticomimetic agent or after iontophoresis of pilocarpine.[117] A method for sodium determination by application of a glass electrode upon the skin has also been devised.[120] "General" sweating, as obtained, for instance, by wrapping the patient in a plastic bag, is most dangerous and can result in death by hyperthermia.

Among patients, sweat chloride concentration ranges between 50 and 120 mEq/liter, whereas in controls it is almost always under 40. Although the variations are quite large, there is minimal overlap.[284] However, cases of CF with normal concentration of chloride in sweat have been reported.[112,211] The concentration is not, or is only slightly, modified by aldosterone or 9-α-fluorohydrocortisone, in contrast to the findings in patients with adrenal insufficiency.[124,199,306] Secretion of adrenal hormones and excretion of their metabolites are normal.[55] Potassium concentration is somewhat increased; other solutes are normal.[57,111]

The concentrations of chloride and sodium are also increased in mixed saliva. However, due to the large variation and overlap, the differences between patients and controls are not so definite. From analysis of separate parotid and submaxillary saliva, and despite some contradictory results, it can be concluded that sodium and chloride concentrations are increased in both.[21,51,53,207,208] The concentration of electrolytes appears to be normal in body fluids other than sweat and saliva. Sodium and potassium levels are raised in hair and nails.[168]

Indirect evidence gained from the measurement of sweat urea concentration, and computation by extrapolation of the quantity of reabsorbed sodium, suggest that neither excessive reabsorption of water, nor insufficient sodium reabsorption would account for the high sodium concentration in sweat; this abnormality must be due to a disturbance of the secretion of precursor solution by the coil of the gland.[53,119,197]

Direct analysis by cryoscopy demonstrates that the fluid in the coil is isotonic or even hypertonic, and no difference can be demonstrated between patients and controls.[41,309] Confirmation of these results has been obtained by determination of osmolarities in samples withdrawn directly from sweat gland coils by micropuncture.[288] The precursor solution is slightly hypertonic in both patients and controls. It seems that the disturbance must affect the sweat duct. However, it cannot be said exactly where the disturbance is located or what its precise nature is. The microscopic appearance and electron-microscopic structure of the sweat glands are normal.[223] Therefore, the defect must be a functional one. It does not result from excessive water reabsorption, which has been calculated to be markedly decreased.[46,92] It is more likely due to a defective sodium reabsorption, which may be reduced to 60–75 % of its normal value.[92] This defective sodium reabsorption seems to result from a disturbance of passive diffusion rather than of active sodium transport.[122,284]

As a matter of fact, no abnormality has been found among the several enzymatic activities which have been examined by histochemical or biochemical techniques on frozen dried slices of sweat glands, e.g., acid and alkaline phosphatases, dehydrogenases, and ouabain-sensitive ATPase.[113-116]

## Glycoprotein Abnormalities

Hyperviscosity of mucous secretions is a striking feature of cystic fibrosis. Since 1957 several attempts have been made to investigate systematically the composition of the carbohydrate moiety of glycoproteins.

First of all, di Sant'Agnese et al.[283] showed that after treatment with ethanol benzene a precipitate insoluble in water is found in the duodenal juice of almost all patients. Later it was shown that the ratio of fucose to sialic acid was higher in this insoluble fraction than in other fractions of the same sample of duodenal juice, a phenomenon which could account for the excessive viscosity of the secretion by an increase of molecular size and decreased solubility.[79]

Consistent results have been obtained independently, and similar ratios with increased fucose and decreased sialic acid have been found in sweat, submaxillary saliva, tracheobronchial secretions, rectal mucus (normal sialic acid), meconium, and urine.[52,80,155,209,233,258] Contradictory data have been published by others.[24,156,207,246]

Postulating the occurrence of an abnormal glycoprotein, immunochemical techniques have been devised in an attempt to find out some differences between the antigenic determinants of this glycoprotein and its normal counterpart. Until now such differences have not been convincingly proved,[284,318] although sometimes claimed.[202]

More recently, interesting work has been performed on the influence of ion concentrations—notably calcium. The work began from the observation that submaxillary saliva from patients is turbid, with a higher content of calcium, total proteins, and glycoproteins than that of controls, and that parasympatheticomimetic stimulation in normal children induces an appearance and composition of the saliva similar to that found in the patients.[51] Further investigation of this phenomenon led to finding that the pattern of glycoproteins after electrophoresis on polyacrylamide gel is different in patients and controls, but that it is possible to transform the pattern of the latter to a pattern similar to that of the former simply by increasing calcium concentration in controls to levels found in CF. Having found no immunological differences, the authors concluded that "the saliva of patients and controls contain probably identical glycoproteins that combine or polymerize with calcium present in high concentration to form a reversible precipitate of high molecular weight."[131]

This work gives a first insight into the possible relationship between the electrolyte abnormalities and the mucous abnormalities. For many years a malfunction of the autonomic nervous system has been postulated to have a role in the genesis of the cystic fibrosis. Although some suggestive evidence has been obtained, the matter remains open to discussion.[51,54,81,256]

Another fascinating observation which is difficult to reconcile with the preceding one concerns the effect of sera of patients on human and animal respiratory tract epithelium in tissue culture: the induction, after 10–15 min of exposure, of a kind of asymmetrical or jerky ciliary beat. This effect was consistently found with serum from 50 patients, but never with serum from 50 controls. The fraction responsible for the phenomenon was found to reside in the euglobulin fraction of the serum, in the $19S$ macroglobulins. Interestingly enough, the euglobulin fractions from 25 parents—but not the whole serum—also altered the ciliary activity. Only one of 25 control sera produced the same phenomenon.[314]

## Genetics

**Incidence.** CF appears to be the most frequent lethal hereditary disease among white children, as was pointed out in early estimates based on autopsy records and examination of hospital files. However, these methods were too indirect to give accurate results, as stressed by Steinberg and Brown[316] and Danks et al.[71] The high figure of Goodman and Reed (0.7–1/1000)[121] has also been discussed by Steinberg and Brown.[316] New and more reliable estimates have come in the last few years from retrospective population studies (see Table II). An alternative method of deriving incidence figure

TABLE II.   Incidence of Cystic Fibrosis of Pancreas in Various Series

| Author | Location | Incidence per live births |
|---|---|---|
| Baumann[25] | Switzerland (Arrau) | 1/1400 |
| Steinberg and Brown[316] | USA (Ohio) | 1/3700 |
| Selander[292] | Sweden | 1/8000 |
| Kramm et al.[170] | USA (Massachusetts) | 1/2400 |
| Simankova et al.[307] | Czechoslovakia | 1/2600 |
| Merritt et al.[216] | USA (Indiana) | 1/1900 |
| Danks et al.[71] | Australia | 1/2000–1/2500 |
| Pickup and Pugh[a] | Britain (Yorkshire) | 1/2900 |
| Carter and Watson[a] | Britain | 1/3000 |
| Kramm[b] | USA (South) | 1/3400 |

[a] Cited by Carter.[49]
[b] Cited by di Sant'Agnese and Talamo.[284]

is to ascertain the proportion of affected individuals found among first cousins of index cases. Assuming no consanguinity in the relevant unions, the gene frequency, i.e., the square root of incidence, is simply $q = 4 \times$ proportion of first cousins affected.[317] This approach has been used by Danks et al.,[71] who found consistent results from it and the direct counting method. From the currently available data it seems that 1/2000 is a conservative and acceptable figure in a population of Caucasian extraction with a frequency of heterozygotes of the order of 1/25. A very remarkable exception is provided by Selander's estimate,[292] which is considerably lower. Regional variations in the incidence of the disease have also been found by Kramm et al.[170] within the United States. In addition, the rarity of the disease among Negro and Oriental populations has been pointed out.

**Mechanism of Inheritance.**   CF is a recessive disease, and the proportion of cases in the sibships of index cases has been seen not to differ from the expected proportion of 0.25 when proper methods of analysis are applied, taking into account the mode of ascertainment. For instance, using the method of quasimaximum of likelihood, after Bailey,[20] and assuming multiple incomplete ascertainment, we found an estimate of $p = 0.20 \pm 0.05$ for proved cases and $p = 0.28 \pm 0.05$ for proved and likely cases. Assuming the same kind of ascertainment, Danks et al.[71] gave an estimate of $p = 0.243 \pm 0.016$. By the proband method and supposing incomplete single ascertainment, Steinberg et al.[316] found $p = 0.24 \pm 0.03$.

Finally, Crow[67] has analyzed Lobeck's data by Morton's segregation ratio-method; again, his estimate is very close to 0.25 ($p = 0.2485 \pm 0.05$); furthermore, he pointed out that there is no evidence for sporadic cases according to Morton's terminology (mutations, phenocopies, etc,...). On the other hand, other authors claimed that the proportion of affected cases in families was too high to be consistent with the recessive hypothesis.[25,257] It seems likely that these conclusions were drawn from improper use of methods and miscalculations, as stressed by Steinberg and Brown[316] and by Bulmer.[42]

Considering the protean aspects of the disease and the possibility of intrafamilial correlations in symptomatology, the hypothesis has been put forward that CF could be genetically heterogeneous, depending either on a system of multiple alleles at the same locus, or on genes at different loci. Such hypothesis remains difficult to prove or to exclude, the phenotypic expression representing, in all likelihood, a remote consequence of the primary effect of the gene(s). However, two arguments point against such a hypothesis from a formal point of view. In the first place, the consanguinity rates which have been recorded are quite low, as could be expected from a common condition, and in contrast what should be found if CF were indeed a heterogeneous group of rarer diseases. Furthermore, the incidence of the disease among the first cousins of the index cases gives no indication for more than one locus.[61,67] However, as there is considerable uncertainty in incidence figures, and until better data are available, the question must remain open.

**Heterozygote Detection.** Di Sant'Agnese *et al.*[280] demonstrated that a significant number of relatives of patients had excessive sweat chloride values, although not as high as in the patients themselves. This observation has been repeatedly confirmed and the conclusion drawn that the mean of a group of (heterozygous) parents or of sibs differs significantly from the mean of controls, although there is a considerable overlapping of the distributions. However, it must be noticed that the increased electrolyte level observed in some of them after stimulation of sweating by heat[161,310] has not been found to be reproducible by "local" techniques.[7,120,198,211,228] These discrepancies are due in part to the differences in the rates of sweating obtained by different methods. They are also explained by the fact that the chloride content is higher in the adult than in the child, and that this has not always been taken into account in comparing results. Better discrimination should be achieved by sets of four simultaneous sweat chloride tests, according to Sproul and Huang,[315] who devised discriminant functions between parents and controls (children or adults).

It has been suggested that carriers of the CF gene were more susceptible to various acquired diseases, particularly of the respiratory and the gastrointestinal tracts.[9,132,228,307] This has not been confirmed by careful studies. Furthermore, while some authors have found a higher sweat electrolyte level among adults suffering from chronic bronchopulmonary conditions, diabetes, or allergy, many have not found any significant differences. Even if such a difference should exist—which the present authors are reluctant to admit— it could not necessarily be inferred that the individuals concerned are heterozygous for the CF gene; to reach such a conclusion, it would still have to be proved that the character—excessive chloride content in the sweat—behaves in a Mendelian way and that there exists a relationship between its appearance and the occurrence of CF in the families concerned.

**Heterozygote Advantage.** The high frequency of CF in Caucasians has been attributed to a very high mutational rate or to a selective advantage of heterozygotes. The first hypothesis was favored by Goodman and Reed.[121] However, beside the very unusual value of the mutation rate required to assure equilibrium, on the order of 1/2500 per gene per generation, that is, at least 40 times the more commonly accepted values, this hypothesis leaves no explanation for the implied difference in mutation rates among populations, e.g., among Negroes or Orientals and Whites.

On the other hand, a selective advantage of heterozygotes which could maintain the incidence of the disease at its actual level through generations remains difficult to prove. It is worthwhile to notice that the magnitude of this advantage would need to be only about 2 %. Two studies have been devoted to this question. Danks et al.[71] have compared against three different control groups the size of families of grandparents of cases of the disease. They found considerable variations among the control group. However, in all the comparisons made, the CF grandparents had the larger families. Consistent results have been observed by Knudson et al.[166] The difference was still significant among survivors despite a higher infant mortality in the cystic fibrosis group.

These results must be considered with considerable caution and great reservation about their biological significance. As a matter of fact, the magnitude of the heterozygote advantage apparently shown in these studies is very much greater than would be needed to maintain the gene at the same frequency. Indeed, if the calculated advantage is real and still operating, the necessary conclusion—a very hazardous one—would be that the gene frequency will continue to rise.

### Congenital Hypoplasia of the Exocrine Pancreas

Congenital hypoplasia of the exocrine pancreas, which is also referred to as "lipomatosis of the pancreas," is an anatomical lesion which was first observed at post-mortem examination of adults. Cases were subsequently reported in children and presumed—soundly, in our opinion—to be congenital in origin.[33,225]

Clinical features are strikingly reminiscent of CF, but this diagnosis can be excluded by the normal electrolyte content of sweat. The first manifestations appear in the neonatal period or in infancy. They consist of failure to thrive and diarrhea, which can be attributed, based on biochemical studies, to exocrine pancreatic deficiency. Respiratory infections are not uncommon. These children experience episodes of pneumonia, but very rarely any of the residual emphysema which is so characteristic of CF. Final diagnosis requires histological examination of the pancreas. Unfortunately, the biopsy is hardly justified for the patient's sake. On gross examination, the pancreas is of yellow, fatty appearance. On section, the pancreas consists mainly of fat in which there are several isolated, but normal, islets of Langerhans and clumps of small ducts. Scattered clusters of acini can be sometimes observed. The liver shows a focal steatosis, fibrosis, and cellular infiltration.

The significance of the association of hematological abnormalities has been stressed by Shwachman et al.[303] The clinical onset of these hematological changes may sometimes date from birth, or they may appear later in life. They are of varying severity and consist, in the first place, of a more or less pronounced neutropenia. In most cases, neutropenia is associated with hypoplastic anemia. Thrombocytopenia is less common. These abnormalities of the peripheral blood are correlated with hypocellularity of the bone marrow affecting one or all of the stem lines.

It remains difficult to assess the true frequency of the occurence of the hematological disturbances among the cases of congenital hypoplasia of the exocrine pancreas, and so to state whether this association constitutes a genuine and discrete entity.[153,222] It is worthy of note that Ozsoylu and Argun[231] found a significant decrease in tryptic activity of the duodenal juice in five out of six patients with aplastic anemia. This finding needs confirmation.

Another curious association has been mentioned by Burke et al.[45] In three of their cases they observed irregular areas of varying density of long bones, consistent with the radiological diagnosis of metaphysial dysostosis. These associated features are of interest in relation to the description of the so-called cartilage-hair hypoplasia syndrome (CHHS) by McKusick et al.[212] They claimed that some of their patients experienced diarrhea, supposed, but not convincingly proved, to be due to malabsorption. Furthermore, it must be borne in mind that it is by no means certain that the topographical distribution of the bone lesions is similar in CHHS and in Burke's cases. Here again, the precise classification of these cases, in relationship to hypoplasia of the exocrine pancreas on one hand, and to the several forms of metaphysial dysostosis in the other, has to await further, thoroughly planned investigations of patients, including examinations of digestive and hematological functions, and X-ray examination of the entire skeleton.

In the present, unsettled state of the matter, it seems difficult to put forward any hypothesis about the etiology of hypoplasia of the exocrine pancreas. One can just mention that three families have been described with several affected sibs [two by Lumb and Beautyman (cited by Bodian et al.[33]), three in a sibship of five by Shwachman et al.[303] and three in a sibship of four by Burke et al.[45]], a significant finding with regard to the rarity of cases, and suggestive of a recessive trait. However, we favor the idea that the hypoplasias of the exocrine pancreas with or without associated features form a clinically, and probably etiologically, heterogeneous group.

### Lipase Deficiency

Pancreatic lipase deficiency is a very rare condition; six cases have been published.[251,296] The clinical onset may date from birth, or the digestive disturbances may appear later (see below) The unique symptom is a chronic diarrhea of a very particular kind. The stools are bulky, but not so frequent— once or twice a day. They contain a great amount of fat, which segregates from the solid part of the feces. The patients are handicapped by soiling their clothes with this liquid oil, which they are unable to restrain. Otherwise, growth is satisfactory, the abdomen is not enlarged, the hair and skin are not altered as in the malabsorption syndromes. Finally, there is no anemia, no vitamin (folic acid) deficiency, no osteoporosis, and no hypoproteinemia.

Steatorrhea amounts to 50–80 % of ingested fats. The increase of neutral fats and the pattern of fatty acids in the stools are suggestive of a disturbance of hydrolysis of fats as in CF. Analysis of duodenal juice confirms this point; lipase activity is as low as 10 % of normal, and does not increase after stimulation, whereas amylase and trypsin activities are only a little below the normal values. Digestion of proteins, estimated by nitrogen balance, and digestion of starch appear to be normal. Furthermore, the pancreas was normal at histologic examination in the one case so studied.

Oral administration of a lipase preparation noticeably improves the fat absorption, although it does not restore it to normal. Therefore, dietary restriction of fat intake remains necessary in order to control the diarrhea. Medium-chain triglycerides (MCT) also normalize fat absorption, a finding which demonstrates that lysosomal lipase of intestinal cells is different from pancreatic lipase. The practical use of MCT requires the same reservations as in CF.

The fact that both children of the two families studied by Sheldon[296] were affected suggests an inherited factor, and, according to Carter, the condition is probably due to an autosomal recessive gene. However, it is interesting to note that a similar clinical picture, with deficiency of pancreatic lipase, developed as a temporary phenomenon following an attack of chickenpox in a further case also described by Sheldon. In our case the clinical onset was retarded until the patient was three years old; however, the lipase deficiency persists unchanged at 12 years, so that we are prone to think that this case is more like the persistent cases of Sheldon[296] than his further case.

From a clinical point of view, deficiency of bile salts reported in one case by Ross et al.[267] appears indistinguishable from lipase deficiency.

### Trypsinogen Deficiency

Three cases (two males, one female) of trypsinogen deficiency disease have been reported so far, in unrelated children.[221,322,323] The symptomatology exhibited a striking parallelism in the three patients. They presented in the first months of life with severe failure to thrive hypoproteinemic edema and hypochromic anemia, sparse hair, and no evidence either of hepatic or renal disease or of protein-losing gastroenteropathy (serum albumin half-life and albumin loss in stool were normal, as was the PVP [131]I test). The anemia is due to protein as well as to iron deficiency. It was associated in one case with neutropenia, which is of interest with regard to the problem discussed with hypoplasia of the exocrine pancreas. Hypocalcemia was also manifest.

Nitrogen-balance studies provided evidence for an impaired capacity to hydrolyze proteins, for they indicated that 60 % of the nitrogen ingested as intact casein was excreted in the stools, whereas only 18 % was excreted when the nitrogen was ingested as a hydrolysate.

Fat absorption was normal in two cases, but impaired, curiously enough, in the other. Since the fat malabsorption was corrected in parallel with the general improvement during treatment, it was presumed to have been secondary to the prolonged malnutrition. No data are available on the lipase activity of the duodenal juice in this case.

All symptoms were dramatically corrected within some weeks by dietary administration of protein hydrolysate. Body weight increased strikingly, and the growth response was of the impressive catch-up type observed, for instance, in treated malabsorption syndromes.

Specific assays performed on duodenal juice demonstrate that lipase and amylase activities were in the normal range in two cases. In none of the three patients was there proteolytic activity, i.e., no trypsin, chymotrypsin, or carboxypeptidase. Addition of a trace amount of trypsin activates chymotrypsinogen and procarboxypeptidase in a normal fashion.

In contrast, added trypsin does not result in activation of trypsinogen. Therefore, the apparent total lack of trypsin activity seems truly due to defective synthesis of trypsinogen rather than to lack of enterokinase.

However Hadorn *et al.*[131a,245a] have demonstrated in two apparently similar cases that lack of activity of proteolytic enzymes was not the consequence of trypsinogen deficiency but of enterokinase deficiency in the duodenal juice and mucosa.

Distribution of cases in reported families is suggestive of recessive inheritance.

### Amylase Deficiency

Amylase deficiency has been observed in the duodenal juice of a thirteen-year-old boy by Lowe and May.[201] The trypsin activity was very much reduced. Lipase activity was normal. So far no similar case has been reported. If we consider that amylase activity is the most sensitive to variation in pH, followed by trypsin activity, the reality of the defect remains questionable and needs confirmation.

## MALABSORPTION SYNDROMES

### Celiac Disease

The main features of the celiac affections were described by Gee.[108a] Since then a better knowledge has been gained of the clinical variants, and

many advances have been achieved concerning the biochemical and pathological aspects of the disease. Finally, the etiology of the symptoms has been
clarified. Celiac disease appears as a precise and discrete entity characterized
by malabsorption, atrophy of the villi, infiltration, and epithelial cell damage;
a clinical, biochemical, and histological response to gluten-free diet; and
relapse when the diet is relaxed, demonstrating that the gluten itself can induce
mucosal damage.

Celiac disease is a rather uncommon disease with a familial tendency. It
is presumed to be due to an underlying constitutional defect which has not
yet been unveiled. It is also referred to as gluten-induced enteropathy,
nontropical sprue, idiopathic sprue, or celiac sprue.

## Natural History

The symptoms have an insidious onset, appearing earlier or later after
the ingestion of cereals. In most cases the clinical disturbances are manifest
in two or three months. Typically, celiacs are fair-haired, pale, miserable-
looking, and depressed children with short stature, muscle wasting, hypotonia, and abdominal distension. Anorexia and vomiting are not infrequent.
Diarrhea is the principal symptom; the stools are bulky, pale, and loose.
Subjects can occasionally be constipated. In some cases digestive disturbances
are not so prominent. The presenting symptoms could be failure to thrive,
severe hypotrophy, or idiopathic hypoproteinemia.[12,180,295,337]

In other cases infancy and childhood are uneventful, or the disturbances
are unremarkable or neglected. Patients which have not been seen or have
not been treated may be referred to a physician in their teens for stunted
growth or delay in sexual development.[101,109] They are often misdiagnosed
for "endocrine disorder," with unfortunate consequences, since no recovery
can be expected from anabolic or sex-hormone therapy.

It seems that celiac disease follows a general pattern: poor health in
childhood, good health in early adult life, and a tendency to relapse between
35 and 55—a period when most adult patients come under care. Here again,
even if the patients are first seen at this time, a careful history can reveal that
the majority of them had symptoms very suggestive of the disease in early
childhood. They complain of asthenia and loss of weight as well as bone
tenderness, and sometimes they develop the classical waddling and sore-
footed gait of osteomalacia. X-rays demonstrate rarefaction of bones. Skin
changes, i.e., desquamation rash or eczema, and recurrent glossitis are
common, as is mild anemia, which is usually hypochromic and only rarely
has megaloblastic features.[28,59,76,152]

Emphasis has been placed on the occurrence of neuropathy, the features
of which suggest subacute combined degeneration of the cord, commencing

with a picture of peripheral neuritis and posterior column disturbance affecting the lower limbs.[60] Although in nearly all patients steatorrhea preceded neurological changes by months or many years, the relationship between steatorrhea and neuropathy was not thought to be explained simply as cause and effect.

In summary, clinical aspects of celiac diseases are numerous, depending on the age at onset, on the intensity of gastrointestinal symptoms, and on the nutritional disturbances.

## Biochemical Features

Steatorrhea is a constant symptom of celiac disease. It is, as a rule, of moderate degree, and 15–20 % of ingested lipids are recovered in the stools. Malabsorption chiefly affects saturated fats. Patients absorb unsaturated fats quite efficiently. They may indeed have a normal coefficient of fat absorption and improve clinically if all of the fat in their diet is unsaturated.[36,180,336] Fat malabsorption causes secundary hypolipemia—blood lipid levels range between 300 and 400 mg %—involving cholesterol, phospholipids, and triglycerides. It is associated with symptoms of essential fatty acid deficiency, evidencing endogenous synthesis, as in all steatorrheas. Vitamin A and carotene levels are low in adult patients, in contrast with children who are given carrots for the symptomatic treatment of diarrhea.[250]

Fecal nitrogen is about twice its normal value. This feature is accounted for, first of all, by a failure of amino acid absorption, as demonstrated by isotopic studies with ingested [131]I albumin or [15]N protein,[63] and secondly by exudative enteropathy, as shown after injection of labeled proteins. All proteins, even intravenous macroglobulin, can be excreted into the intestine. The intestinal loss of proteins can result in a deficiency of serum immunoglobulins when the losses outbalance the capacity of synthesis; in such states, the IgG and IgA levels are lowered more than that of IgM, which has a shorter half-life.[333] However, severe combined IgA and IgM deficiencies, or isolated IgA or IgM deficiencies have been described.[138,226] In contrast, Immonen et al.[148] noticed, on immunoelectrophoresis, an early appearance or accentuation of IgA which, in their opinion, reflects an immunological process taking place in the damaged mucosa.

Sugar malabsorption induces fermentation, with an increase of volatile acids in the stools and lowering of their pH. In some circumstances, during acute phases of the disease or when the lactose intake is excessive, fermentation is more marked and lactic acid is excreted into the stools.[180,342] Fermentation disappears when lactose is withdrawn from the diet, suggesting a superimposed deficiency of its hydrolysis. In contrast, substitution of glucose by α-glucosides results in no change in symptomatology, absorption rate being the limiting factor in this case.[127,128,214] Sugar malabsorption can be confirmed by glucose tolerance test (GTT), xylose test, or 3-o-methylglucose tolerance test. The results of these tests are not always consistent; a normal GTT points strongly against the diagnosis, whereas a flat curve can be occasionally observed in normal subjects. On the other hand, a low xylose excretion favors the diagnosis of malabsorption; however, contrary to others, we have found normal xylose excretion in a few patients with proved malabsorption.

Malabsorption also affects minerals and vitamins. Iron deficiency is common and often refractory. Serum calcium is commonly low, as a consequence of vitamin D deficiency and of binding of calcium by unabsorbed fats. Phosphate is often low, and alkaline phosphatase raised. Vitamin K deficiency results in hypoprothrombinemia and hypoconvertinemia. Folic acid deficiency can be documented either by determination of blood "folic acid" levels or by measure of FIGLU in urine following a loading dose of histidine.[105] Some degree of vitamin $B_{12}$ deficiency is noted in many patients, though this does not necessarily correlate with changes in the ileal mucosa, and the cause of impaired vitamin $B_{12}$ absorption is not always apparent.[76]

Increased urinary excretion of tryptophan metabolites has been found, with large amounts of 5-hydroxy-indoleacetic acid (5-HIAA), indole-3-acetic acid, kynurenine, and xanthurenic acid;[28] contradictory results have also been reported.[59] The abnormal excretion of degradation products after a tryptophan load was corrected with intramuscular vitamin $B_6$. On the other hand, the high indole excretion is probably due to colonic degradation of unabsorbed tryptophan, and is reduced by feeding antibiotics. Finally, the increase in urinary excretion of 5-HIAA is more closely related to excessive 5-hydroxytryptamine production in patients with diarrhea.[76]

## Histopathology

Anatomical changes in untreated celiac disease are constant and characteristic. They usually consist, in their most severe type, of a strictly flat appearance of the intestinal fragment, sometimes divided, under dissecting microscopy, into round or polygonal shapes, in striking contrast to the beautiful slender villi which normally appear.[35] On histological section the mucosa is of normal or reduced width and the surface flattened, with no normal villi present. The epithelial cells undergo severe alterations, and the brush border is reduced in width and sometimes not visible. The lamina propria is infiltrated by inflammatory cells, mainly lymphocytes and plasmocytes. The depth of the Lieberkühn crypts is increased, and the mitotic index is high, suggesting either an increased rate of cell turnover or simply a change in the ratio of immature to mature cells.[47,65,181,269,298,346] On electron microscopy the microvilli are short, sparse, and frequently distorted. Ribonucleoprotein granules are abnormally abundant and cytoplasmic vacuoles are decreased in number. Mitochondria are altered. The basement membrane is often disrupted.[270] Morphologic abnormalities are associated with histochemical changes. Enzymatic deficiencies involve mainly ATPase, 5-nucleotidase, glucose-6-phosphatase, monoamine-oxidase, leucine-amino-peptidase, and lactase. Alkaline phosphatase may also be affected.[158,232,254,279]

In rare cases the lesions of the duodenum and jejunum are milder. Under the dissecting microscope the mucosa displays convoluted ridges or a leaf like pattern. On histological examination the villi are broad, short, and blunted. They tend to fuse together. Infiltration of the lamina propria is noticeable. Alterations of the epithelial cells are not so conspicuous and can be absent. Rubin[270] has stressed that the mild abnormality is very difficult to differentiate from nonspecific abnormalities as observed, for instance, in blind loop syndrome, after neomycin therapy, or in ileojejunitis.

If fragments are taken in several parts of the small intestine, it appears that duodenum and jejunum are most severely and diffusely affected, whereas the lesions can be of a mild degree in the ileum. This difference could be related to the higher exposure to gluten of the proximal part of the gut.[270]

The observed lesions are referred to as villous atrophy, total or subtotal in the severe form, partial in the mild one. Although these expressions are commonly used for convenience, the exact mechanism which leads to the disappearance of the villi is not properly understood, and the term "atrophy" is probably misleading.[273] It has been suggested that the villous shape is plastic and remolds to a more simple and economical shape as adult cells become fewer, and that there are two abnormal patterns of cell turnover associated with the diminution of adult epithelial cells, one analogous with "hemolysis" and the other with hypoplasia.[66] This hypothesis is rather verbal and gives no clue as to the infiltration of the mucosa. It seems very unlikely that the lesions of epithelial cells are simply the consequence of the extension into and encroachment upon the epithelium by the inflammatory cells.[15] Complete loss of a villous pattern with a flat mucosa could result from adhesion between adjacent ridges or from inflammatory cell infiltration and edema within the lamina propria.[286] The generalized decrease observed in enzyme activity would be due to the damaging action of lysosomal enzymes, which may well also account for the breakdown of the cyto-architecture.[254]

## Influence of the Diet

Patients, particularly children, respond dramatically to the complete withdrawal of gluten from the diet. In a few days or a few weeks they enjoy a general improvement, with a profound change in temper, a sensation of better health, and more appetite. Their weight begins to increase. The digestive disturbances progressively disappear. The stools are less bulky and more solid, although they remain somewhat loose for some weeks. The most extraordinary sign of the clinical recovery in childhood is the resumption of growth at a catch-up rate until the patients have reached their normal height. This is a constant feature if therapy is begun at an early age and if patients stick stricktly to the regimen.[110,180,295,337]

Clinical improvement is correlated with biochemical progress. Fecal fat excretion progressively decreases in two or three weeks, but does not completely return to normal until after several months. Nitrogen and volatile acids excretion fall proportionately with the reduction in weight of the stools. Tests of sugar absorption normalize within several weeks. Excretion of 5-HIAA is reduced, while steatorrhea disappears. Calcium absorption increase. However, the bone lesions need months for repair.[28,76,152,180,276,337]

The clinical and biochemical improvement is related to changes in the appearance of the mucosa. The first modification which has been observed in the few cases adequately studied from that point of view consists in a restoration of the height and shape of the epithelial cells within approximately ten days or less.[346] Some enzymatic activities also reappear very quickly (e.g., 5-nucleotidase, leucine aminopeptidase, ATPase), and may be restored in a few days.[158,254,279]

In contrast, the return of villi is not indisputably apparent until the third or fourth month after the start of dietary treatment. At that time the villi are short and broad, with a corresponding convoluted or leaflike pattern seen with the dissecting microscope. Complete repair requires more than one year.[6,15,28,34,181,297,346]

However, for complete appreciation of the anatomoclinical correlations attention must be given not only to the restoration of the functional capacity of the epithelial cells as demonstrated by histochemical studies, but also to the rapid reversibility of distal lesions, which are, as already mentioned, milder.[273]

Is the repair of the mucosal lesions, either complete or incomplete, a constant feature of celiac disease? We are inclined to answer that it surely is, at least in our experience with the disease in children. Persistance of the lesions after one year, with or without clinical disturbances, can be explained either by regular violation of the diet, or by a superimposed secondary intolerance. In the latter event, symptoms subside and the mucosa is repaired with the proper alteration of the diet.[59,180] These factors being excluded, lack of response to gluten-free diet requires that the diagnosis of celiac disease be discarded.

The clinical consequences of the regular ingestion of gluten by patients in complete remission—i.e., with no symptoms, normal tests of absorption, no steatorrhea, and normal appearance of mucosa under light microscope—are diverse. The very first ingestion could exceptionally, produce acute symptoms of intolerance.[4,171,326] In other patients the relapse is rapidly progressive, and in some weeks or months the clinical picture of the disease is complete. However, even in young children, and more often in teenagers, the relaxation from the gluten-free diet does not provoke any apparent digestive disturbance, and one is tempted to conclude that patients gain tolerance to gluten. However, careful examination often demonstrates that in many cases the stools are not entirely normal. Results of biochemical tests are also variable and, although somewhat correlated with the clinical state, they are more sensitive; at least in our experience, it is very rare that the absorption tests are entirely normal, even in asymptomatic subjects, if they regularly ingest wheat cereals.

The point is that in every case histological studies show the reappearance of the mucosal lesions. The mucosal damage can be demonstrated in some cases in the hours following the ingestion of gluten. It is delayed in others, until the seventh day or even later, giving a clear indication of the differences in sensitivity among patients. If the intake is stopped again, as in acute experiments, the lesions are temporary and almost disappear within one to two days.[26,271,272] It is interesting to add that wheat or gliadin, when given as an enema, produces characteristic changes of the rectal mucosa.[242,273]

In our opinion, the certain diagnosis of celiac disease can only be made in patients who first recover with a gluten-free diet, then have histological relapse when they are again put on a normal diet.

Finally, from a practical point of view, an indication of strict dietary control cannot be derived from histological data, but from the long-term effect of normal diet, which is variable, particularly with regard to growth and sexual maturation.

Consideration should perhaps also be given to the possible occurrence of abdominal lymphomas which have been reported in patients with proven celiac disease and which seem to be more than a chance association. This should be suspected when a patient with well-controlled celiac disease develops a relapse or a change in symptomatology.[123,134,186]

## Pathogenesis

The harmful effects of wheat and rye and barley cereals were demonstrated by Dicke, who later, with Weijers and Van de Kamer,[18,326] made clear that toxicity was not due to starch but to gluten, the protein moiety of wheat flour, and, more precisely, to gliadin, which is the alcohol-soluble fraction of the former.

The action of pepsin trypsin, or pancreatic extract does not modify the toxicity of gliadin, but this disappears following digestion with fresh hog intestinal mucosa or complete hydrolysis with HCl.[4,102,172,339] Complete breakage of disulfide bonds by performic acid or bromine also does not affect toxic action, suggesting that the toxic substance is a straight-chain peptide including proline and glutamine.[259] The role of the latter was suspected by Van de Kamer and Weijers,[327] who demonstrated that deamidation with dilute HCl reduces the toxic effect. The same result was observed by Krainick and Mohn[172] using crude papain, which yields $NH_3$. Messer et al.[218] demonstrated that it was not papain by itself which was involved, but another enzyme, glutamine cyclotransferase, which is not endowed with peptidase action but which reacts with N-glutaminyl peptides to form cyclic (pyrrolidone carboxylic) compounds.[219] The latter data suggest that the celiac-active component is an N-glutaminyl-peptide, but they do not imply either that there exists an enzyme similar to glutamine cyclotransferase in the normal intestinal mucosa, or that such an enzyme and a process are operative in gluten digestion.[218] However, cyclic peptides were demonstrated in the course of hydrolysis of gluten by the intestinal mucosa.[32,40]

Many uncertainties remain about the true nature of the toxic peptide. It is worth remarking that the investigations so far have been made on patients in remission, the effects being assessed on clinical and biochemical grounds (abdominal distension, steatorrhea). It is desirable that new methods be devised to provide more and better-defined fractions and to allow one to test more conveniently and accurately either by in vitro or in vivo techniques.[234,272]

One might have guessed that the problem would have been approached by the analysis of plasma changes after a load of gluten.[338] However, such studies give inconsistent results, probably due to the inaccuracy of the methods.[339] In any case, detection of one or several "abnormal" peptides in the blood[130,160,169] would not enable one to make a choice between the two hypotheses currently proposed about the mechanism whereby gliadin exerts its harmful effect, i.e., the toxic and allergic hypotheses. According to the toxic hypothesis, celiac disease would be an inborn error of metabolism with a deficient peptidase, which could account for the presence of an unhydrolyzed peptide in the blood. According to the allergic hypothesis, the disease finds its basis in an immunologic response of the gut to gluten. In this event, it could be supposed that the damaged mucosa provokes the leakage of native or incompletely degraded proteins into the blood stream.

Although the hypothesis of the enzymatic deficiency is most popular at the present time, one must be aware that proof is lacking. Pittman and Pollitt,[243] by means of fingerprint peptide maps, found that, in contrast to normal mucosa, homogenates from celiac patients failed to liberate proline from gliadine peptides. This work does not, however, distinguish primary from secondary peptidase deficiency. The latter hypothesis is suggested in the first place by the demonstration by Van de Kamer[328] that incubation of "nontoxic" dietary proteins with celiac mucosal homogenates gives the same results. Second, if the enzymatic assays are performed on a specimen obtained from a patient on a gluten-free diet with a normal appearing mucosa, no significant difference is found between controls and patients in their ability to hydrolyze a number of peptides.[192,217,275] However, these investigations are still preliminary, and more details may be expected in the future.

Several arguments suggest, on the other hand, that an immunologic mechanism may be involved in the pathogenesis of the disease.[29,103] The first argument is drawn from the possible occurrence of an acute response, named gliadin shock, to ingestion of small quantities of gluten in patients treated with a gluten-free diet.[4,171,326] Another indication is given by the finding that steroid therapy may relieve the symptoms of adult celiac disease.[76,152] Also, an increase of the number of plasma cells has been found in the lamina propria. Immunofluorescence techniques suggest that they are mainly of the IgA-secreting type,[274] but conflicting results have been published.[226] Finally, antibodies to gluten have been demonstrated, by several techniques, in the serum of many, but not all, patients.[1,135,245,268,319] However, although gliadin is bound by epithelial cells of patients, but not by those of controls, neither complement-fixing antigen–antibody complexes nor immunoglobulin aggregates could be identified in the mucosa.[206,274] Moreover, conventional allergic tests (skin tests) are negative.[169] The significance of the antibodies found in the sera of patients deserves discussion. Antigliadin antibodies are directed against the native protein, but not against peptides, which are devoid of antigenic properties, although they still retain the toxicity of gliadin.[2,30] If one considers that it is common to detect other antibodies, such as milk protein antibodies, in the sera of patients, the possibility arises that the antibodies are the consequence of the transfer of undigested proteins through the mucosa. It could be that such antibodies are responsible for secondary intolerances. In short, the allergic hypothesis is not supported by any conclusive arguments. However, the pattern of the restoration of mucosa, which takes months, is suggestive.

## Genetics

There are several studies of celiac disease and nontropical sprue. Most of them, as well as isolated case reports, antedate current concepts of the role of gluten sensitivity. Furthermore, they are based on insufficient evidence, lacking the support of modern biochemical investigations and of histological techniques. Hence, their value is limited. In any case, although they all indicate a familial aggregation of the disease, a Mendelian pattern of inheritance is not apparent.

Davidson and Foutain[73] obtained a history of steatorrhea in a relative in 9.2 % of 130 cases of celiac disease and in 4 % of 75 cases of idiopathic steatorrhea. In her series of 104 patients, Thompson[321] found 15 of 117 sibs and 11 of 189 parents affected. Boyer and Andersen[38] reported that five of 100 parents had the disease. In addition, 29 complained of unexplained recurrent diarrhea. Also, 14 of 59 sibs from 25 patients with severe celiac disease and 25 with mild disease and so-called starch intolerance were affected. In these surveys, it has been claimed that the incidence of diabetes is higher in these families than in the general population. However, due to the pitfalls and bias inherent to such estimations, one is very reluctant to accept a conclusion which has not been confirmed by others. Carter *et al.*[48] studied relatives of clinic patients only taking as positive clinical stories that had been proven elsewhere by fecal fat studies. They estimated the risk in the general population to be about one in 3000. In contrast, five of 205 brothers and sisters, two of 85 fathers, one of 580 aunts and uncles, and one of 806 cousins were definitely affected. However, as no biopsies were performed at the time of the study, they probably missed milder cases. MacDonald *et al.*[205] performed 207 biopsies on 96 relatives of 17 selected cases. Among 62 sibs of index cases (recalculated from the data with the omission of one monozygotic twin), 32 were biopsied, and the specimens of four showed the histologic appearance of celiac. Twelve of 34 parents were biopsied, and none had the lesion. Seventeen of the children of 37 probands were biopsied, and two had the intestinal lesion. Celiac sprue was demonstrated by biopsy in four nieces or nephews of the probands. Five of the affected relatives were virtually asymptomatic, and the four of these, who were tested, had normal fecal fat excretion. In two asymptomatic cases the intestinal mucosa returned to normal with a gluten-free diet. Finally, several other relatives presented nonspecific abnormalities which could be "partial expression of the trait." Anderson[12] briefly mentions that sibs of seven probands and one parent of three others were affected. In our own series only one proven case has been ascertained in the families of 50 patients. In no instance has evidence of consanguinity been mentioned.

The general impression drawn from these studies and from the occurrence of celiac disease in successive generations is that it could be considered as a dominant character with "low penetrance and irregular expressivity." As a matter of fact, such an irregular pattern was not unexpected from a character which is so variable in its manifestation and so strongly influenced by environment. In our opinion, such a familial pattern appears difficult to reconcile with the concept of an inborn error resulting from some unknown enzymatic deficiency, although one cannot exclude it. For instance, clinical manifestation of G-6-P-D deficiency, e.g., favism, are also very irregularly distributed.

At present, it would be unwise to accept the conclusion that celiac disease is primarily related to a single gene effect. Among three pairs of identical twins,[48,139,205] carefully and recently studied, only one has been found to be concordant. In view of what has been said about the compulsory anatomical relapse when patients are again fed gluten, often without any clinical or even biochemical signs, it does not seem very likely that one would observe such a discordancy between MZ twins on a single-gene hypothesis. If genetic factors are at work, they would more probably be multifactorial and constitute at most a predisposition in which additional unknown factors (threshold effect?) determine whether intolerance to gluten develops.

### Milk Protein Intolerance

Cow's milk has long been invoked as an etiologic factor in certain infants and children with digestive disturbances and malabsorption syndromes. However, in very few instances are the cases documented well enough to allow such a conclusion.

### Clinical and Biochemical Features

The onset of symptoms takes place very early, sometimes at the very first ingestion of cow's milk. They consists of diarrhea, enlarged abdomen, and poor growth. Vomiting may be the presenting and prominent symptom. Watery diarrhea is more common than typical celiac steatorrhea, but, as a rule, one finds a large increase of fecal lipids and nitrogen and fermentation as well. Multiple nutritional deficiencies are likely to appear if the condition is allowed to persist. Lesions of intestinal mucosa are ussually milder although, in rare cases, indistinguishable from that of celiac disease.[75,93,104,173,330]

Complete withdrawal of cow's milk from the diet is followed by the disappearance of symptoms, and recovery. Vomiting stops at once, appetite improves, and the patient starts to gain weight. Diarrhea and malabsorption may disappear in a few days if histological lesions were minimal. They subside more slowly when the intestinal lesions were severe, i.e., when they consisted of a total or subtotal atrophy of the mucosa. As in celiac patients, these lesions are slow to repair.

In a number of cases, one in ten in Visakorpi's series,[330] in one in two of our own group of patients,[104] the response to ingestion of cow's milk is delayed and the gastrointestinal upsets appear slowly. In other cases ingestion of even a very minute amount of cow's milk results, quite immediately, in a severe state of collapse, with vomiting and profuse diarrhea. Examination of stools shows heavy steatorrhea, and lactic and volatile acids.[75,104,330] If exposure to cow's milk is prolonged, or even if the amount ingested is progressively increased, intensity of symptoms diminishes, and vomiting ceases. Diarrhea, steatorrhea, and fermentation become milder. However, the absorption coefficient of fats remains definitely below the normal range. Generalized malabsorption and intestinal atrophy continue steadily. Therefore, in a few weeks, as the general condition of the patient worsens, one is led to again prescribe a diet free of cow's milk.[104] A most interesting feature of cow's milk intolerance which is quite different from what happens in celiac disease is its transient nature. After some weeks or some months, the patients become tolerant to cow's milk, the ingestion of which no longer induces either acute symptoms or intestinal atrophy.[75,104,330]

Another peculiarity is the frequency of associated intolerance to various proteins such as rice, soya bean, egg, or beef proteins. These associated intolerances are manifested by the same acute symptoms, i.e., shock and vomiting after exposure, and thereafter by malabsorption. They raise difficulties for the feeding of infants, who must be given breast milk or casein hydrolysate formulas. Scandinavian authors[93,330] stress that gluten intolerance may sometimes develop later; in approximately half of the cases this is progressive; in the remaining cases the reaction after ingestion of flour is acute and very similar to an anaphylactic reaction. These cases of gluten intolerance were transient. They have not been observed either by Davidson or ourselves.

## Pathogenesis

The offending factors are the protein of cow's milk. The point is easy to prove in the cases of acute intolerance, by short-term experiments with small doses of pure milk protein fractions, although even in these circumstances one has to take into account the possibility of progressive desensitization of patients in the interpretation of results. On the other hand, the causative role of protein fractions is quite impossible to demonstrate when acute symptoms are absent and intolerance only results in a delayed reaction.

Intolerance may involve one or several fractions of the cow-milk proteins, among which one distinguishes two groups, caseins and lacto-serum proteins. Caseins represent 80 % of the total proteins. They precipitate after acidification to pH 4.6. Caseins are very heterogeneous and are made of many components, the main ones being the $\alpha$, $\beta$, and $\kappa$ components; several genetic variants have been described from each of them. Lactoserum proteins or soluble proteins account for the remaining 20 %; 80 % of this fraction is represented by albumins, which can be resolved into $\beta$-lactoglobulins (50 %), several genetic allotypes of which have been described; $\alpha$-lactalbumin (20 %), two types of which have been isolated; and serum albumin. The remaining fractions are the immunoglobulins (mainly IgA), proteoses, peptones, and minor components like the red protein and enzymes. All these fractions may be separated by chromatographic technique or precipitation.

Some of them, chiefly $\beta$-lactoglobulin and $\alpha$-lactalbumin, may be purified by repeated precipitation and solubilization and finally obtained in a reasonably pure crystalline form which can be used for tests. Finally, it is worth noticing that some of these proteins are antigenically species-specific, whereas others share common antigenic properties with similar fractions from other species, e.g., cow and goat caseins. This phenomenon should account for cross-intolerances.

In Davidson's case[75] the patient was intolerant just to $\beta$-lactoglobulin. In one of our cases[104] we were able to demonstrate an intolerance both to $\beta$-lactoglobulin and $\alpha$-lactalbumin; acute symptoms were provoked with 1 mg of the latter and 3 mg of the former, and an associated intolerance has been noticed to soya bean and rice in one patient and to casein and rice in another. In Visakorpi's experience[330] the patients reacted to several of the proteins. The mechanism of intolerance is not yet defined. There is no evidence for an enzymatic defect. It seems more likely that some immunologic process is involved. Circulating antibodies have been found in a number of patients against whole milk proteins or lactoserum proteins, a trivial finding commonly present also in controls, and against $\beta$-lactoglobulin, more likely to be significant evidence.[176] Caution has been urged in the interpretation of these data.[239,285] One could perhaps suggest that they have some significance in relation to the immediate acute reaction, whereas one might guess that the delayed response is conditioned by a local immunologic process, i.e., the induction of antibodies in the intestinal mucosa. Sensitization could arise from the passing of undegraded proteins through the intestinal wall, a normal phenomenon in newborn and young infants which might be enhanced by lesions of the intestinal epithelium. The possibility of sensitization *in utero* or during lactation has also been suggested, and could explain the occurence of acute accidents at the time of weaning.

## Genetics

No information is available on this point.

### Malabsorption Syndromes and Immunologic Deficiencies

Gastrointestinal disorders have been described in association with immunoglobulin deficiencies. Although the disturbances are often referred to as malabsorption or spruelike syndromes, their true pattern is not well documented in many observations. Furthermore, although they appear to be most common in so-called acquired hypogammaglobulinemia, they have been mentioned as well in other types of immunoglobulin deficiencies. The causal relationship between the two kinds of disorders cannot always be settled with certainty. First of all, in many instances it is difficult to assess which disorder was antecedent. Second, the type of hypogrammaglobulinemia remains doubtful in the absence of data of [131]I albumin and [131]I PVP tests, which are necessary to distinguish between hyposynthetic hypogammaglobulinemia and associated excessive intestinal protein loss. Finally, investigation of absorption has not often been conducted systematically.

## Congenital Agammaglobulinemia

In congenital agammaglobulinemia so-called sex-linked recessive, or Bruton-type, gastrointestinal disturbances have been reported. They consist mainly of an infectious diarrhea with bloody and purulent liquid stools and, in many cases, bacteria and protozoa, suggestive of ileocolitis.[3] Malabsorption is usually absent. Duodenojejunal biopsies display no atrophy of the villi, but infiltration of the lamina propria, mainly by polymorphonuclear neutrophils. In these cases the causal role of infection in the occurence of diarrhea is suggested by the fact that it subsides with antibiotic and immunoglobulin replacement therapy. It is worth noticing that some cases referred to as congenital agammaglobulinemia must be discarded from this category because they are females.[31] Other cases remain difficult to classify. For instance, in the often-quoted observation of Pelkonen et al.[236] it is claimed that the family study disclosed the hereditary sex-linked nature of the disease. As a matter of fact, if one accepts the authors suggestion that the patient's only child also has hypogammaglobulinemia, this pattern of inheritance is, of course, excluded. Finally, severe ileocolitis has also been mentioned in the Swiss type of agammaglobulinemia.

## Acquired Hypogammaglobulinemias

Gastrointestinal disorders are frequent in acquired hypogammaglobulinemias and have been noticed in more than 50 % of adult cases.[146,210,260,344] They consist either of ileocolitis or of a spruelike syndrome. In the latter cases malabsorption is conspicuous, with low excretion of xylose, a flat glucose test, and definite steatorrhea. Hypoalbuminemia may be present, due either to defective synthesis or to excessive loss.[331] In many cases the mucosa is normal, as far as the villi are concerned. In some the duodenal mucosa displays a flat appearance and epithelial impairment indistinguishable from celiac disease. In addition, lymphocytic infiltration of the lamina propria and scarcity of IgA plasma cells have been noted. These disturbances do not appear to respond to a gluten-free diet and they are likely to be due to chronic enteric infections.

Gastrointestinal disturbances have been observed in all kinds of hypogammaglobulinemias, in cases secondary to neoplastic diseases such as myelomas, chronic lymphocytic leukemias, or Hodgkin's disease, and in hypogammaglobulinemia with thymoma. They have also been noted in primary or idiopathic acquired hypogammaglobulinemia, a disease of obscure origin, in which it is often claimed that genetic factors are involved, owing to the occurrence of immunoglobulin deficiencies of several types, often poorly defined, in the relatives of patients.

In some of the primary cases the hypoglobulinemia was associated with an enteric loss of protein.[329,332] These cases are difficult to distinguish from excessive enteric protein loss due to primary bowel disease, in which the hypoalbuminemia and hypogammaglobulinemia are due solely to the exudative enteropathy, and in which reversal of the abnormal protein loss restores the concentration of both proteins to normal. However, this excessive loss has also been demonstrated in one case of agammaglobulinemia.[331]

## Dysgammaglobulinemias

A syndrome has been described[136] in adult patients which is characterized by dysgammaglobulinemia, consisting of virtual absence of the IgA and IgM immunoglobulins and a moderately decreased level of IgG immunoglobulin in the serum, called type II of Rosen and Janeway[260] or type I of Hobbs.[137] It is associated with an unusual susceptibility to infection, diarrhea, sometimes with steatorrhea, the presence of Giardia lamblia in the stools, and nodular lymphoid hyperplasia of the small intestine.

Most interesting are the cases of diarrhea associated with IgA deficiency, to which attention has been called by Crabbé.[61] In nearly every case diarrhea was symptomatic of malabsorption and was said to respond to a gluten-free diet,[61,137] although it seems doubtful that all the criteria required for the diagnosis of celiac disease were fulfilled. So far, in one single case the histological appearance has been followed up.[61] In this case clinical improvement was associated with partial repair of intestinal lesions, which relapsed when the patient was again fed gluten. Therefore, it would seem that, at least in some cases, the patients are affected with gluten-induced enteropathy, and if this is so, the IgA deficiency should be considered either as secondary to malabsorption or as coincidental. Both hypotheses remain difficult to accept. On the one hand, in most cases of celiac disease the IgA level is not depressed, but actually increased, and the IgA cells in the mucosa are numerous, in striking contrast with the cases just mentioned.[149] On the other hand, the frequency of cases seems rather too high for the coincidence of celiac disease and IgA deficiency to be simply considered as a chance association.[61]

The hypothesis of a primary immunologic deficiency has been considered along with the current theory of IgA synthesis by submucosal plasma cells, secretion through epithelial cells onto the mucous surface, and their role in the immunologic defense of these surfaces. However, it appears that gastrointestinal disturbances are not a constant feature of IgA deficiency as would be expected from this hypothesis. First of all, IgA deficiency has been observed in healthy individuals. Second, IgA deficiency in serum and secretions (saliva) is common in ataxia telangiectasia, in which, although respiratory tract infections are frequent, no gastrointestinal disturbance has been reported so far.[313] Whatever the true relationship may be between these two disorders, the cause of the IgA deficiency by itself is also obscure. Since many patients had onset of symptoms in adult life, either they acquired their IgA deficiency or lived for many years in good health with it.

A genetic basis of IgA deficiency has been suggested after the finding of similar deficiencies in relatives, but the pattern of inheritance is not apparent from the scanty data available. So far, ataxia telangiectasia is the only known anomaly associated with IgA deficiency to be likely transmitted as a Mendelian autosomal recessive.

## FAILURES OF CHYLOMICRON FORMATION

### Congenital Absence of β-Lipoproteins

Twenty four cases of congenital absence of $\beta$-lipoproteins have been described[182] since Bassen and Kornzweig's publication.[23] Besides the absence of $\beta$-lipoproteins, the syndrome is characterized by intestinal malabsorption, acanthocytosis, retinopathy, ataxia, mental retardation, and a very low level of plasma lipids.[177,204,278]

### Clinical Features

Digestive disturbances begin in the first weeks of life and worsen when the lipid content of the diet is progressively increased. They consist of diarrhea, vomiting, loss of appetite, and abdominal enlargement with distension of the loops, coarsening of the folds, and dilution and fragmentation of the barium meal on X-ray films of the small intestine. The digestive disturbances provoke a failure to thrive and hypothrepsia. They are not influenced by gluten-free diet.[179] Acanthocytosis is characteristic. The red cells take a sea-urchin shape. There is no rouleau formation. ESR is low. Hemolysis is increased, as demonstrated by isotopic studies with $^{51}$Cr or after incubation at 37°C for 48 hr.[308] The onset of neurological symptoms is delayed. They develop when the patients are about five years old and consist of an abolition of deep reflexes and ataxia rather like that observed in Friedreich's disease. Mental retardation is often associated.[182] Retinal degeneration has a course parallel to that of the neurological symptoms. Early detection of the retinal involvement is possible with electroretinograms. Later the lesions may be seen on fundal examination where they have appearance of atypical retinitis pigmentosa with myriads of bright silvery spots. Retinopathy provokes a progressive diminution of visual acuity and night blindness. Later, pigmentary deposits may be observed.[345]

## Biochemical Features

The prominent anomaly is the absence of low-density lipoproteins ($d < 1.063$). Immunochemical techniques demonstrate that their concentration is lower than 1/10,000 of normal values.[189] The presence of B-protein (apoprotein) would have been detectable by immunological techniques, although its antigenic properties differ from that of the native lipoprotein.[187] Concentration of high-density lipoproteins is slightly decreased and their electrophoretic mobility slowed.[157,179,189] Their density is somewhat lower than usual, and on preparative ultracentrifugation a part of them float in the density region 1.019–1.063, probably as a result of an overloading of α-protein by lipids; otherwise, the HDL seems to be perfectly normal, based on immunochemical characteristics and amino acid composition.[189]

Absence of β-lipoprotein is responsible for the very low concentration of plasma lipids. Total lipid level is below 100–150 mg %, cholesterol ranges between 20 and 90 %, and phospholipids from 25 to 95 %. Triglycerides are practically undetectable. Cholesterol esterification ratio is unmodified.[179,278] In contrast, the composition pattern of phospholipids is changed, with a relative increase of sphingomyelin and a decrease of lecithin. Such an anomaly seems to be rather paradoxical if one considers the higher lecithin/sphingomyelin ratio in α- as compared to β-lipoproteins. It is also found in the phospholipids of cell membranes.[240,334]

The fatty acid pattern is modified. The observed anomalies are identical with those noted in severe deficiencies of essential fatty acids, i.e., low concentration of the linoleic family (ω6) and raised concentration of the oleic family (ω9) and of palmitoleic acid (ω7).[179,241,334] These alterations are not the consequence of a specific malabsorption of linoleic acid, but reflect an increase of lipogenesis from carbohydrates and proteins. Reduction of fat intake, which is commonly prescribed in these patients in order to improve the digestive disturbances, further worsens the deficiency of essential fatty acids. Carotenoid, vitamin A, and vitamin E concentrations are also extremely low.[162,179,278]

## Anatomical Study

Villi are of normal length and shape. Epithelial cells are unusually enlarged, with a seemingly "empty" cytoplams. Staining with Sudan of frozen sections or of sections fixed with osmic acid shows that they are filled with lipid droplets. The accumulated lipids are essentially glycerides, the amount being about 10 times the normal value. No fat is observed either in lamina propria (but in macrophages as in normal subjects) or in the lacteals.[179,204,278,335]

On electron microscopy the microvilli appear normal; however, the cytoplasmic matrix is coarse and granular. Mitochondria are impaired. Endoplasmic reticulum is not readily apparent and ribosomes are difficult to identify. Nucleic and intercellular areas are squashed by the lipid overload. The basement membrane is also modified. All these changes are likely to be secondary to the accumulation of fats within the cells. Most of the lipid droplets are located within the endoplasmic reticulum, which occasionally seems to be broken by large droplets of fat dispersed in the cytoplasm. Golgi apparatus, intercellular areas, and the lacteals are definitely clear of chylomicrons. Also, the intercellular areas and lacteals do not contain the very minute particles (0.01–0.1 $\mu$) which are found in normal subjects.[83]

### Pathogenesis

In all likelihood, the defect is concerned with protein synthesis by ribosomes of the endoplastic reticulum. Similar lesions of the intestinal cells can be reproduced experimentally in rats fed with puromycin or ethionine, which inhibit protein synthesis, but which do not interfere either with fatty acid acylation or incorporation into glycerides.[277] Furthermore, analysis of intracellular lipids[335] and study of palmitate [14]C incorporation[150] demonstrate that the synthesis of glycerides proceeds normally in the cells of patients. However, from the aforementioned results of immunochemical studies, it could be inferred that a nonsense protein is synthesized which is no longer able to prevent lipid particles from fusing together. This aggregation of lipids would then be unable to pass through the Golgi apparatus and from there into the intercellular areas.

### Genetics

Bassen–Kornzweig's disease has been found more frequently among males than among females (17 males and 7 females). It is due to a mutant gene which manifests itself in the homozygous state. In four families, two sibs, a boy and a girl, were affected. Consanguinity rate is 25 %.[182] In most cases heterozygotes are undetectable. They experience no digestive disturbances and the histological appearance of their intestinal mucosa is normal.[335] Red-cell shape is unmodified, and, as a rule, $\beta$-lipoprotein levels are normal. A significant lowering to about half the normal value has, however, been noticed in two families.[182,278] In our opinion, such a finding is not by itself a reliable index of the heterozygous state in the absence of the complete form of the disease in relatives. Occurrence of asymptomatic forms manifested solely by a reduction of $\beta$-lipoproteins seems to us to be very questionable.

### Type II

A failure of fat transport without any deficit of blood $\beta$-lipoproteins has been briefly described by Anderson et al.[8] Since then, two more families have been reported. [181a,306a] The diagnosis can only be ascertained by intestinal biopsy, for intestinal malabsorption is not associated with any other symptoms. There is neither acanthocytosis nor neuroocular symptoms, and low-density lipoproteins are present in the plasma.

The impairment of intestinal absorption is similar to that observed in abetalipoproteinemia. From birth, the patients had bulky liquid stools, abdominal distension, and failure to thrive. Vomiting was usual. The absorption coefficient of fats ranged between 50 and 70%. Fecal nitrogen was slightly increased, as was excretion of volatile acids. Tests of sugar absorption gave normal results. Red cells had a normal discoid shape, and there was normal rouleaux formation and no hyperhemolysis. Hypochromia and hyposideremia were present and responded well to iron therapy. Neurological and ophtalmologic examination revealed no abnormality. In our case the developmental quotient was rather low. Blood lipid levels were not so low as in abetalipoproteinemia (total lipids: 215–350 mg; cholesterol: 55–85 mg; phospholipids: 65–95; glycerides: 35–75). On electrophoresis all lipoprotein fractions were diminished. Carotene and vitamin A were lowered. Vitamin E was not detectable.

The pathogenesis of the defect is not elucidated. It can be supposed that it consists of another structural modification of B-protein which might be able to bind circulating lipids but no longer to form chylomicrons. One could also invoke a failure in the intracellular synthesis of phospholipids, which could affect one of the reactions which lead to lecithin formation.

Type II failure of chylomicrons formation is very likely a recessive character. Two brothers were affected in a sibship. Parental consanguinity has been recorded in Silberberg's case.[306a]

## DISTURBANCES IN CARBOHYDRATE HYDROLYSIS AND SUGAR TRANSPORT

### Sucrose and Isomaltose Intolerance

### Clinical and Biochemical Features

Since its original description by Weijers et al.[340] more than ninety cases have been published in the literature.[248,252] Diarrhea is the presenting symptom of the disease, which appears, in virtually all cases, as soon after birth as sucrose or dextrin and starch are added to cow's milk formula. In breast-fed infants the onset of diarrhea is delayed until sucrose is introduced into the diet. The severity of the diarrhea is roughly proportional to the amount of the ingested disaccharide. With a high sucrose intake the weight of the stools may reach 300–500 g per day or more. Their appearance is very suggestive of the fermentative nature of the diarrhea. They are liquid and frothy, with a sour smell. Their pH is usually very low, between 3.8 and 5.2, in contrast to 6.2–7.4 in normal cow's-milk-fed infants. Considerable amounts of lactic acid are found, in many cases up to several grams per day. The lactic acid is produced by the bacterial fermentation of sugar in the large intestine. The bacterial flora consists, almost exclusively, of gram-positive organisms (*Bacillus acidophilus*). Besides lactic acid, important amounts of volatile acids are recovered, 90 % of which is acetic acid.[341] Sucrose, as well as glucose and fructose, are detected in the stools. Sucrosuria is constant.[252]

There is no evidence of malabsorption. The fecal fat excretion is normal, as are xylose absorption, glucose tolerance, and lactose tolerance, when these tests are performed on treated patients without diarrhea. As a rule, the digestive disturbances have no effect on the nutritional state. There is no vitamin deficiency, no anemia, no osteoporosis, etc. Finally, the morphological appearance of the intestinal mucosa has been found to be normal with very few exceptions.[10,43,165,249]

Diarrhea persists as long as children are fed a normal diet. Removal of sucrose and starch from the diet brings about a dramatic improvement of the child's condition. The fermentation disappears and the stools become solid again; the children gain weight. If sucrose is given, one at once notices abdominal pains and distention and watery fermentative diarrhea. Lactic acid and volatile acids are recovered in the stools, the pH of which is reduced. Furthermore, a sucrose load does not induce any rise in blood glucose level, in contrast with what happens in controls.[341] Addition of starch or dextrins to the diet provokes more progressive changes, but they are somewhat variable from case to case.[16,247] In almost every case fecal volatile acids increase and the pH decreases, but the diarrhea is delayed until the pH of the stools falls below 5 and the lactic acid excretion rises sharply.[252] In contrast, some patients are able to tolerate moderate amounts of starch, namely, those from rice and corn, which contain fewer $\alpha$-1,6 bonds. However, even in such cases the defect of hydrolysis can be demonstrated by a careful analysis of stools and direct assay of enzymatic activities.[17,43,165,252,294,324]

The differences observed in the apparent tolerance of sucrose and starch may be explained by the fact that oligosaccharides with $\alpha$-1,6 bonds represent at most 10 % of the starch molecule; under these conditions it would be necessary to give a very large load of starch to get symptoms comparable to those obtained with sucrose. The degree of hydrolysis of straight chains by α-amylase is also involved in the occurrence and severity of starch intolerance.[19] It could account for the fact that after some months children seem to be able to tolerate a certain amount of flour in their diet.

The long-term evolution of the disease is poorly known. It appears that the intensity of the clinical disorder decreases as the patients grow up. Several cases have, however, been detected in adolescents and adults, suggesting that disturbances persists throughout life and that there is no enzymatic adaptation.[151,224,312,343]

## Pathogenesis

Sucrose and isomaltose intolerance is due to a deficit in two α-glucosidases, namely, isomaltase (maltase Ia) and sucrase (maltase Ib), which share, besides their main activity, 50 and 25 %, respectively, of total maltase activity. Maltases Ia and Ib can only be separated from each other by heat inactivation at 45°C. In contrast, thermoresistant maltases (maltases II and III from Dahlqvist, or 1 and 2 from Semenza et al.) are unchanged; in patients they represent almost all of the remaining maltase activity, as against 20–25 % in normal subjects. Maltases II and III can be separated from each other only by heat inactivation. In contrast, thermoresistant maltases can be distinguished from thermosensitive maltases by column chromatography on Sephadex.[17,18,69,70,293,294] All the evidence just mentioned suggests that there exist only two proteins, each with at least two active sites. The defect is not due to the action of an inhibitor.[224,294,312] It must be the consequence either of a lack of synthesis of the enzyme(s) or of an alteration of its structure.

## Genetics

The intolerance to sucrose and isomaltose behaves as a recessive character. Males and females are equally affected (50 males, 38 females). They are born to normal parents. The proportion of affected among the sibs of the propositi is consistent with the hypothesis. Parental consanguinity is mentioned in two families.[252] Some parents are reported to have suffered from digestive disturbances in infancy and childhood;[247] however, such hearsay evidence has not been corroborated by actual observation. Maltase, isomaltase, and sucrase activities are significantly diminished in heterozygous parents.[17,43,165,252] The level of isomaltase and sucrase activity is, on the average, 50 % of normal. The proportion of thermoresistant maltase and the ratio of total maltase activity to isomaltase (or sucrase) activity are increased to the extent expected if synthesis of thermoresistant maltases is unimpaired, sucrase and isomaltase activities being reduced to 50 %.

*Lactose Intolerance*

## Clinical and Biochemical Features

Lactose intolerance was described by Durand[89] and by Holzel et al.[141] It is characterized by a fermentative diarrhea beginning within a few days after birth, as soon as milk feeding is well established, which can lead to hypotrophy, dehydration, and, eventually, to death, particularly in infants who are fed on breast milk. Lactosuria is common, and is related to the lactose intake, and even if it is not found in every case, it is not justified, in our opinion, to distinguish two forms of lactose intolerance, according to its occurrence or its absence. Sometimes hyperaminoaciduria and acidosis are present. All symptoms subside when lactose is removed from the diet.

## Pathogenesis

Congenital lactose intolerance is due to a deficit of lactase 1, whereas lactase 2 activity is normal.[17,74,184,190,311] The former is located on the brush border and active upon cellobiose as well as upon lactose; in contrast, the latter is a lysosomal enzyme which mainly splits other substrates, such as 6-bromo-2-naphtyl-$\beta$-galactoside.[84,144,167,293] A similar enzymic defect has been found in cases of definitely acquired deficiencies.[185,348] Therefore, the type of the defect gives no indication about its etiology. Furthermore, the same clinical disturbances may be observed in infants associated with histological changes of mucosa consisting of a villous atrophy with an alteration of the epithelium very akin to that observed in celiac patients; the fermentative diarrhea disappears on feeding with a lactose-free formula, and weight gain follows; repeated biopsies demonstrate that the mucosa returns to normal; however, the lactase level may remain at a low level for a long period.[44] The natural history of this disease is very informative, demonstrating how easy it may be to evoke a primary disorder in such circumstances. In Burke's opinion,[44] and we fully agree with her, it is likely that a number of so-called congenital lactase deficiencies actually are of this temporary variety.

## Genetics

The best type of argument to favor the existence of congenital lactase deficiency would be to find a familial pattern. Occurrence in sibs has been ascertained in some families. Consanguinity of parents is not mentioned, except in Durand's case. In one report the father of a patient demonstrated malabsorption of lactose. In another one the father and the mother were involved. However, the significance of these findings is doubtful, due to the frequent occurrence of acquired lactase deficiency.[27,58,68,145,213]

## Lactase Deficiency in Adults

The cause of lactase deficiency in adults remains unclear. The first explanation proposed was that it is secondary to milk deprivation.[68] However, contrary to what is observed in animals after weaning, the lactase activity seems to persist at the same level throughout life in human beings. Furthermore, lactase activity can be demonstrated in patients who have avoided milk, for instance, in patients treated for milk allergy or galactosemia. It has been shown that in animals it is possible to increase the tolerance to lactose by feeding it. However, this phenomenon was not shown to be accompanied by any increase of the specific enzymatic activity except in the experiments of Girardet et al.[118] Clinical observations have also demonstrated that it is possible to progressively increase the lactose intake without trouble, that is, to increase lactose absorption, without any significant modification of lactase activity.[97,129]

Cook and Kajubi,[58] using lactose tolerance tests and enzymatic assays, found significant differences in the incidence of lactase deficiency among African tribes, differences which could not be explained by dietary habits and were thought to have a hereditary basis. The difference between levels of lactase activities in Negroes and white adults has been confirmed by Bayless et al.[27] and by McMichael et al.[213] At present it is difficult to draw any definite conclusion from these observations. First of all, it would be necessary to have family studies demonstrating a Mendelian pattern of inheritance. It is possible that other genetic factors than the $\beta$-galactosidase genes are involved. For instance, one is aware of the relationship between the ABO groups and the serum level of intestinal alkaline phosphatase. Furthermore, some ill-defined environmental factors could be involved. The possibility remains that lactase deficiency in adults is acquired and represents the sequelae of some kind of damage to the mucosa, e.g., by a gastroenteritis, the lack of lactase becoming permanent. In conclusion, we think that all these factors must be considered before making a diagnosis of congenital lactase deficiency.

## Glucose-Galactose Malabsorption

## Clinical and Biochemical Features

Glucose-galactose malabsorption has been described by Laplane et al.[183] and by Lindquist and Meeuwisse.[193] The clinical symptoms closely resemble those of patients with lactose intolerance: when the monosaccharides glucose and galactose are fed (or disaccharides or polysaccharides such as lactose, sucrose, dextrins, or starch, which give rise to them), osmotic and fermentative diarrhea quickly develops, which can be severe enough to cause death in early infancy. If fructose replaces all other sugars, the diarrhea subsides and the patient grows normally.

Polysaccharides and disaccharides are normally split into mono-saccharides, but glucose and galactose are poorly and slowly absorbed. As a consequence, they can be recovered in the stools (but not the disaccharides), along with lactic and volatile acids. Otherwise, fructose, sorbose (a ketosugar with furanose configuration), and mannose are absorbed in a normal way. Furthermore, the intermediary metabolism of glucose does not seem to be impaired.

## Pathogenesis

The defect is concerned with the transport of carbohydrates, which are absorbed by an active mechanism, i.e., against a concentration gradient, using energy. This hypothesis has been demonstrated by intubation studies *in vivo*[194] and isotopic experiments *in vitro*.[90,215,287]

Intubation studies also show that the absorption rate for fructose is faster than those for glucose and galactose. This finding, which could not be explained on the basis of passive diffusion of fructose, favors the hypothesis of facilitated diffusion for this monosaccharide.[194] Another point of interest is connected with xylose absorption, which has been found to be at the lower end of the normal range. In the light of current hypotheses regarding xylose absorption, one wonders if the mutation responsible for the disorder results in a quantitative decrease of synthesis of "mobile carrier for active transport," or, rather, in a qualitative alteration of its structure, with a change of respective affinities for sugars. Finally, glucosuria is a common feature of the disease, a finding which suggests that intestinal absorption of glucose and renal transfer share common mechanisms. Some authors claimed that they found evidence of a disturbance of intestinal absorption of glucose in patients affected with renal glucosuria. At this time, proof is completely lacking.

## Genetics

The disease has been observed in male and female infants. Consanguinity has been recorded in three families.[195,227] Several sibs have been affected who were born from normal parents.[11,183,195] In all likelihood, we are dealing with a recessive character manifesting itself in patients homozygous for a mutant gene.

## DISORDERS OF AMINO ACID TRANSPORT

### Cystinuria

### Clinical and Biochemical Features

Cystinuria is characterized by an excessive urinary excretion of cystine, which leads to the formation of cystine stones; the excreted amount ranges between 500 mg and 1 g per day. Cystinuria is associated with an excessive excretion of dibasic aminoacids, lysine, arginine, and ornithine, as well as the excretion of the disulfides L-cysteine and L-homocysteine. A single observation of isolated cystinuria appears in the literature.[39]

A defect in the intestinal transport has been demonstrated both *in vivo* and *in vitro*,[13,320] and, from that of view, three types of cystinuria have been defined by Rosenberg *et al.*[264] In type I the intestinal mucosa completely lacks the mechanisms for mediated or active transport of cystine, lysine, and arginine; cystine blood level is decreased, and no rise is observed after an oral load. In type II the uptake of cystine by intestinal mucosa is normal, whereas the level of plasma cystine is deficient. Finally, intestinal transport of cystine, lysine, and arginine is normal in mucosa of patients with type III cystinuria, and plasma cystine rises almost normally after oral cystine loads.

### Pathogenesis

It is generally assumed, after Dent and Rose,[77] that cystinuria results from an impairment in the renal tubular reabsorption of cystine and dibasic amino acids associated with a similar defect in intestinal absorption. The mechanism of the underlying defect is poorly understood due to insufficient knowledge of the systems of amino acid transport. It has been postulated that two types could be distinguished in human kidney.[290] The first one is a high-capacity group-specific system. The second would have a far greater specificity, but low capacity for substrate. Evidence for two systems has been provided for lysine, but not for cystine.[290] In cystinuria the affected system would be the group-specific one. In contrast, the defect in isolated cystinuria would be involved with an unknown substrate-specific carrier. However, several findings remain difficult to explain. For instance, in type I cystinuria the mediated transport of cystine and dibasic amino acids is completely abolished, in contrast to the partial transport defect in the kidney. No difference is observed in the uptake of labeled cystine by kidney tissue *in vitro* between biopsies from controls and patients.[100,261] Cystine uptake is not inhibited by dibasic amino acids, which are mutually competitive. Conversely, the uptake of the dibasic amino acids is not inhibited by cystine. Therefore, it has not been demonstrated *in vitro* that cystine and the dibasic amino acids share a common transport mechanism in kidney. Another question concerns the lowered cysteine blood level; in contrast to results with cystine, cysteine uptake is not defective in the gut of cystinuric patients and no cysteine is recovered in the urine.[266] An abnormal cystine–cysteine relationship has been postulated, in view of high renal arteriovenous difference for cysteine but not for cystine. However, these results have not been confirmed.[107,262]

## Genetics

Harris *et al.* demonstrated that two types of cystinuria could be differentiated on genetic grounds.[133] The first type is the recessive form; the patients are homozygous for the mutant gene; the heterozygote parents are normal. In the second type, the incompletely recessive form, the homozygotes are indistinguishable from those of the recessive form; the heterozygotes excrete excessive amounts of cystine, lysine, and arginine. It is difficult to ascribe a peculiar genotype to one individual on the ground of cystine and lysine excretion, as a continuous range of values can be observed.[64] Arginine could be a more significant marker.

According to Rosenberg *et al.*,[264] type I corresponds to the recessive form, whereas in type II, heterozygotes excrete markedly increased, and in type III, heterozygotes excrete slightly increased, quantities of cystine. Both are then incompletely recessive forms. In the majority of published observations one single type of heterozygote—i.e., normal or intermediate—has been found within a single family. In some, two types of heterozygote have been observed. For instance, in one of the families studied by Christiaens *et al.*[56] and in one described by Boström and Tottie[37] only one parent had abnormal aminoacid excretion. Recently, Rosenberg[263] described four stone-forming cystinuric subjects from three unrelated pedigrees. Each was heterozygous for two of the three described mutant genes producing cystinuria, i.e., I–II, II–III, and I–III. These doubly heterozygous patients were almost phenotypically indistinguishable from cystinuric homozygotes of genotypes I–I, II–II, and III–III. However, a patient whose genotype appears to be I–III responded to an oral cystine tolerance test with findings intermediate between those observed with homozygotes of type I and type III. These data suggest that all of the known mutations responsible for the genetic heterogeneity in cystinuria are allelic.

Finally, little data is available on the incidence of the disease. In their recent survey Crawhall *et al.*[64] found an apparent incidence of detectable heterozygotes of 1/200, and gave an incidence of heterozygotes of both types approaching 1/100.

### Familial Protein Intolerance with Deficient Transport of Basic Amino Acids

Familial protein intolerance with deficient transport of basic amino acids was described by Perheentupa *et al.*[238] in 1965. The authors recently added seven new cases to their description.[163,238]

A few months after weaning, vomiting and diarrhea appeared, and the patients lost appetite and ceased to thrive. In addition, some of them experienced episodes of ammonia intoxication, with loss of consciousness and alkalosis. Once able to select their food, all patients systematically rejected cow's milk, as well as protein-containing foods. On this self-restricted diet, the tendency to diarrhea subsided. All continued to have occasional vomiting. At examination the patients were thin and markedly retarded in growth. Bone maturation was delayed. Hepatomegaly was constant without any detectable impairment of liver function. On biopsy, signs of portal inflammation were found. Some patients also had enlarged spleens.

Plasma protein content, plasma aminonitrogen, and blood ammonia concentrations were normal in the fasting state. Plasma urea was low. In some patients there was slight evidence of intestinal malabsorption, but the intestinal mucosa displayed a normal appearance at histological examination. The patients had a characteristic renal aminoaciduria, with excessive leakage of lysine and less of arginine. In contrast, cystine excretion was mostly normal. Therefore, it is suggested that there is a renal transport defect of basic amino acids with normal cystine reabsorption. The transport defect is apparently shared by the intestine. The rate of urea production has been found to be subnormal in spite of the normality of the activities of the associated enzymes. The relationship between the defects of transport and urea synthesis has not been solved. The pattern of familial occurrence corroborates the possibility of an autosomal recessive mode of inheritance.

### Hartnup Disease

Hartnup disease was first described by Baron *et al.*[22] in 1956. Since that time some 20 cases have been published in the literature.[142,230]

### Clinical Features

The disease is characterized by rashes, episodes of cerebellar ataxia, and mental retardation. The most usual skin lesion consists of a pellagra-like photosensitive rash, localized to the exposed skin surfaces, which are dry, red, scaly, and hyperpigmented. The rash is frequent, but not constant. It worsens during spring and summer. It is sometimes associated with stomatitis and glossitis. In addition, most cases show recurrent episodes of cerebellar ataxia which involve upper and lower limbs and are associated with intention tremor, nystagmus, and pyramidal tract involvement. Neurological disturbances usually develop during acute phases of the disease, then disappear. They are transient and reversible. The psychiatric features of Hartnup disease are also transient, and more or less severe, consisting mainly of emotional lability. Mental retardation was reported in less than half the cases.

The course is usually mild, and the disease displays a tendency to gradually improve with age.

## Biochemical Features

The most characteristic biochemical finding is a marked and permanent increase of urinary amino acids and indole derivatives with otherwise normal renal function. Aminoaciduria involves mainly the neutral amino acids and tryptophan with the exception of glycine, proline, and hydroxyproline, which are not excreted in excessive amounts. Aminoacidemia is normal and tryptophanemia rather low.

Indican and indole-3-acetic acid excretion are grossly increased.[14] Kynureninuria and N-methylnicotinamide excretion are reduced. Indole derivatives disappear from the urine if patients are treated with neomycin. A gross fecal loss of amino acids, similar in its pattern to the aminoaciduria, has been reported,[289] but it is not constant.[291]

Effects of amino acid loads have been studied in some patients. After ingestion of L-tryptophan there is delayed and incomplete absorption of the amino acid from the gut. Some is recovered in the feces. There is also an increased and sustained excretion of indican, indoleacetic and indolelactic acid, acetylglutamine, and indolylacroyl-glycine. In contrast, intravenously administered tryptophan is metabolized normally with normal indoluria. After ingestion tyrosine is also poorly absorbed compared with controls, and considerably impairs the absorption of other neutral amino acids. No difference has been found in fecal histidine excretion between one patient and a control, although his renal tubular reabsorption was impaired. Oddly enough, lysine loads resulted in the fecal excretion of large amounts of this basic amino acid.

## Pathogenesis

It is generally agreed that Hartnup's disease is due to a defect of the active transport of a group of neutral amino acids through the renal tubule and the intestinal cells.[175,220,289] Unabsorbed tryptophan is partly converted by intestinal bacteria to indole and other products of bacterial tryptophan metabolism. According to de Laey et al.,[176] indole or indican inhibit tryptophan-pyrrolase and kynurenine formamidase in the liver and could produce a relative nicotinamide deficiency. They claim that nicotinic acid therapy enhances the absorption of tryptophan and other amino acids in the intestine and renal tubule and leads to a disappearance of all the biochemical features of the disease. However, these results have not been confirmed. It is likely that skin lesions are the consequence of the relative nicotinamide deficiency. The pathogenesis of the neurological disturbances is poorly understood. They could be due to the diffusion in the systemic circulation of amines formed during bacterial degradation of tryptophan and other amino acids.

## Genetics

The 19 published cases belong to ten separate kindreds. Parents are normal. Consanguinity has been mentioned in three instances. Therefore, it is likely that Hartnup's disease behaves as a recessive character. The pattern of excretion of amino acids and indole has been found to be normal in most parents and asymptomatic investigated sibs. Some of them had indicanuria and generalized aminoaciduria.[230]

### Blue Diaper Syndrome

The blue diaper syndrome was described by Drummond et al.[88] in 1964 in two sibs. It was characterized by failure to thrive, recurrent unexplained fever, infections, marked irritability, and constipation. Each patient had hypercalcemia, nephrocalcinosis, and elevated blood urea nitrogen level. In each case an unusual bluish discoloration of the diaper was observed, which had been present since infancy. No renal aminoaciduria was noted.

It was presumed that the patients had a decreased ability to absorb tryptophan from the gastrointestinal tract. The stools before and after tryptophan loading contained tryptophan in amounts far in excess of those of the control subjects. There was excessive urinary excretion of indolic metabolites, such as indican, indole acetic acid, and indigotin, the product of the oxidative conjugation of two molecules of indican, which is responsible for the blue coloration of the diapers. These excretions diminish after neomycin therapy. As there is no aminoaciduria, the defect is probably restricted to the gut. In relation to the findings made in Hartnup disease, it would have been of interest to know about the intestinal absorption of other neutral amino acids. Finally, the relationship between hypercalcemia and defective transport of tryptophan remains unsettled.

### Methionine Malabsorption Syndrome

Hooft et al.[143] reported the observation of a girl with mental retardation, diarrhea, convulsions, and polypnea. The patient had blue eyes and strikingly white hair. Her urine had a peculiar smell, due to the presence of α-hydroxy-butyric acid. α-Ketoacids were excreted. Aminoaciduria was normal. Examination of the feces revealed large quantities of methionine and other amino acids, particularly with branched chains, serine, and N-α-aminobutyric acid. After an oral load of methionine the patient developed diarrhea and the fecal excretion of methionine and other amino acids was slightly increased. α-Hydroxybutyric acid was recovered. The patient's condition improved on a methionine-restricted diet, and α-hydroxybutyric acid, methionine, and branched-chain amino acids disappeared from the stools. No family study is available.

It has been suggested that the primary defect lies in the malabsorption of methionine. The unabsorbed methionine is degraded into α-hydroxybutyric acid by bacteria. Malabsorption of other amino acids would be secondary to methionine malabsorption. It is remarkable that the intestinal defect is not associated with a renal tubular disturbance. Furthermore, it seems that most neutral amino acids are normally absorbed.

## MISCELLANEOUS

### Chloride Diarrhea with Alkalosis

Gamble *et al.*[108] and Darrow[72] described simultaneously in 1945 a new and apparently distinct syndrome called congenital alkalosis with diarrhea. Less than 20 cases have appeared in the literature since that time. The condition is now preferably called chloride diarrhea with alkalosis.

### Clinical and Biochemical Features

The disorder is probably present during fetal life. Pregnancy is sometimes complicated by hydramnios, and some patients are born prematurely.[237,347] From the first few hours of life the infants pass voluminous watery stools leading to significant weight loss and severe dehydration. The diarrhea persists, unrelated to diet, for months and years. In some cases the onset is somewhat delayed. Besides the diarrhea and its consequences for growth, which is stunted, with a retarded mental development, no other symptom is noticed. The patients enjoy good appetite and are very thirsty. Vomiting is uncommon.

The outcome has been fatal in most cases, due to infections, acute episodes of dehydration, or surgical exploration.[108,237,347] In one patient the troubles subsided when he was two and a half years old.[229]

The main disturbance in the blood is a metabolic alkalosis with hypochloremia and hypokalemia. Blood pH is, as a rule, higher than 7.50, and can reach 7.70 at some stages of the disease. Bicarbonate level is above 35 or 40 mM, whereas $pCO_2$ is normal. Chloremia ranges between 50 and 70 mEq/liter and kalemia between 1.5 and 3 mEq/liter. Natremia is normal or moderately low.

Urinary excretion of chloride is extremely reduced or absent. It does not increase after a parenteral load of either NaCl or KCl. Kaluria is high relative to the kalemia. So-called paradoxical aciduria has been observed, which disappears when Cl and K deficits are corrected. Urinary excretion of 17-keto and 17-hydroxy steroids are normal, as is excretion of precursors or metabolites of epinephrine. Aldosterone excretion has been found to be normal but more often increased; the rate of secretion of this hormone was high in the one case so far studied.[154]

In the stools, chloride concentration greatly surpasses that of sodium, in contrast with what happens in normals or in loose or watery "ordinary" stools. The chloride concentration averages 150 mEq/liter and remains remarkably constant, whatever the chloride intake or the blood Cl level. Extra intake of chloride or parenteral load with this electrolyte results in a huge increase of stool volume and aggravation of electrolyte loss.

Measurements of body composition have been undertaken in a few cases, by means of isotopic dilution technique. They display a reduction in exchangeable K and Cl, as well as a slight contraction of extracellular volume. Exchangeable Na does not seem to be significantly modified.[50,154]

Intestinal absorption of fats, carbohydrates, and proteins is not impaired. The pH of stools varies between 5 and 7; secondary deficient lactose hydrolysis has been noticed twice, with a deficit of enzymatic activity demonstrated in a fragment of duodenal mucosa.[229,325]

## Pathology

Anatomical examination performed either at surgical exploration or at necropsy failed to reveal any abnormality, such as the presence of gastric mucosal heterotopy. The most interesting findings are related to the kidney, which has been studied in some cases after biopsy. Typical potassium-losing nephropathy has been observed. In every patient studied so far, except one case, juxtaglomerular hyperplasia was present; sequential biopsies demonstrate that this lesion is secondary.[235]

## Pathogenesis

The mechanism of the chloride diarrhea is still obscure. It has been demonstrated that absorption of chloride in the proximal intestine is normal, and it is suggested that the primary defect lies in a failure of Cl transfer through the mucosa of the lower part of the intestine. The suggestion, originally made by Gamble et al.,[108] of an acid–base imbalance has been rejected. However, the chloride loss does not appear to be directly responsible for the whole picture, and, notably, for the metabolic alkalosis. This is more likely due to potassium depletion consequent on the intestinal losses and hyperaldosteronism induced through the sequence: hypovolemia, juxtaglomerular hyperplasia, increased renin-angiotensin release. Potassium depletion would further account for the paradoxical aciduria and might also aggravate chloride loss and diarrhea, as has been shown experimentally.

## Genetics

Chloride diarrhea has been observed in both sexes. In three families two sibs were definitely or very probably affected.[164,237] Parents were normal. Consanguinity is not mentioned. It can be suggested that the disease behaves as a recessive character.

## Specific Malabsorption of Vitamin $B_{12}$

Specific malabsorption of vitamin $B_{12}$ is a rare disease which has been described independently by Imerslund[147] and by Gräsbeck et al.[125] More than twenty cases have been reported.[126,178] The disease must be distinguished from the other forms of pernicious anemia in childhood, e.g., true Addison–Biermer anemia, the juvenile from of pernicious anemia which is characterized by inadequate production of gastric intrinsic factor, normal gastric mucosa, and normal acid secretion.

## Clinical and Biochemical Features

Patients are referred to physicians in infancy or early childhood for pallor, failure to thrive, and various symptoms like anorexia, vomiting, abdominal pains, edema, mild icterus, and fever. Besides the signs of anemia, examination sometimes reveals ecchymoses, petechiae, and glossitis. Neurological symptoms like hypotonia, ataxia, paresthesia, and diminished deep tendon reflexes can also be encountered in older cases. Liver and spleen are not enlarged. Anemia is usually severe, macrocytic with megaloblastic maturation in the bone marrow. It is associated with leucopenia and often pronounced thrombocytopenia. Mild proteinuria is an almost constant feature. It is usually permanent and not influenced by posture. It is isolated and not associated either with other changes of urinary sediment or with symptoms of renal failure. In some cases Imerslund[147] found anomalies of the urinary tract. Kidney biopsies have been reported in two cases, demonstrating in one case a slight subacute glomerulitis.

Evidence of vitamin $B_{12}$ deficiency is provided either by serum bioassays or by Schilling's test demonstrating a low urinary excretion remaining uncorrected after oral administration of vitamin $B_{12}$. In contrast, the symptoms rapidly subside if the vitamin is administered parenterally. Volume of gastric secretion, HCl secretion after histamine, and pepsin secretion after stimulation are usually normal. However, Lamy et al.[178] and Lillibridge et al.[191] found in some instances an achlorhydria or hypochlorhydria during acute phases. The gastric mucosa is normal. Intrinsic factor secretion measured after stimulation is also normal, a feature which excludes a diagnosis of juvenile pernicious anemia. Furthermore, ingestion of exogenous intrinsic factor does not restore the absorption of vitamin $B_{12}$ to normal.

The capacity of the serum of these patients to bind vitamin $B_{12}$ has been found unimpaired, and no antibodies against either intrinsic factor or gastric parietal cells can be found, in contrast with what happens frequently in true Addison–Biermer disease.

All these features point to a defect of absorption of vitamin $B_{12}$, which normally takes place in the ileum. The most common cause of such a defect is general malabsorption. Therefore, it is necessary to demonstrate that absorption of fat, nitrogen, glucose, etc. as well as the histological appearance of the intestinal mucosa and the X-ray appearance of the gut is normal to retain the diagnosis.

## Pathogenesis

Absorption of vitamin $B_{12}$ is an active process which normally takes place in the ileum. It is generally accepted that intrinsic factor, which is required for efficient absorption of physiological doses of vitamin $B_{12}$, forms a macromolecular complex with the vitamin. According to Donaldson et al.,[86] intrinsic factor is essential for this attachment to take place, and their results provide further support for the presence of a specific receptor for the complex at the microvillous surface of the intestinal cell. It can be assumed that specific malabsorption of vitamin $B_{12}$ results either from a lack of or an alteration of the receptor, or from a defect in hypothetical releasing factor which sets free the vitamin from the complex after absorption, or from a defect of a cellular carrier. The pathogenesis of the associated proteinuria is unclear.

## Genetics

Several cases have been observed, and both sexes were affected in sibships born from healthy parents. The proportion of cases does not differ significantly from the expected 0.25 among the sibs of propositi. Consanguinity of parents has been recorded several times. All these features point strongly to an auto-somal recessive mode of inheritance.

## Specific Malabsorption of Folic Acid

A case of relapsing megaloblastic anemia has been described in an infant by Luhby *et al.*[203] which subsided when upon daily treatment by pharmacological doses of 5/10 mg of folic acid orally. The infant's urinary formiminoglutamic acid (FIGLU) excretion was high. There was no abnor-mality in the gastrointestinal absorption of vitamin A or glucose. Stool fat was normal. X-ray examination of the gastrointestinal tract showed no abnor-malities. Peak serum folic after 10 mg of folic acid orally for 10 days was 5.2 m$\mu$g/ml; normal values under these conditions should have been 100–500 m$\mu$g/ml. The authors concluded that the relapsing anemia was due to a specific defect in the gastrointestinal absorption of folic acid, which probably represents a new inborn error.

## BIBLIOGRAPHY

1. Alarcón-Segovia, D., T. Herskovic, K. G. Wakim, P. A. Green, and H. H. Scudamore, Presence of circulating antibodies to gluten and milk fractions in patients with nontropical sprue, *Amer. J. Med.* **36**:485 (1964).
2. Alarcón-Segovia, D., K. G. Wakim, and E. E. Wollaeger, Antigenicity of various gluten fractions, *Amer. J. Dig. Dis.* **9**:72 (1964).
3. Allen, G. E., and D. R. Hadden, Congenital hypogammaglobulinaemia with steatorrhoea in two adult brothers, *Brit. Med. J.* **ii**:486 (1964).
4. Alvey, C., C. M. Anderson, and M. Freeman, Wheat gluten and coeliac disease, *Arch. Dis. Childh.* **32**:434 (1957).
5. Andersen, D. H., Cystic fibrosis of the pancreas and its relation to celiac disease: a clinical and pathologic study, *Amer. J. Dis. Child.* **56**:344 (1938).
6. Anderson, C. M., Histological changes in the duodenal mucosa in coeliac disease. Reversibility during treatment with a wheat gluten-free diet, *Arch. Dis. Childh.* **35**:419 (1960).
7. Anderson, C. M., and M. Freeman, Sweat test results in normal persons of different ages compared with families with fibrocystic disease of the pancreas, *Arch. Dis. Childh.* **35**:581 (1960).
8. Anderson, C. M., R. R. W. Townley, M. Freeman, and P. Johansen, Unusual causes of steatorrhoea in infancy and childhood, *Med. J. Aust.* **ii**:617 (1961).
9. Anderson, C. M., M. Freeman, F. Allan, and L. Hubbard, Observations on (i) sweat sodium levels in relation to chronic respiratory disease in adults and (ii) the incidence of respiratory and other disease in parents and siblings of patients with fibrocystic disease of the pancreas, *Med. J. Aust.* **i**:965 (1962).
10. Anderson, C. M., M. Messer, R. R. W. Townley, and M. Freeman, Intestinal sucrase and isomaltase deficiency in two siblings, *Pediatrics* **31**:1003 (1963).

11. Anderson, C. M., K. R. Kerry, and R. R. W. Townley, An inborn defect of intestinal absorption of certain monosaccharides, *Arch. Dis. Childh.* **40**:1 (1965).
12. Anderson, C. M., Intestinal malabsorption in childhood, *Arch. Dis. Childh.* **41**:571 (1966).
13. Asatoor, A. M., B. W. Lacey, D. R. London, and M. D. Milne, Amino acid metabolism in cystinuria, *Clin. Sci.* **23**:285 (1962).
14. Asatoor, A. M., J. Craske, D. R. London, and M. D. Milne, Indole production in Hartnup disease, *Lancet* i:126 (1963).
15. Ashworth, C. T., and W. C. Chears, Jr., Follow-up of intestinal biopsy in nontropical sprue after gluten-free diet and remission, *Fed. Proc.* **21**:880 (1962).
16. Auricchio, S., A. Dahlqvist, G. Mürset, and A. Prader, Isomaltose intolerance causing decreased ability to utilize dietary starch, *J. Ped.* **62**:165 (1963).
17. Auricchio, S., A. Rubino, A. Prader, J. Rey, J. Jos, J. Frézal, and M. Davidson, Intestinal glycosidase activities in congenital malabsorption of disaccharides, *J. Ped.* **66**:555 (1965).
18. Auricchio, S., G. Semenza, and A. Rubino, Multiplicity of human intestinal disaccharidases. II. Characterization of the individual maltases, *Biochim. Biophys. Acta* **96**:498 (1965).
19. Auricchio, S., D. Della Pietra, and A. Vegnente, Studies on intestinal digestion of starch in man. II. Intestinal hydrolysis of amylopectin in infants and children, *Pediatrics* **39**:853 (1967).
20. Bailey, N. T. J., The estimation of the frequencies of recessives with incomplete multiple selection, *Ann. Eugen. (Camb.)* **16**:215 (1951).
21. Barbero, G. J., Diagnosis of cystic fibrosis of the pancreas, *Pediatrics* **24**:658 (1959).
22. Baron, D. N., C. E. Dent, H. Harris, E. W. Hart, and J. B. Jepson, Hereditary pellagra-like skin rash with temporary cerebellar ataxia, constant renal aminoaciduria, and other bizarre biochemical features, *Lancet* ii:421 (1956).
23. Bassen, F. A., and A. L. Kornzweig, Malformation of the erythrocyte in a case of atypical retinitis pigmentosa, *Blood* **5**:381 (1950).
24. Bauer, U., A biochemical study of the mucopolysaccharides present in several body fluids of children suffering from fibrocystic disease of the pancreas and normal controls, *Ann. Paediat. (Basel)* **194**:236 (1960).
25. Baumann, T., Die Mucoviscidosis als rezessives und irregulär dominantes Erbleiden; eine klinische und genetische Studie, *Helv. Paed. Acta* **13**(*suppl.* 8):102 (1958).
26. Bayless, T. M., J. H. Yardley, J. H. Norton, and T. R. Hendrix, Adult celiac disease: rapid sequential changes in jejunal mucosa with alterations of dietary gluten. (Abstract), *J. Clin. Invest.* **41**:1344 (1962).
27. Bayless, T. M., and N. S. Rosensweig, Incidence and implications of lactase deficiency and milk intolerance in white and negro populations, *Johns Hopkins Med. J.* **121**:54 (1967).
28. Benson, G. D., O. D. Kowlessar, and M. H. Sleisenger, Adult celiac disease with emphasis upon response to the gluten-free diet, *Medicine* **43**:1 (1964).
29. Berger, E., Zur allergischen Pathogenese der Cöliakie, *Ann. Paediat. (Basel)* **1958**(*suppl.* 67).
30. Berger, E., and E. Freudenberg, Gibt es peptisch-tryptische Abbaustufen des Gliadins mit Antigencharakter, *Experientia* **18**:264 (1962).
31. Bernheim, M., R. Creyssel, R. Gilly, and P. Fournier, Agammaglobulinémie congénitale avec stéatorrhée chez deux jumeaux hétérozygotes de sexe différent, *Pédiatrie* **14**:881 (1959).

32. Biserte, G., and K. Han, Peptides résiduels de l'hydrolyse enzymatique de la gliadine du blé, *Bull. Soc. Chim. Biol. (Paris)* **47**:597 (1965).
33. Bodian, M., W. Sheldon, and R. Lightwood, Congenital hypoplasia of the exocrine pancreas, *Acta Paediat. (Uppsala)* **53**:282 (1964).
34. Bolt, R. J., J. A. Parrish, A. B. French, and H. M. Pollard, Adult coeliac disease. Histologic results of long-term low gluten diet, *Ann. Intern. Med.* **60**:581 (1964).
35. Booth, C. C., J. S. Stewart, R. Holmes, and W. Brackenbury, Dissecting microscope appearances of intestinal mucosa, *in*: Intestinal Biopsy. Ciba Foundation Study Group No. 14, G. E. W. Wolstenholme and M. P. Cameron, eds., Churchill, London (1962), p. 2.
36. Borgström, B., and B. Lindquist, Favorable effect of liquid formula-feeding high in fat to coeliac children, *Acta Paediat. (Uppsala)* **46**:449 (1957).
37. Boström, H., and K. Tottie, Cystinuria in Sweden. II. The incidence of homozygous cystinuria in Swedish school children, *Acta Paed. Scand.* **48**:345 (1959).
38. Boyer, P. H., and D. H. Andersen, A genetic study of celiac disease. Incidence of celiac disease, gastrointentinal disorders, and diabetes in pedigrees of children with celiac disease, *Amer. J. Dis. Child.* **91**:131 (1956).
39. Brodell, J., K. Gellissen, and S. Kowalewski, Isolierter Defekt der tubulären Cystin-Rückresorption in einer Familie mit idiopathischen Hypoparathyroïdismus, *Klin. Wschr.* **45**:38 (1967).
40. Bronstein, H. D., L. J. Haeffner, and O. D. Kowlessar, The nature of the toxic peptides of gliadin and their effects in celiac disease. (Abstract), *Clin. Res.* **13**:251 (1965).
41. Brusilow, S. W., and E. H. Gordes, Solute and water secretion in sweat, *J. Clin. Invest.* **43**:477 (1964).
42. Bulmer, M. G., Fibrocystic disease of the pancreas: a comment, *Ann. Hum. Genet.* **25**:163 (1961).
43. Burgess, E. A., B. Levin, D. Mahalanabis, and R. E. Tonge, Hereditary sucrose intolerance: levels of sucrase activity in jejunal mucosa, *Arch. Dis. Childh.* **39**:431 (1964).
44. Burke, V., K. R. Kerry, and C. M. Anderson, The relationship of dietary lactose to refractory diarrhoea in infancy, *Aust. Paediat. J.* **1**:147 (1965).
45. Burke, V., J. H. Colebatch, C. M. Anderson, and M. J. Simons, Association of pancreatic insufficiency and chronic neutropenia in childhood, *Arch. Dis. Childh.* **42**:147 (1967).
46. Cage, G. W., R. L. Dobson, and R. Waller, Sweat gland function in cystic fibrosis, *J. Clin. Invest.* **45**:1373 (1966).
47. Cameron, A. H., R. Astley, M. Hallowell, A. B. Rawson, C. G. Miller, J. M. French, and D. V. Hubble, Duodeno-jejunal biopsy in the investigation of children with coeliac disease, *Quart. J. Med.* **31**:125 (1962).
48. Carter, C., W. Sheldon, and C. Walker, The inheritance of coeliac disease, *Ann. Hum. Genet.* **23**:266 (1959).
49. Carter, C. O., Genetical aspects of cystic fibrosis of the pancreas, *Mod. Probl. Pediat.* **10**:372 (1967).
50. Chaptal, J., R. Jean, D. Dossa, F. Meylan, G. Morel, and D. Rieu, Diarrhée chlorée congénitale. Étude clinique et biologique d'une observation de l'enfant, *Sem. Hôp. Paris* **43**:1086 (1967).
51. Chernick, W. S., G. J. Barbero, and F. H. Parkins, Studies on submaxillary saliva in cystic fibrosis, *J. Ped.* **59**:890 (1961).
52. Chernick, W. S., and G. J. Barbero, Studies on human tracheobronchial and

submaxillary secretions in normal and pathophysiological conditions, *Ann. N.Y. Acad. Sci.* **106**:698 (1963).

53. Chernick, W. S., H. J. Eichel, and G. J. Barbero, Submaxillary salivary enzymes as a measure of glandular activity in cystic fibrosis, *Pediatrics* **65**:694 (1964).
54. Chernick, W. S., and G. J. Barbero, Reversal of submaxillary salivary alterations in cystic fibrosis by guanethidine, *Mod. Probl. Pediat.* **10**:125 (1967).
55. Chodos, D. D. J., R. S. Ely, G. A. Limbeck, and V. C. Kelley, Corticosteroid metabolism in cystic fibrosis, *Amer. J. Dis. Child.* **110**:76 (1965).
56. Christiaens, L., G. Biserte, G. Fontaine, and C. Debussche, La cystinurie (Étude clinique, biochimique et génétique), *Sem. Hôp. Paris* **36**:225 (1960).
57. Clarke, J. T., E. Elian, and H. Shwachman, Components of sweat. Cystic fibrosis of the pancreas compared with controls, *Amer. J. Dis. Child.* **101**:490 (1961).
58. Cook, G. C., and S. K. Kajubi, Tribal incidence of lactase deficiency in Uganda, *Lancet* i:725 (1966).
59. Cooke, W. T., D. J. Fone, E. V. Cox, M. J. Meynell, and R. Gaddie, Adult coeliac disease, *Gut* **4**:279 (1963).
60. Cooke, W. T., and W. T. Smith, Neurological disorders associated with adult coeliac disease, *Brain* **89**:683 (1966).
61. Crabbé, P., Signification du Tissu Lymphoïde des Muqueuses Digestives, Arscia, Bruxelles (1967).
62. Craig, J. M., H. Haddad, and H. Shwachman, The pathological changes in the liver in cystic fibrosis of the pancreas, *Amer. J. Dis. Childh.* **93**:357 (1957).
63. Crane, C. W., and A. Neuberger, Absorption and elimination of $^{15}$N after administration of isotopically labeled yeast protein and yeast protein hydrolysate to adult patients with coeliac disease. I. Rate of absorption of $^{15}$N yeast protein and yeast protein hydrolysate, *Brit. Med. J.* ii:815 (1960).
64. Crawhall, J. C., E. P. Saunders, and C. J. Thompson, Heterozygotes for cystinuria, *Ann. Hum. Genet.* **29**:257 (1966).
65. Creamer, B., Variations in small-intestinal villous shape and mucosal dynamics, *Brit. Med. J.* ii:1371 (1964).
66. Creamer, B., Small-intestinal mucosal dynamics and the environment, *Brit. Med. J.* ii:1373 (1964).
67. Crow, J. F., Problems of ascertainment in the analysis of family data, *in*: Genetics and the Epidemiology of Chronic Diseases, J. V. Neel, M. W. Shaw, and W. J. Schull, eds., Public Health Service Publ. No. 1163, Washington (1965), p. 23.
68. Cuatrecasas, P., D. H. Lockwood, and J. R. Caldwell, Lactase deficiency in the adult; a common occurrence, *Lancet* i:14 (1965).
69. Dahlqvist, A., Specificity of the human intestinal disaccharidases and implications for hereditary disaccharide intolerance, *J. Clin. Invest.* **41**:463 (1962).
70. Dahlqvist, A., S. Auricchio, G. Semenza, and A. Prader, Human intestinal disaccharidases and hereditary disaccharide intolerance. The hydrolysis of sucrose, isomaltose, palatinose (isomaltulose), and a 1,6-α-oligosaccharide (-isomalto-oligosaccharide) preparation, *J. Clin. Invest.* **42**:556 (1963).
71. Danks, D. M., J. Allan, and C. M. Anderson, A genetic study of fibrocystic disease of the pancreas, *Ann. Hum. Genet.* **28**:323 (1965).
72. Darrow, D. C., Congenital alkalosis with diarrhea, *J. Ped.* **26**:519 (1945).
73. Davidson, L. S. P., and J. R. Fountain, Incidence of sprue syndrome with some observations on natural history, *Brit. Med. J.* **1**:1157 (1950).
74. Davidson, M., E. H. Sobel, M. M. Kugler, and A. Prader, Intestinal lactase deficiency

of presumed congenital origin in two older children. (Abstract), *Gastroenterology* **46**:737 (1964).

75. Davidson, M., R. C. Burnstine, M. M. Kugler, and C. H. Bauer, Malabsorption defect induced by ingestion of beta-lactoglobulin, *J. Ped.* **66**:545 (1965).

76. Dawson, A. M., Malabsorption, *Abstr. World Med.* **38**:361 (1965).

76a. Dehaey,

77. Dent, C. E., and G. A. Rose, Aminoacid metabolism in cystinuria, *Quart. J. Med.* **20**:205 (1951).

78. Dicke, W. K., H. A. Weijers, and J. H. Van De Kamer, Coeliac disease. II. The presence in wheat of a factor having a deleterious effect in cases of coeliac disease, *Acta Paediat. (Uppsala)* **42**:34 (1953).

79. Dische, Z., P. A. di Sant'Agnese, C. Pallavicini, and J. Youlos, Composition of mucoprotein fractions from duodenal fluid of patients with cystic fibrosis of the pancreas and from controls, *Pediatrics* **24**:74 (1959).

80. Dische, Z., J. C. Pallavicini, N. Smirnow, and P. A. di Sant'Agnese, Abnormalities in composition of urinary nondialyzable glycoproteins in cystic fibrosis of pancreas (CFP). (Abstract), *Amer. J. Dis. Child.* **102**:733 (1961).

81. Dische, Z., C. Pallavicini, L. J. Cizek, and S. Chien, Changes in control of secretion of mucus glycoproteins as possible pathogenic factor in cystic fibrosis of pancreas, *Ann. N.Y. Acad. Sci.* **93**:526 (1962).

82. Dobbins, W. O., III, and C. E. Rubin, Studies of the rectal mucosa in celiac sprue, *Gastroenterology* **47**:471 (1964).

83. Dobbins, W. O., III, An ultrastructural study of the intestinal mucosa in congenital $\beta$-lipoprotein deficiency with particular emphasis upon the intestinal absorptive cell, *Gastroenterology* **50**:195 (1966).

84. Doell, R. G., and N. Kretchmer, Studies of small intestine during development. II. The intracellular location of intestinal $\beta$-galactosidase, *Biochim. Biophys. Acta* **67**:516 (1963).

85. Doershuk, C. F., L. W. Matthews, A. S. Tucker, and S. Spector, Evaluation of a prophylactic and therapeutic program for patients with cystic fibrosis, *Pediatrics* **36**:675 (1965).

86. Donaldson, R. M., Jr., I. L. Mackenzie, and J. S. Trier, Intrinsic factor-mediated attachment of vitamin $B_{12}$ to brush borders and microvillous membranes of hamster intestine, *J. Clin. Invest.* **46**:1215 (1967).

87. Donnison, A. B., H. Shwachman, and R. E. Gross, A review of 164 children with meconium ileus seen at the Children's Hospital Medical Center, Boston, *Pediatrics* **37**:833 (1966).

88. Drummond, K. N., A. F. Michael, R. A. Ulstrom, and R. A. Good, The blue diaper syndrome: familial hypercalcemia with nephrocalcinosis and indicanuria, *Amer. J. Med.* **37**:928 (1964).

89. Durand, P., Lattosuria idiopatica in una paziente con diarrhea cronica ed acidosi, *Minerva Pediat.* **10**:706 (1958).

90. Eggermont, E., and H. Loeb, Glucose-galactose intolerance (letter to the editor), *Lancet* **ii**:343 (1966).

91. Elian, E., H. Shwachman, and W. H. Hendren, Intestinal obstruction of the newborn infant. Usefulness of the sweat electrolyte test in differential diagnosis, *New Engl. J. Med.* **246**:13 (1961).

92. Emrich, H. M., E. Stoll, B. Friolet, J. P. Colombo, E. Rossi, and R. Richterich, Excretion of different substances in the sweat of children with cystic fibrosis and controls, *Mod. Probl. Pediat.* **10**:58 (1967).

93. Fällström, S. P., J. Winberg, and H. J. Andersen, Cow's milk-induced malabsorption as a precursor of gluten intolerance, *Acta Paed. Scand.* **54**:101 (1965).

94. Fanconi, G., E. Uehlinger, and C. Knauer, Das Coeliakie Syndrom bei angeborener zystischer Pankreasfibromatose und Bronchiektasien, *Wien. Med. Wschr.* **86**:753 (1936).

95. Farber, S., Some organic digestive disturbances in early life, *J. Mich. Med. Soc.* **44**:587 (1945).

96. Fernandes, J., J. H. Van De Kamer, and H. A. Weijers, Differences in absorption of the various fatty acids studied in children with steatorrhea, *J. Clin. Invest.* **41**:488 (1962).

97. Fischer, J. E., Effect of feeding a diet containing lactose upon β-D-galactosidase activity and organ development in the rat digestive tract, *Amer. J. Physiol.* **188**:49 (1957).

98. Fleisher, D. S., A. M. Di George, L. A. Barness, and D. Cornfeld, Hypoproteinemia and edema in infants with cystic fibrosis of the pancreas, *J. Ped.* **64**:341 (1964).

99. Fleisher, D. S., A. M. Di George, V. H. Auerbach, N. N. Huang, and L. A. Barness, Protein metabolism in cystic fibrosis of the pancreas, *J. Ped.* **64**:349 (1964).

100. Fox, M., S. Thier, L. Rosenberg, W. Kiser, and S. Segal, Evidence against single renal transport defect in cystinuria, *New Engl. J. Med.* **270**:556 (1964).

101. Frazer, A. C., Discussion on some problems of steatorrhoea and reduced stature, *Proc. Roy. Soc. Med.* **49**:1009 (1956).

102. Frazer, A. C., R. F. Fletcher, C. A. C. Ross, B. Shaw, H. G. Sammons, and R. Schneider, Gluten-induced enteropathy. The effect of partially digested gluten, *Lancet* **ii**:252 (1959).

103. Frazer, A. C., The present state of knowledge on the celiac syndrome, *J. Ped.* **57**:262 (1960).

104. Frézal, J., and J. Rey, L'intolérance à la β-lactoglobuline, *in: Journées pédiat.*, R. Debré, ed., Lanord, Paris (1964), p. 91.

105. Frézal, J., J. Rey, H. Jarlier, and M. Lamy, L'excrétion de l'acide formiminoglutamique (FIGLU) chez le nourrisson "normal" et dans les stéatorrhées par trouble de l'absorption intestinale, *Rev. Franc. Etudes Clin. Biol.* **9**:38 (1964).

106. Frézal, J., and J. Rey, Inborn errors of digestive enzymes, *in*: Proceedings of the Third International Congress of Human Genetics, Chicago, 1966, J. F. Crow and J. V. Neel, eds., The Johns Hopkins Press, Baltimore (1967), p. 153.

107. Frimpter, G. W., M. Horwith, E. Furth, R. E. Fellows, and D. O. Thompson, Inulin and endogenous amino acid renal clearances in cystinuria: evidence for tubular secretion, *J. Clin. Invest.* **41**:281 (1962).

108. Gamble, J. L., K. R. Fahey, J. Appleton, and E. MacLachlan, Congenital alkalosis with diarrhea, *J. Ped.* **26**:509 (1945).

108a. Gee, S., On the coeliac affection, *St. Bart's Hosp. J.* **24**:17 (1888).

109. Gerrard, J. W., C. A. C. Ross, R. Astley, J. M. French, and J. M. Smellie, Coeliac disease: is there a natural recovery?, *Quart. J Med.* **24**:23 (1955).

110. Gerrard, J. W., C. A. C. Ross, and J. M. Smellie, Coeliac disease. Results of late treatment with gluten-free wheat diet, *Lancet* **i**:587 (1955).

111. Ghadimi, H., M. Stern, and H. Shwachman, A study of the free amino acids in sweat from patients with cystic fibrosis, *Amer. J. Dis. Child.* **99**:333 (1960).

112. Gharib, R., H. A. Joos, and L. B. Hilty, Sweat chloride concentration. A comparative study in children with bronchial asthma and with cystic fibrosis, *Amer. J. Dis. Child.* **109**:66 (1965).

113. Gibbs, G. E., K. Reimer, R. L. Kollmorgen, and P. G. Young, Quantitative micro-

determination of enzymes in sweat gland. I. Alkaline phosphatase, acid phosphatase, adenosine triphosphatase, cholinesterases, and carbonic anhydrase in cystic fibrosis patients and controls, *Amer. J. Dis. Child.* **105**:249 (1963).

114. Gibbs, G. E., and K. Reimer, Quantitative microdetermination of enzymes in the sweat gland. II. Dehydrogenases in patients with cystic fibrosis and in control subjects, *J. Ped.* **65**:540 (1964).

115. Gibbs, G. E., K. Reimer, and J. Adams, Quantitative microdetermination of enzymes in sweat gland. IV. Phosphatidic acid cycle in cystic fibrosis, *Amer. J. Dis. Child.* **110**:81 (1965).

116. Gibbs, G. E., and K. Reimer, Quantitative microdetermination of enzymes in sweat gland. III. Succinic dehydrogenase in cystic fibrosis, *Proc. Soc. Expt. Biol.* **119**:470 (1965).

117. Gibson, L. E., and R. E. Cooke, A test for concentration of electrolytes in sweat in cystic fibrosis of the pancreas utilizing pilocarpine by iontophoresis, *Pediatrics* **23**:545 (1959).

118. Girardet, P., R. Richterich, and I. Antener, Adaptation de la lactase intestinale à l'administration de lactose chez le rat adulte, *Helv. Physiol. Pharmacol. Acta* **22**:7 (1964).

119. Gochberg, S. H., and R. E. Cooke, Physiology of the sweat gland in cystic fibrosis of the pancreas, *Pediatrics* **18**:701 (1956).

120. Goldbloom, R. B., and P. Sekelj, Cystic fibrosis of the pancreas. Diagnosis by application of a sodium electrode to the skin, *New Engl. J. Med.* **269**:1349 (1963).

121. Goodman, H. O., and S. C. Reed, Heredity of fibrosis of the pancreas. Possible mutation rate of the gene, *Amer. J. Hum. Genet.* **4**:59 (1952).

122. Gordon, R. S., Jr., and G. W. Cage, Mechanism of water and electrolyte secretion by eccrine sweat gland, *Lancet* **1**:1246 (1966).

123. Gough, K. R., A. E. Read, and J. M. Naish, Intestinal reticulosis as a complication of idiopathic steatorrhoea, *Gut* **3**:232 (1962).

124. Grand, R. J., P. A. di Sant'Agnese, R. C. Talamo, and J. C. Pallavicini, The effects of exogenous aldosterone on sweat electrolytes. II. Patients with cystic fibrosis of the pancreas, *J. Ped.* **70**:357 (1967).

125. Gräsbeck, R., R. Gordin, I. Kantero, and B. Kuhlbach, Selective vitamin $B_{12}$ malabsorption and proteinuria in young people A syndrome, *Acta Med. Scand.* **167**:289 (1960).

126. Gräsbeck, R., and G. Kvist, La malabsorption congénitale et sélective de la vitamine $B_{12}$ avec protéinurie, *Europ. Med.* **1967**(3):3.

127. Gray, G. M., and F. J. Ingelfinger, Intestinal absorption of sucrose in man: interrelation of hydrolysis and monosaccharide product absorption, *J. Clin. Invest.* **45**:388 (1966).

128. Gray, G. M., and N. A. Santiago, Disaccharide absorption in normal and diseased human intestine, *Gastroenterology* **51**:489 (1966).

129. de Groot, A. P., and P. Hoogendoorn, The detrimental effect of lactose. II. Quantitative lactase determinations in various mammals, *Neth. Milk Dairy J.* **11**:290 (1957).

130. Grüttner, R., R. Mellin, and F. Bramstedt, Untersuchungen über das Auftreten von Serumpeptiden bei der Cöliakie, *Klin. Wschr.* **37**:237 (1959).

131. Gugler, E., J. C. Pallavicini, H. Swerdlow, and P. A. di Sant'Agnese, The role of calcium in submaxillary saliva of patients with cystic fibrosis, *J. Ped.* **71**:585 (1967).

131a. Hadorn, B., M. J. Tarlow, J. K. Lloyd, and O. H. Wolff, Intestinal enterokinase deficiency, *Lancet* **i**:812.

132. Hallett, W. Y., A. G. Knudson, Jr., and F. J. Massey, Jr., Absence of detrimental effect of the carrier state for cystic fibrosis gene, *Amer. Rev. Resp. Dis.* **92**:714 (1965).

133. Harris, H., U. Mittwoch, E. B. Robson, and F. L. Warren, Phenotypes and genotypes in cystinuria, *Ann. Hum. Genet.* **20**:57 (1955).
134. Harris, O. D., W. T. Cooke, H. Thompson, and J. A. H. Waterhouse, Malignancy in adult coeliac disease and idiopathic steatorrhoea, *Amer. J. Med.* **42**:899 (1967).
135. Heiner, D. C., M. E. Lahey, J. F. Wilson, J. W. Gerrard, H. Shwachman, and K. T. Khaw, Precipitins to antigens of wheat and cow's milk in celiac disease, *J. Ped.* **61**:813 (1962).
136. Hermans, P. E., K. A. Huizenga, H. N. Hoffman, A. L. Brown, Jr., and H. Markowitz, Dysgammaglobulinemia associated with nodular lymphoid hyperplasia of the small intestine, *Amer. J. Med.* **40**:78 (1966).
137. Hobbs, J. R., Immune imbalance in dysgammaglobulinaemia type IV, *Lancet* i:110 (1968).
138. Hobbs, J. R., and G. W. Hepner, Deficiency of $\gamma_M$-globulin in coeliac disease, *Lancet* i:217 (1968).
139. Hoffman, H. N., II, E. E. Wollaeger, and E. Greenberg, Discordance for nontropical sprue (adult celiac disease) in a monozygotic twin pair, *Gastroenterology* **51**:36 (1966).
140. Holsclaw, D. S., H. B. Eckstein, and H. H. Nixon, Meconium ileus; a 20-year review of 109 cases, *Amer. J. Dis. Child.* **109**:101 (1965).
141. Holzel, A., V. Schwarz, and K. W. Sutcliffe, Defective lactose absorption causing malnutrition in infancy, *Lancet* i:1126 (1959).
142. Hooft, C., P. de Laey, J. Timmermans, and J. Snoeck, La maladie de Hartnup, *Acta Paediat. Belg.* **16**:281 (1962).
143. Hooft, C., J. Timmermans, J. Snoeck, I. Antener, W. Oyaert, and C. van den Hende, Methionine malabsorption syndrome, *Ann. Paediat. (Basel)* **205**:73 (1965).
144. Hsia, D. Y. Y., M. Makler, G. Semenza, and A. Prader, $\beta$-galactosidase activity in human intestinal lactases, *Biochim. Biophys. Acta* **113**:390 (1966).
145. Huang, S. S., and T. M. Bayless, Lactose intolerance in healthy children, *New Engl. J. Med.* **276**:1283 (1967).
146. Huizenga, K. A., E. E. Wollaeger, P. A. Green, and B. F. McKenzie, Serum globulin deficiencies in nontropical sprue, with report of two cases of acquired agammaglobulinemia, *Amer. J. Med.* **31**:572 (1961).
147. Imerslund, O., Idiopathie chronic megaloblastic anemia in children, *Acta Paediat. (Uppsala)* **49**(suppl. 119) (1960).
148. Immonen, P., K. Kouvalainen, and J. K. Visakorpi, The immunoelectrophoretic gamma-A-globulin in malabsorption, *Ann. Paediat. (Basel)* **207**:269 (1966).
149. Immonen, P., Levels of the serum immunoglobulins $\gamma_A$, $\gamma_G$, and $\gamma_M$ in the malabsorption syndrome in children, *Ann. Paediat. Fenn.* **13**:115 (1967).
150. Isselbacher, K. J., R. Scheig, G. R. Plotkin, and J. B. Caufield, Congenital $\beta$-lipoprotein deficiency: an hereditary disorder involving a defect in the absorption and transport of lipids, *Medicine* **43**:347 (1964).
151. Jansen, W., G. S. Que, and W. Veeger, Primary combined saccharase and isomaltase deficiency. Report of two adult siblings of consanguineous parentage, *Arch. Intern. Med.* **116**:879 (1965).
152. Jeffries, G. H., E. Weser, and M. H. Sleisenger, Malabsorption, *Gastroenterology* **46**:434 (1964).
153. Jeune, M., M. Hermier, D. Germain, C. Collombel, M. Mathieu, H. Duc, and B. Ponson, L'insuffisance pancréatique externe avec insuffisance médullaire hématopoiétique chez le nourrisson et l'enfant. "Syndrome de Shwachman," *Pédiatrie* **22**:551 (1967).

154. Jeune, M., M. Hermier, E. Hartemann, B. Loras, F. Haour, J. B. Cotton, and C. Collombel, Diarrhée chlorée congénitale avec alcalose métabolique, *Pédiatrie* **22**:663 (1967).
155. Johansen, P. G., Some observations on mucous secretions in cystic fibrosis of the pancreas, *Ann. N.Y. Acad. Sci.* **106**:755 (1963).
156. Johansen, P. G., Physicochemical investigations on two unusual sialic acid-rich mucoids from the intestinal tract of patients with fibrocystic disease of the pancreas, *Biochem. J.* **87**:63 (1963).
157. Jones, J. W., and P. Ways, Abnormalities of high-density lipoproteins in abetalipoproteinemia, *J. Clin. Invest.* **46**:1151 (1967).
158. Jos, J., J. Frézal, J. Rey, and M. Lamy, Etude histochimique de la muqueuse duodénojéjunale dans la maladie coeliaque, *Pediat. Res.* **1**:27 (1967).
159. Jos, J., J. Rey, J. Frézal, C. Nézelof, and M. Lamy, La biopsie intestinale chez l'enfant. Acquisitions récentes, *Arch. Franc. Pédiat.* **24**:1159 (1967).
160. Jupilet, M., Gliadine et maladie coeliaque. Contribution à l'étude des gliadines. Rapports avec la maladie coeliaque de l'enfant, Thèse de Doctorat en pharmacie, Lille, 1962.
161. Karlish, A. J., and A. L. Tarnoky, Mucoviscidosis and chronic lung disease, *Proc. Roy. Soc. Med.* **54**:980 (1961).
162. Kayden, H. J., and R. Silber, The role of vitamin E deficiency in the abnormal autohemolysis of acanthocytosis, *Trans. Ass. Amer. Phys.* **78**:334 (1965).
163. Kekomäki, M., J. K. Visakorpi, J. Perheentupa, and L. Saxén, Familial protein intolerance with deficient transport of basic amino acids. An analysis of 10 patients, *Acta Paed. Scand.* **56**:617 (1967).
164. Kelsey, W. M., Congenital alkalosis with diarrhea, *Amer. J. Dis. Child.* **88**:344 (1954).
165. Kerry, K. R., and R. R. W. Townley, Genetic aspects of intestinal sucrase-isomaltase deficiency, *Aust. Paediat.* **1**:223 (1965).
166. Knudson, A. G., Jr., L. Wayne, and W. Y. Hallett, On the selective advantage of cystic fibrosis heterozygotes, *Amer. J. Hum. Genet.* **19**:388 (1967).
167. Koldovsky, O., R. Noack, G. Schenk, V. Jirsova, A. Heringova, H. Brana, F. Chytil, and M. Fridrich, Activity of $\beta$-galactosidase in homogenates and isolated microvilli fraction of jejunal mucosa from suckling rats, *Biochem. J.* **96**:492 (1965).
168. Kopito, L., A. Mahmoodian, R. R. W. Townley, K. T. Khaw, and H. Shwachman, Studies in cystic fibrosis. Analysis of nail clippings for sodium and potassium, *New Engl. J. Med.* **272**:504 (1965).
169. Kowlessar, O. D., and M. H. Sleisenger, The role of gliadin in the pathogenesis of adult celiac disease. (Editorial), *Gastroenterology* **44**:357 (1963).
170. Kramm, E. R., M. M. Crane, M. G. Sirken, and M. L. Brown, A cystic fibrosis pilot survey in three New England states, *Amer. J. Public Health* **52**:2041 (1962).
171. Krainick, H. G., F. Debatin, E. Gautier, R. Tobler, and J. A. Velasco, Weitere Untersuchungen über den schädlichen Weizenmehleffekt bei der Cöliakie. 1. Die akute Gliadinreaktion (Gliadinschock), *Helv. Paed. Acta* **13**:432 (1958).
172. Krainick, H. G., and G. Mohn, Weitere Untersuchungen über den schädlichen Weizenmehleffekt bei der Cöliakie. 2. Die Wirkung der enzymatischen Abbauprodukte des Gliadin, *Helv. Paed. Acta* **14**:124 (1959).
173. Kuitunen, P., J. K. Visakorpi, and N. Hallman, Histopathology of duodenal mucosa in malabsorption syndrome induced by cow's milk, *Ann. Paediat. (Basel)* **205**:54 (1965).
174. Kuo, P. T., and N. N. Huang, The effect of medium-chain triglyceride upon fat absorption and plasma lipid and depot fat of children with cystic fibrosis of the pancreas, *J. Clin. Invest.* **44**:1924 (1965).

175. de Laey, P., C. Hooft, J. Timmermans, and J. Snoeck, Biochemical aspects of the Hartnup disease. I. Results of intravenous and oral tryptophan loading tests in a case of Hartnup disease, *Ann. Paediat. (Basel)* **202**:145 (1964).

176. Lalande, J. A., J. Frézal, J. Rey, M. Lamy, B. N Halpern, and N. T. Ky, Etude immunologique de la maladie coeliaque et de l'intolérance au lait de vache chez l'enfant (A propos de 35 cas), *Méd. et Hyg. (Genève)* **24**:51 (1966).

177. Lamy, M., J. Frézal, J. Polonovski, and J. Rey, L'absence congénitale de β-lipoprotéines, *Compt. Rend. Soc. Biol. (Paris)* **154**:1974 (1960).

178. Lamy, M., F. Besançon, A. Loverdo, and F. Afifi, La malabsorption spécifique de la vitamine $B_{12}$ avec protéinurie. L'anémie mégaloblastique d'Imerslund–Najman–Grasbeck. Etude de quatre cas, *Arch. Franc. Pédiat.* **18**:1109 (1961).

179. Lamy, M., J. Frézal, J. Polonovski, G. Druez, and J. Rey, Congenital absence of beta-lipoproteins, *Pediatrics* **31**:277 (1963).

180. Lamy, M., J. Frézal, and J. Rey, with the collaboration of C. Nézelof, M. Fortier-Beaulieu, and J. Jos, Les stéatorrhées par troubles de l'absorption intestinale, Rapport au XIXe Congrès des Pédiatres de Langue Française, Expansion, Paris (1963), Vol. I, p. 160.

181. Lamy, M., C. Nézelof, J. Jos, J. Frézal, and J. Rey, La biopsie de la muqueuse intestinale chez l'enfant. Premiers résultats d'une étude des syndromes de malabsorption, *Presse méd.* **71**:1267 (1963).

181a. Lamy, M., J. Frézal, J. Rey, J. Jos, C. Nézelof, A. Herrault, and J. Cohen-Salal, Diarrhée chronique par trouble du transfert intra-cellulaire des lipides, *Arch. Franc. Pédiat.* **24**:1079 (1967).

182. Lamy, M., P. Royer, J. Frézal, and J. Rey, Maladies Héréditaires du Métabolisme chez l'Enfant, Masson, Paris (1968), 2nd ed.

183. Laplane, R., C. Polonovski, M. Etienne, P. Debray, J.-C. Lods, and B. Pissarro, L'intolérance aux sucres à transfert intestinal actif (ses rapports avec l'intolérance au lactose et le syndrôme coeliaque), *Arch. Franc. Pédiat.* **19**:895 (1962).

184. Launiala, K., P. Kuitunen, and J. K. Visakorpi, Disaccharidases and histology of duodenal mucosa in congenital lactose malabsorption, *Acta Paed. Scand.* **55**:257 (1966).

185. Launiala, K., Intestinal β-galactosidase and β-glucosidase activities in congenital and acquired lactose malabsorption, *Scand. J. Clin. Lab. Invest.* **19**(suppl. 95):69 (1967).

186. Lee, F. D., Nature of the mucosal changes associated with malignant neoplasms in the small intestine, *Gut* **7**:361 (1966).

187. Lees, R. S., Presence of B-protein (apoprotein of β-lipoprotein) in normal plasma and in abetalipoproteinemia. (Abstract), *J. Clin. Invest.* **46**:1083 (1967).

188. Le Tan, V., D. Alagille, J. Penot, and M. Lelong, Les cirrhoses biliaires avec concrétions de la maladie fibro-kystique du pancréas, *Rev. Int. Hépat.* **9**:111 (1959).

189. Levy, R. I., D. S. Fredrickson, and L. Laster, The lipoproteins and lipid transport in abetalipoproteinemia, *J. Clin. Invest.* **45**:531 (1966).

190. Lifshitz, F., Congenital lactase deficiency, *J. Ped.* **69**:229 (1966).

191. Lillibridge, C. B., L. L. Brandborg, and C. E. Rubin, Childhood pernicious anemia. Gastrointestinal secretory and electron microscopic aspects, *Gastroenterology* **52**:792 (1967).

192. Lindberg, T., Dipeptidase activity in small intestinal mucosa in patients with gluten-induced enteropathy. (Abstract), *Acta Paed. Scand.* **1967**(suppl. 177):23.

193. Lindquist, B., and G. W. Meeuwisse, Chronic diarrhoea caused by monosaccharide malabsorption, *Acta Paediat.* **51**:674 (1962).

194. Lindquist, B., and G. W. Meeuwisse, Intestinal transport of monosaccharides in generalized and selective malabsorption, *Acta Paediat.* **1963**(suppl. 146):110.

195. Lindquist, B., G. Meeuwisse, and K. Melin, Osmotic diarrhoea in genetically transmitted glucose-galactose malabsorption, *Acta Paediat.* **52**:217 (1963).

196. Lindquist, B., Blockage of active transport of glucose, *in*: Group panel discussions, XIe Congrès Intern. de Pédiatrie, Tokio, 1965, The University of Tokio Press, p. 85.

197. Lobeck, C. C., and D. Huebner, The importance of age and rate of sweating in the evaluation of sweat test results. (Abstract), *Amer. J. Dis. Child.* **102**:488 (1961).

198. Lobeck, C. C., and D. Huebner, Effect of age, sex, and cystic fibrosis on the sodium and potassium content of human sweat, *Pediatrics* **30**:172 (1962).

199. Lobeck, C. C., and N. R. McSherry, Response of sweat electrolyte concentrations to 9 alpha-fluorohydrocortisone in patients with cystic fibrosis and their families, *J. Ped.* **62**:393 (1963).

200. Lowe, C. U., C. D. May, and S. C. Reed, Fibrosis of the pancreas in infants and children. A statistical study of clinical and hereditary features, *Amer. J. Dis. Child.* **78**:349 (1949).

201. Lowe, C. U., and C. D. May, Selective pancreatic deficiency: absent amylase, diminished trypsin, and normal lipase, *Amer. J. Dis. Child.* **82**:459 (1951).

202. Lowe, C. U., W. Adler, O. Broberger, J. Walsh, and E. Neter, Mucopolysaccharide from patients with cystic fibrosis of pancreas, *Science* **153**:1124 (1966).

203. Luhby, A. L., F. J. Eagle, E. Roth, and J. M. Cooperman, Relapsing megaloblastic anemia in an infant due to a specific in gastrointestinal absorption of folic acid. (Abstract), *Amer. J. Dis. Child.* **102**:482 (1961).

204. Mabry, C. C., A. M. Di George, and V. H. Auerbach, Studies concerning the defect in a patient with acanthrocytosis, *Clin. Res.* **8**:371 (1960).

205. MacDonald, W. C., W. O. Dobbins, III, and C. E. Rubin, Studies of the familial nature of celiac sprue using biopsy of the small intestine, *New Engl. J. Med.* **272**:448 (1965).

206. Malik, G. B., W. C. Watson, D. Murray, and B. Cruickshank, Immunofluorescent antibody studies in idiopathic steatorrhoea, *Lancet* **i**:1127 (1964).

207. Mandel, I. D., R. H. Thompson, Jr., S. Wotman, M. Taubman, A. H. Kutscher, E. V. Zegarelli, C. R. Denning, J. T. Botwick, and B. S. Fahn, Parotid saliva in cystic fibrosis. II. Electrolytes and protein-bound carbohydrates, *Amer. J. Dis. Child.* **110**:646 (1965).

208. Marmar, J., G. J. Barbero, and M. S. Sibinga, The pattern of parotid gland secretion in cystic fibrosis of the pancreas, *Gastroenterology* **50**:551 (1966).

209. Maxfield, M., and W. Wolins, A molecular abnormality of urinary mucoprotein in cystic fibrosis of the pancreas, *J. Clin. Invest.* **41**:455 (1962).

210. McCarthy, C. F., W. I. Austad, and A. E. A. Read, Hypogammaglobulinemia and steatorrhea, *Amer. J. Dig. Dis.* **32**:945 (1965).

211. McKendrick, T., Sweat sodium levels in normal subjects, in fibrocystic patients and their relatives, and in chronic bronchitic patients, *Lancet* **i**:183 (1962).

212. McKusick, V. A., R. Eldridge, J. A. Hostetler, V. Ruangwit, and J. A. Egeland, Dwarfism in the Amish. II. Cartilage-hair hypoplasia, *Bull. Johns Hopkins Hosp.* **116**:285 (1965).

213. McMichael, H. B., J. Webb, and A. M. Dawson, Jejunal disaccharidases and some observations on the cause of lactase deficiency, *Brit. Med. J.* **2**:1037 (1966).

214. McMichael, H. B., J. Webb, and A. M. Dawson, The absorption of maltose and lactose in man, *Clin. Sci.* **33**:135 (1967).

215. Meeuwisse, G., and A. Dahlqvist, Glucose-galactose malabsorption. (Letter to the editor), *Lancet* **ii**:858 (1966).

216. Merritt, A. D., B. L. Hanna, C. M. Todd, and T. L. Myers, Incidence and mode of inheritance of cystic fibrosis. (Abstract), *J. Lab. Clin. Med.* **60**:998 (1962).

217. Messer, M., C. M. Anderson, and R. R. W. Townley, Peptidase activity of biopsies of the duodenal mucosa of children with and without coeliac disease, *Clin. Chim. Acta* 6:768 (1961).
218. Messer, M., C. M. Anderson, and L. Hubbard, Studies on the mechanism of destruction of the toxic action of wheat gluten in coeliac disease by crude papain, *Gut* 5:295 (1964).
219. Messer, M., and M. Ottesen, Isolation and properties of glutamine cyclotransferase of dried papaya latex, *Biochim. Biophys. Acta* 92:409 (1964).
220. Milne, M. D., M. A. Crawford, C. B. Girao, and L. W. Loughridge, The metabolic disorder in Hartnup disease, *Quart. J. Med.* 29:407 (1960).
221. Morris, M. D., and D. A. Fisher, Trypsinogen deficiency disease, *Amer. J. Dis. Child.* 114:203 (1967).
222. Mozziconacci, P., J. Boisse, C. Attal, Pham-Huu-Trung, D. Guy-Grand, and C. Griscelli, Hypoplasie du pancreas exocrine avec troubles hématologiques. Absence de cellules A dans les îlots de Langerhans, *Arch. Franc. Pédiat.* 24:741 (1967).
223. Munger, B. L., S. W. Brusilow, and R. E. Cooke, An electron microscope study of eccrine sweat glands in patients with cystic fibrosis of the pancreas, *J. Ped.* 59:497 (1961).
224. Neale, G., M. L. Clark, and B. Levin, Intestinal sucrase deficiency presenting as sucrose intolerance in adult life, *Brit. Med. J.* ii:1223 (1965).
225. Nézelof, C., and M. Watchi, L'hypoplasie congénitale lipomateuse du pancréas exocrine chez l'enfant, *Arch. Franc. Pédiat.* 18:1136 (1961).
226. Nordio, S., C. Borrone, A. G. Marchi, and G. Vignola, The immunoglobulins of intestinal mucosa of children in celiac disease and other pathological conditions, *Helv. Paed. Acta* 22:320 (1967).
227. Nusslé, D., and E. Gautier, Malabsorption congénitale du glucose et du galactose, *Helv. Paed. Acta*, to be published.
228. Orzalesi, M. M., D. Kohner, C. D. Cook, and H. Shwachman, Anamnesis, sweat electrolyte and pulmonary function studies in parents of patients with cystic fibrosis of the pancreas, *Acta Paediat.* 52:267 (1963).
229. Owen, G. M., Metabolic alkalosis with diarrhea and chloride-free urine, *J. Ped.* 65:849 (1964).
230. Oyanagi, K., M. Takagi, M. Kitabatake, and T. Nakao, Hartnup disease, *Tohoku J. Exp. Med.* 91:383 (1967).
231. Ozsoylu, S., and G. Argun, Tryptic activity of the duodenal juice in aplastic anemia, *J. Ped.* 70:60 (1967).
232. Padykula, H. A., E. W. Strauss, A. J. Ladman, and F. H. Gardner, A morphologic and histochemical analysis of the human jejunal epithelium in nontropical sprue, *Gastroenterology* 40:735 (1961).
233. Pallavicini, J. C., O. Gabriel, P. A. di Sant'Agnese, and E. R. Buskirk, Isolation and characterization of carbohydrate-protein complexes from human sweat, *Ann. N.Y. Acad. Sci.* 106:330 (1963).
234. Parkins, R. A., The metabolic activity of human small intestinal biopsies in health and celiac sprue. The effect of wheat gliadin, *Gastroenterology* 51:345 (1966).
235. Pasternack, A., J. Perheentupa, K. Launiala, and N. Hallman, Kidney biopsy findings in familial chloride diarrhoea, *Acta Endocr. (Kbh.)* 55:1 (1967).
236. Pelkonen, R., M. Siurala, and P. Vuopio, Inherited agammaglobulinemia with malabsorption and marked alterations in the gastrointestinal mucosa, *Acta Med. Scand.* 173:549 (1963).
237. Perheentupa, J., J. Eklund, and N. Kojo, Familial chloride diarrhoea ("congenital alkalosis with diarrhoea"), *Acta Paed. Scand.* 1965(*suppl.* 159):119.
238. Perheentupa, J., and J. K. Visakorpi, Protein intolerance with deficient transport

of basic aminoacids. Another inborn error of metabolism, *Lancet* **ii**:813 (1965).

239. Peterson, R. D. A., and R. A. Good, Antibodies to cow's milk proteins—their presence and significance, *Pediatrics* **31**:209 (1963).

240. Phillips, G. B., Quantitative chromatographic analysis of plasma and red blood cell lipids in patients with acanthocytosis, *J. Lab. Clin. Med.* **59**:357 (1962).

241. Phillips, G. B., and J. T. Dodge, Evidence for essential fatty acid deficiency in patients with abetalipoproteinemia. (Abstract), *J. Clin. Invest.* **46**:1104 (1967).

242. Pittman, F. E., and J. C. Pittman, A light and electron microscopic study of sigmoid colonic mucosa in adult celiac disease, *Scand. J. Gastroent.* **1**:21 (1966).

243. Pittman, F. E., and R. J. Pollitt, Studies of jejunal mucosal digestion of peptic-tryptic digests of wheat protein in coeliac disease, *Gut* **7**:368 (1966).

244. Playoust, M. R., and K. J. Isselbacher, Studies on the intestinal absorption and intramucosal lipolysis of a medium-chain triglyceride, *J. Clin. Invest.* **43**:878 (1964).

245. Pokorná, M., J. Šourek, and J. Švejcar, Die Bedeutung der Präzipitine gegenüber Gliadin im Serum von Kindern mit Cöliakie, *Helv. Paed. Acta* **18**:393 (1963).

245a. Polonovski, C., B. Hadorn, and H. Bier, unpublished observations.

246. Potter, J. L., L. W. Matthews, J. Lemm, and S. Spector, Human pulmonary secretions in health and disease, *Ann. N.Y. Acad. Sci.* **106**:692 (1963).

247. Prader, A., S. Auricchio, and G. Mürset, Durchfall infolge hereditären Mangels an intestinaler Saccharaseaktivität (Saccharoseintoleranz), *Schweiz. Med. Wschr.* **91**:465 (1961).

248. Prader, A., and S. Auricchio, Defects of intestinal disaccharide absorption, *Ann. Rev. Med.* **16**:345 (1965).

249. Rey, J., J. Frézal, J. Jos, P. Bauche, and M. Lamy, Diarrhée par trouble de l'hydrolyse intestinale du saccharose, du maltose et de l'isomaltose, *Arch. Franc. Pédiat.* **20**:381 (1963).

250. Rey, J., J. Frézal, J. Polonovski, and M. Lamy, Modifications des lipides plasmatiques dans les troubles de l'absorption intestinale chez l'enfant, *Rev. Franc. Etudes Clin. Biol.* **10**:488 (1965).

251. Rey, J., J. Frézal, P. Royer, and M. Lamy, L'absence congénitale de lipase pancréatique, *Arch. Franc. Pédiat.* **23**:5 (1966).

252. Rey, J., and J. Frézal, Les anomalies des disaccharidases, *Arch. Franc. Pédiat.* **24**:65 (1967).

253. Rey, J., J. Frézal, and M. Lamy, Influence of an oil containing equal amounts of six fatty acids on the composition of fecal lipids in cystic fibrosis, *Mod. Probl. Pediat.* **10**:269 (1967).

254. Riecken, E. O., J. S. Stewart, C. C. Booth, and A. G. E. Pearse, A histochemical study on the role of lysosomal enzymes in idiopathic steatorrhoea before and during a gluten-free diet, *Gut* **7**:317 (1966).

255. Riggs, L. K., and A. Beaty, Some unique properties of lactose as a dietary carbohydrate, *J. Dairy Sci.* **30**:939 (1947).

256. Roberts, G. B. S., Fundamental defect in fibrocystic disease of the pancreas, *Lancet* **ii**:964 (1959).

257. Roberts, G. B. S., Familial incidence of fibrocystic disease of the pancreas, *Ann. Hum. Genet.* **24**:127 (1960).

258. Roelfs, R. E., G. E. Gibbs, and G. D. Griffin, The composition of rectal mucus in cystic fibrosis, *Amer. J. Dis. Child.* **113**:419 (1967).

259. van Roon, J. H., and A. J. C. Haex, Clinical and biochemical analysis of gluten-toxicity—No. II. Clinical experiments on patients suffering from idiopathic steatorrhoea after the administration of bromine-treated performic acid oxidized polypeptides originating from wheat gluten, *Gastroenterologia (Basel)* **94**:227 (1960).

260. Rosen, F. S., and C. A. Janeway, The gamma globulins. III. The antibody deficiency syndromes, *New Engl. J. Med.* **275**:709 (1966).
261. Rosenberg, L. E., S. J. Downing, and S. Segal, Competitive inhibition of dibasic aminoacid transport in rat kidney, *J. Biol. Chem.* **237**:2265 (1962).
262. Rosenberg, L. E., J. L. Durant, and J. M. Holland, Intestinal absorption and renal excretion of cystine and cysteine in cystinuria, *New Engl. J. Med.* **273**:1239 (1965).
263. Rosenberg, L. E., Cystinuria: genetic heterogeneity and allelism, *Science* **154**:1341 (1966).
264. Rosenberg, L. E., S. Downing, J. L. Durant, and S. Segal, Cystinuria: biochemical evidence for three genetically distinct diseases, *J. Clin. Invest.* **45**:365 (1966).
265. Rosenberg, L. E., I. Albrecht, and S. Segal, Lysine transport in human kidney: evidence for two systems, *Science* **155**:1426 (1967).
266. Rosenberg, L. E., J. C. Crawhall, and S. Segal, Intestinal transport of cystine and cysteine in man: evidence for separate mechanisms, *J. Clin. Invest.* **46**:30 (1967).
267. Ross, C. A. C., A. C. Frazer, J. M. French, J. W. Gerrard, H. G. Sammons, and J. M. Smellie, Coeliac disease. The relative importance of wheat gluten, *Lancet* i:1087 (1955).
268. Roy, C., J. Lalande, J. Frézal, J. Rey, M. Lamy, and B. Halpern, Etude immunologique de la maladie coeliaque (à propos de 38 cas), *Path. Biol.* **15**:384 (1967).
269. Rubin, C. E., L. L. Brandborg, P. C. Phelps, and H. C. Taylor, Jr., Studies of celiac disease. I. The apparent identical and specific nature of the duodenal and proximal jejunal lesion in celiac disease and idiopathic sprue, *Gastroenterology* **38**:28 (1960).
270. Rubin, C. E., Malabsorption: celiac sprue, *Ann. Rev. Med.* **12**:39 (1961).
271. Rubin, C. E., L. L. Brandborg, A. L. Flick, P. Phelps, C. Parmentier, and S. Van Niel, Studies of celiac sprue. III. The effect of repeated wheat instillation into the proximal ileum of patients on a gluten-free diet, *Gastroenterology* **43**:621 (1962).
272. Rubin, C. E., L. L. Brandborg, A. L. Flick, W. C. MacDonald, R. A. Parkins, C. M. Parmentier, P. Phelps, S. Sribhibhadh, and J. S. Trier, Biopsy studies on the pathogenesis of coeliac sprue, in: Intestinal Biopsy. Ciba Foundation Study Group No. 14, G. E. W. Wolstenholme and M. P. Cameron, eds., Churchill, London (1962), p. 67.
273. Rubin, C. E., and W. O. Dobbins, III, Peroral biopsy of the small intestine. A review of its diagnostic usefulness, *Gastroenterology* **49**:676 (1965).
274. Rubin, W., A. S. Fauci, M. H. Sleisenger, and G. H. Jeffries, Immunofluorescent studies in adult celiac disease, *J. Clin. Invest.* **44**:475 (1965).
275. Rubino, A., unpublished data.
276. Ruffin, J. M., S. M. Kurtz, J. L. Borland, Jr., C. R. W. Bain, and W. M. Roufail, Gluten-free diet for nontropical sprue. Immediate and prolonged effects, *J. Amer. Med. Ass.* **188**:162 (1964).
277. Sabesin, S. M., and K. J. Isselbacher, Protein synthesis inhibition: mechanism for the production of impaired fat absorption, *Science* **147**:1149 (1965).
278. Salt, H. B., O. H. Wolff, J. K. Lloyd, A. S. Fosbrooke, A. H. Cameron, and D. V. Hubble, On having no beta-lipoprotein. A syndrome comprising A-beta-lipoproteinaemia, acanthocytosis, and steatorrhoea, *Lancet* ii:325 (1960).
279. Samloff, I. M., J. S. Davis, and E. A. Schenk, A clinical and histochemical study of celiac disease before and during a gluten-free diet, *Gastroenterology* **48**:155 (1965).
280. di Sant'Agnese, P. A., R. C. Darling, G. A. Perera, and E. Shea, Abnormal electrolyte composition of sweat in cystic fibrosis of the pancreas. Clinical significance and relationship to the disease, *Pediatrics* **12**:549 (1953).
281. di Sant'Agnese, P. A., Fibrocystic disease of the pancreas with normal or partial pancreatic function. Current views on pathogenesis and diagnosis, *Pediatrics* **15**:683 (1955).

282. di Sant'Agnese, P. A., and W. A. Blanc, A distinctive type of biliary cirrhosis of the liver associated with cystic fibrosis of the pancreas. Recognition through signs of portal hypertension, *Pediatrics* **16**:387 (1956).

283. di Sant'Agnese, P. A., Z. Dische, and A. Danilczenko, Physicochemical differences of mucoproteins in duodenal fluid of patients with cystic fibrosis of the pancreas and controls. Clinical aspects, *Pediatrics* **19**:252 (1957).

284. di Sant'Agnese, P. A., and R. C. Talamo, Pathogenesis and physiopathology of cystic fibrosis of the pancreas. Fibrocystic disease of the pancreas (mucoviscidosis), *New Engl. J. Med.* **277**:1287, 1344, 1399 (1967).

285. Saperstein, S., D. W. Anderson, Jr., A. S. Goldman, and W. T. Kniker, Milk allergy. III. Immunological studies with sera from allergic and normal children, *Pediatrics* **32**:580 (1963).

286. Schenk, E. A., I. M. Samloff, and F. A. Klipstein, Pathogenesis of jejunal mucosal alterations: synechia formation, *Amer. J. Path.* **50**:523 (1967).

287. Schneider, A. J., W. B. Kinter, and C. E. Stirling, Glucose-galactose malabsorption. Report of a case with autoradiographic studies of a mucosal biopsy, *New Engl. J. Med.* **274**:305 (1966).

288. Schultz, I. J., and G. Peter, Micropuncture studies of the abnormality in sweat formation in cystic fibrosis (CF). (Abstract), *Fed. Proc.* **26**:287 (1967).

289. Scriver, C. R., Hartnup disease. A genetic modification of intestinal and renal transport of certain neutral alpha-aminoacids, *New Engl. J. Med.* **273**:530 (1965).

290. Scriver, C. R., and O. H. Wilson, Amino acid transport: evidence for genetic control of two types in human kidney, *Science* **155**:1428 (1967).

291. Seakins, J. W. T., and R. S. Ersser, Effects of amino acid loads on a healthy infant with the biochemical features of Hartnup disease, *Arch. Dis. Childh.* **42**:682 (1967).

292. Selander, P., The frequency of cystic fibrosis of the pancreas in Sweden, *Acta Paediat.* **51**:65 (1962).

293. Semenza, G., S. Auricchio, and A. Rubino, Multiplicity of human intestinal disaccharidases. I. Chromatographic separation of maltases and of two lactases, *Biochim. Biophys. Acta* **96**:487 (1965).

294. Semenza, G., S. Auricchio, A. Rubino, A. Prader, and J. D. Welsh, Lack of some intestinal maltases in a human disease transmitted by a single genetic factor, *Biochim. Biophys. Acta* **105**:386 (1965).

295. Sheldon, W., Celiac disease, *Pediatrics* **23**:132 (1959).

296. Sheldon, W., Congenital pancreatic lipase deficiency, *Arch. Dis. Childh.* **39**:268 (1964).

297. Sheldon, W., and E. Tempany, Small intestine peroral biopsy in coeliac children, *Gut* **7**:481 (1966).

298. Shiner, M., and I. Doniach, Histopathologic studies in steatorrhea, *Gastroenterology* **38**:419 (1960).

299. Shwachman, H., H. Leubner, and P. Catzel, Mucoviscidosis, *in*: Advances in Pediatrics, Vol. 7, S. Z. Levine, ed., The Year Book Publ., Inc., Chicago (1955), p. 249.

300. Shwachman, H., R. R. Dooley, F. Guilmette, P. R. Patterson, C. Weil, and H. Leubner, Cystic fibrosis of the pancreas with varying degrees of pancreatic insufficiency, *Amer. J. Dis. Child.* **92**:347 (1956).

301. Shwachman, H., The sweat test, *Pediatrics* **30**:167 (1962).

302. Shwachman, H., L. L. Kulczycki, H. L. Mueller, and C. G. Flake, Nasal polyposis in patients with cystic fibrosis, *Pediatrics* **30**:389 (1962).

303. Shwachman, H., L. K. Diamond, F. A. Oski, and K. T. Khaw, The syndrome of pancreatic insufficiency and bone marrow dysfunction, *J. Ped.* **65**:645 (1964).

304. Shwachman, H., L. L. Kulczycki, and K. T. Khaw, Studies in cystic fibrosis. A report on sixty-five patients over 17 years of age, *Pediatrics* **36**:689 (1965).

305. Sibinga, M. S., and G. J. Barbero, Studies in the physiology of sweating in cystic fibrosis. I. Experimental sweat gland fatigue, *Pediatrics* **27**:912 (1961).
306. Siegenthaler, P., J. de Haller, R. de Haller, A. Hampaï, and A. F. Muller, Effect of experimental salt depletion and aldosterone load on sodium and chloride concentration in the sweat of patients with cystic fibrosis of the pancreas and of normal children, *Arch. Dis. Childh.* **39**:61 (1964).
306a. Silverberg, M., J. Kessler, P. Z. Neumann, and F. W. Wiglesworth, An intestinal lipid transport defect. A possible variant of hypo-$\beta$-lipoproteinemia. (Abstract), *Gastroenterology* **54**:1271 (1968).
307. Simankova, N., V. Vavrova, and J. Houstek, Etude génétique de la mucoviscidose, *Ann. Génét.* **7**:84 (1964).
308. Simon, E. R., and P. Ways, Incubation hemolysis and red cell metabolism in acanthocytosis, *J. Clin. Invest.* **43**:1311 (1964).
309. Slegers, J. F. G., The mechanism of eccrine sweat-gland function in normal subjects and in patients with mucoviscidosis, *Dermatologica* **127**:242 (1963).
310. Smoller, M., and D. Y. Hsia, Studies on the genetic mechanism of cystic fibrosis of the pancreas, *Amer. J. Dis. Child.* **98**:277 (1959).
311. Sobel, E. H., M. Davidson, M. M. Kugler, K. A. Zuppinger, L. Yu-Feng Hsu, and A. Prader, Growth retardation associated with intestinal lactase deficiency. (Abstract), *J. Ped.* **63**:731 (1963).
312. Sonntag, W. M., M. L. Brill, W. G. Troyer, Jr., J. D. Welsh, G. Semenza, and A. Prader, Sucrose-isomaltose malabsorption in an adult woman, *Gastroenterology* **47**:18 (1964).
313. South, M. A., M. D. Cooper, F. Wollheim, and R. A. Good, The IgA system. II. The clinical significance of IgA deficiency: studies in patients with agammaglobulinemia and ataxia-telangectasia, *Amer. J. Med.* **44**:168 (1968).
314. Spock, A., H. M. C. Heick, H. Cress, and W. S. Logan, Abnormal serum factor in patients with cystic fibrosis of the pancreas, *Pediat. Res.* **1**:173 (1967).
315. Sproul, A., and N. Huang, Diagnosis of heterozygosity for cystic fibrosis by discriminatory analysis of sweat chloride distribution, *J. Ped.* **69**:759 (1966).
316. Steinberg, A. G., and D. C. Brown, On the incidence of cystic fibrosis of the pancreas, *Amer. J. Hum. Genet.* **12**:416 (1960).
317. Steinberg, A. G., Population genetics: special cases, *in*: Methodology in Human Genetics, W. J. Burdette, ed., Holden-Day, San Francisco (1962), p. 76.
318. Talamo, R. C., V. Raunio, O. Gabriel, J. C. Pallavicini, S. Halbert, and P. A. di Sant'Agnese, Immunologic and biochemical comparison of urinary glycoproteins in patients with cystic fibrosis of the pancreas and normal controls, *J. Ped.* **65**:480 (1964).
319. Taylor, K. B., D. L. Thompson, S. C. Truelove, and R. Wright, An immunological study of coeliac disease and idiopathic steatorrhoea. Serologic reactions to gluten and milk proteins, *Brit. Med. J.* **ii**:1727 (1961).
320. Thier, S., M. Fox, S. Segal, and L. E. Rosenberg, Cystinuria: *in vitro* demonstration of an intestinal transport defect, *Science* **143**:482 (1964).
321. Thompson, M. W., Heredity, maternal age, and birth order in the etiology of celiac disease, *Amer. J. Hum. Genet.* **3**:159 (1951).
322. Townes, P. L., Trypsinogen deficiency disease, *J. Ped.* **66**:275 (1965).
323. Townes, P. L., M. F. Bryson, and G. Miller, Further observations on trypsinogen deficiency disease: report of a second case, *J. Ped.* **71**:220 (1967).
324. Townley, R. R. W., K. T. Khaw, and H. Shwachman, Quantitative assay of disaccharidase activities of small intestinal mucosal biopsy specimens in infancy and childhood, *Pediatrics* **36**:911 (1965).
325. Ticker, V. L., D. Wilmore, C. J. Kaiser, and R. M. Lauer, Chronic diarrhea and alkalosis, *Pediatrics* **34**:601 (1964).

326. Van De Kamer, J. H., H. A. Weijers, and W. K. Dicke, Coeliac disease. IV. An investigation into the injurious constituents of wheat in connection with their action on patients with coeliac disease, *Acta Paediat. (Uppsala)* **42**:223 (1953).

327. Van De Kamer, J. H., and H. A. Weijers, Coeliac disease. V. Some experiments on the cause of the harmful effect of wheat gliadin. (Preliminary communication), *Acta Paediat. (Uppsala)* **44**:465 (1955).

328. Van De Kamer, J. H., unpublished data.

329. Vesin, P., De la diarrhée des carences en immuno-globulines aux entéropathies avec perte de protéines. Etude physiopathologique, *Sem. Hôp. Paris* **41**:3014 (1965).

330. Visakorpi, J. K., and P. Immonen, Intolerance to cow's milk and wheat gluten in the primary malabsorption syndrome in infancy, *Acta Paed. Scand.* **56**:49 (1967).

331. Waldmann, T. A., and L. Laster, Abnormalities of albumin metabolism in patients with hypogammaglobulinemia, *J. Clin. Invest.* **43**:1025 (1964).

332. Waldmann, T. A., and P. J. Schwab, IgG (7*S* gamma globulin) metabolism in hypogammaglobulinemia: studies in patients with defective gamma globulin synthesis, gastrointestinal protein loss, or both, *J. Clin. Invest.* **44**:1523 (1965).

333. Waldmann, T. A., Protein-losing enteropathy, *Gastroenterology* **50**:422 (1966).

334. Ways, P., C. F. Reed, and D. J. Hanahan, Red-cell and plasma lipids in acanthocytosis, *J. Clin. Invest.* **42**:1248 (1963).

335. Ways, P. O., C. M. Parmentier, H. J. Kayden, J. W. Jones, D. R. Saunders, and C. E. Rubin, Studies on the absorptive defect for triglyceride in abetalipoproteinemia, *J. Clin. Invest.* **46**:35 (1967).

336. Weijers, H. A., and J. H. Van De Kamer, Coeliac disease. III. Excretion of unsaturated and saturated fatty acids by patients with coeliac disease, *Acta Paediat. (Uppsala)* **42**:97 (1953).

337. Weijers, H. A., J. H. Van De Kamer, and W. K. Dicke, Celiac disease, *Adv. Pediat.* **IX**:277 (1957).

338. Weijers, H. A., and J. H. Van De Kamer, Coeliac disease. VII. Application and interpretation of the gliadine tolerance curve, *Acta Paediat. (Uppsala)* **48**:17 (1959).

339. Weijers, H. A., and J. H. Van De Kamer, Celiac disease and wheat sensitivity, *Pediatrics* **25**:127 (1960).

340. Weijers, H. A., J. H. Van De Kamer, D. A. A. Mossel, and W. K. Dicke, Diarrhoea caused by deficiency of sugar-splitting enzymes, *Lancet* **ii**:296 (1960).

341. Weijers, H. A., J. H. Van De Kamer, W. K. Dicke, and J. Ijsseling, Diarrhoea caused by deficiency of sugar-splitting enzymes. I, *Acta Paediat. (Uppsala)* **50**:55 (1961).

342. Weijers, H. A., and J. H. Van De Kamer, Aetiology and diagnosis of fermentative diarrhoeas, *Acta Paediat. (Uppsala)* **52**:329 (1963).

343. Welsh, J. D., and R. C. Brown, Sucrase-palatinase deficiency. (Letter to the editor), *Lancet* **ii**:342 (1966).

344. West, C. D., R. Hong, and N. H. Holland, Immunoglobulin levels from the newborn period to adulthood and in immunoglobulin deficiency states, *J. Clin. Invest.* **41**:2054 (1962).

345. Wolff, O. H., J. K. Lloyd, and E. L. Tonks, A-beta-lipoproteinaemia; with special reference to the visual defect, *Expt. Eye Res.* **3**:439 (1964).

346. Yardley, J. H., T. M. Bayless, J. H. Norton, and T. R. Hendrix, Celiac disease. A study of the jejunal epithelium before and after a gluten-free diet, *New Engl. J. Med.* **267**:1173 (1962).

347. Yssing, M., and B. Friis-Hansen, Congenital alkalosis with diarrhea, *Acta Paed. Scand.* **55**:341 (1966).

348. Zoppi, G., B. Hadorn, R. Gitzelmann, H. Kistler, and A. Prader, Intestinal $\beta$-galactosidase activities in malabsorption syndromes, *Gastroenterology* **50**:557 (1966).

# Index

# DATE DUE

| | | | |
|---|---|---|---|
| | | | |
| | | | |
| | | | |
| | | | |
| | | | |
| | | | |
| | | | |
| | | | |
| | | | |
| | | | |
| | | | |
| | | | |
| | | | |
| | | | |
| | | | |